Surgical Anatomy and Technique

Springer
New York
Berlin
Heidelberg
Barcelona
Budapest
Hong Kong
London
Milan
Paris
Santa Clara
Singapore
Tokyo

John E. Skandalakis
Panajiotis N. Skandalakis
Lee John Skandalakis

Surgical Anatomy and Technique

A Pocket Manual

With 678 Illustrations

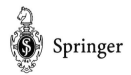

Springer

John E. Skandalakis, M.D., Ph.D.
The Centers for Surgical Anatomy
    and Technique
Emory University School of Medicine
1462 Clifton Road, N.E.
Atlanta, GA 30322
USA

Panajiotis N. Skandalakis, M.D.
The Centers for Surgical Anatomy
    and Technique
Emory University School of Medicine
1462 Clifton Road, N.E.
Atlanta, GA 30322
USA

Lee John Skandalakis, M.D.
The Centers for Surgical Anatomy
    and Technique
Emory University School of Medicine
1462 Clifton Road, N.E.
Atlanta, GA 30322
USA

Library of Congress Cataloging-in-Publication Data
Skandalakis, John Elias, 1920–
    Surgical anatomy and technique: a pocket manual /
    John E. Skandalakis, Panajiotis N. Skandalakis, Lee John
    Skandalakis.
        p. cm.
    Includes bibliographical references and index.
    ISBN 0-387-94081-2. — ISBN 3-540-94081-2 :
    1. Surgery, Operative—Handbooks, manuals, etc.   2. Anatomy,
Surgical and topographical—Handbooks, manuals, etc.
I. Skandalakis, Panajiotis N.   II. Skandalakis, Lee John.
III. Title.
    [DNLM: 1. Surgery, Operative—methods—handbooks.   2. Anatomy—
handbooks.   WO 39 1994]
RD32.S598   1994
617—dc20
DNLM/DLC   94-17332
for Library of Congress   CIP

Printed on acid-free paper.

Production managed by Laura Carlson and Terry Kornak; manufacturing supervised by
Jacqui Ashri.
Typeset by Bytheway Typesetting Services, Inc., Norwich, NY.
Printed and bound by Hamilton Printing Co., Rensselaer, NY.
Printed in the United States of America.

9 8 7 6 5 4

ISBN 0-387-94081-2 Springer-Verlag New York Berlin Heidelberg
ISBN 3-540-94081-2 Springer-Verlag Berlin Heidelberg New York   SPIN 10646769

Dedicated to
Prof. Gregory Skalkeas
with appreciation and gratitude (P.N.S.),
with deep respect (L.J.S.),
and with brotherly love (J.E.S.).

Preface

"Reach what you can, my child. . . . Reach what you cannot!"

Nikos Kazantzakis
(from *Report to Greco*, translated from the
Greek by P.A. Bien, published by
Simon and Schuster, 1965)

Surgical Anatomy and Technique: A Pocket Manual: With this title we want to present the stepchild of basic science, "anatomy," and also to emphasize some of the operative techniques of general surgery. We feel that this combination will take students to the promised surgical land. A good knowledge of anatomy will help surgeons avoid anatomical complications, while a masterful technique will allow them to proceed rapidly and securely in the operating room.

In my 50 years of teaching and practicing surgery, I have observed that residents, in most cases, come into the operating room without preparation or with a minimum of preparation. When I was a resident, the "Bible" was the atlas of my late, respected friend, Prof. Robert M. Zollinger. At the present time, there are several excellent books about surgical technique; among the best are *Operative Strategy in General Surgery* by Jameson L. Chassin, *Atlas of Surgery* by John L. Cameron, and *An Atlas of Head and Neck Surgery* by John M. Loré, Jr.

Several students, residents, and practicing surgeons approached me to write a pocket-sized book that covers both technique and surgical anatomy. Therefore, the philosophy behind this book is to present the anatomical entities involved with each operation and also to present the step-by-step technique of some procedures. We found that there are many huge volumes that describe step-by-step procedures, so, in order to produce a book small and light enough to be carried in the pocket of the white uniforms of students and residents, we selected only the absolutely necessary steps to convey the surgical procedure in continuity; occasionally, it was necessary to present a procedure in toto. This book is designed as a resource about surgical anatomy and technique for residents to read before entering the operating room.

The greatest stimulus for the book was Dr. Panajiotis N. Skandalakis, the senior author, with his hundreds of drawings from Holland, his sound surgicoanatomical notes, and his innumerable discussions of the subject. Most of the kudos belong to him.

We apologize for the steps, details, and procedures (such as the radical mastectomy, internal peritoneal hernias, and several others) that are omitted. With some procedures we do not use any drawings, whereas with some others we give more details. Perhaps our omissions are wrong; we hope the reader will forgive us.

The lack of footnotes and bibliography does not imply any disrespect or lack of appreciation of several authors from whom material has been drawn, but is consistent with our goal of keeping this volume as brief as possible. In our previous publications, *Anatomical Complications in General Surgery, Atlas of Surgical Anatomy for General Surgeons, Embryology for Surgeons*, and *Hernia: Surgical Anatomy and Technique*, we credited all authors to whose material we referred. This handbook should be used in conjunction with the above publications.

This manual is a brief compilation of elements from our previous works, a presentation of our own ideas about technique, and a summary of surgical anatomy lectures given for approximately a half century to the students at Emory University School of Medicine. Anatomy is to be remembered; but surgical anatomy of the entities involved in an operation is to be applied. We hope this handbook helps in that application.

J.E.S.

Acknowledgments

We acknowledge Esther Gumpert, Senior Medical Editor at Springer-Verlag New York, for her guidance, patience, and cooperation in this project from its inception to its completion.

We would like, also, to express our gratitude for the courteous, enthusiastic, and professional assistance throughout the publishing process by Andrea Seils, Associate Editor, Medicine and by the Production Department at Springer-Verlag.

For their dedicated efforts in the preparation of this manuscript, we thank our editors, Phyllis Bazinet and Carol Froman, and Dr. John E. Skandalakis' secretary, Cynthia Painter. We are indebted to Mark Barbaree, Edie Lacy, Sharon Scott, and Beth Simmons, librarians at Piedmont Hospital, Atlanta, for their research assistance.

Special thanks, also, to Brook Fehrenbach Wainwright and Robert Wainwright, Jr., for their outstanding illustrations; and to Tom Fletcher for his excellent photographic and artistic contributions.

We appreciate the advice of Adel Bagh, M.D., regarding the material on the colon and perianal area, and of Patrick M. Battey, M.D., regarding varicose veins of the lower extremity and shunts for portal hypertension.

Contents

1

Skin, Scalp, and Nail

ANATOMY

■ SKIN AND SUBCUTANEOUS TISSUE (Fig. 1.1)

The skin is composed of two layers: the epidermis (superficial) and the dermis (under the epidermis). The thickness of the skin varies from 0.5–3.0 mm.

The epidermis is avascular and is composed of stratified squamous epithelium. It has a thickness of 0.04–0.4 mm. The palms of the hands and the soles of the feet are thicker than the skin of other areas of the human body, such as the eyelids.

The dermis has a thickness of 0.5–2.5 mm and contains smooth muscles and sebaceous and sweat glands. Hair roots are located in the dermis or subcutaneous tissue.

Blood Supply

There are two arterial plexuses: one close to the subcutaneous fat (subdermal) and the second in the subpapillary area. Venous return is accomplished by a subpapillary plexus to a deep plexus and then to the superficial veins.

There is also a lymphatic plexus situated in the dermis which drains into the subcutaneous tissue. For innervation of the skin, there is a rich sensory and sympathetic supply.

Remember:

✓ The epidermis is avascular.

✓ The dermis is tough, strong, and very vascular.

✓ The superficial fascia is the subcutaneous tissue that blends with the reticular layer of the dermis.

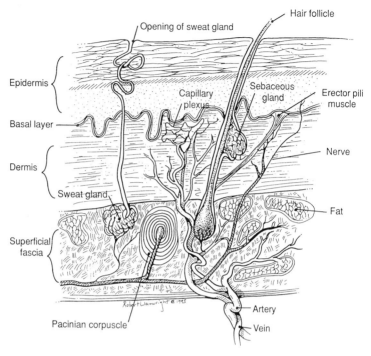

Figure 1.1

✓ The principal blood vessels of the skin lie in subdermal areas.

✓ The basement membrane is the lowest layer of the epidermis.

✓ The papillary dermis is the upper (superficial) layer of the dermis, just below the basement membrane.

✓ The reticular dermis is the lower (deep) layer of the dermis, just above the fat.

■ SCALP

The following mnemonic device will serve as an aid in remembering the structure of the scalp. See also Fig. 1.2.

	Layers	Description	Observations
S	Skin	Hair, sebaceous glands	
C	Connective close subcutaneous tissue	Superficial layer avascular Deep layer vascular (internal and external carotid lymphatic network) Nerves are present (cervical, trigeminal)	Bleeding due to gap and nonvascular contraction
A	Aponeurosis epicardial, galea	Aponeurosis of the occipitofrontalis muscle	Sensation present
L	Loose connective tissue	Emissary veins	Dangerous zone = extracranial and intracranial infections
P	Pericardium–periosteum		No sensation Heavy fixation at the suture lines, so limitation is infection

Surgicoanatomical notes:

✔ The blood supply of the scalp is rich. Arteries are anastomosed very freely.

✔ The arteries and the veins travel together in a longitudinal fashion.

✔ A transverse incision or laceration will produce a gap. Dangerous

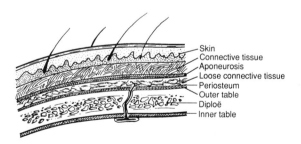

Skin
Connective tissue
Aponeurosis
Loose connective tissue
Periosteum
Outer table
Diploë
Inner table

Figure 1.2

bleeding will take place from both vascular ends due to nonretraction of the arteries by the close, dense, connective layer.

✓ Always repair the aponeurotic galea to avoid hematoma under it.

✓ With elective cases (excision of sebaceous cysts, etc.), whenever possible, make a longitudinal incision.

✓ Drain infections promptly. Use antibiotics to prevent intracranial infections via the emissary veins.

✓ Shave 1–2 cm around the site of the incision or laceration.

✓ After cleansing the partially avulsed scalp, replace it and debride the wound; then suture with nonabsorbable sutures.

✓ Use pressure dressing as required. Sutures may be removed in 3–5 days.

✓ Be sure about the diagnosis. A very common sebaceous cyst could be an epidermoid cyst of the skull involving the outer or inner table, or both, with extension to the cerebral cortex. In such a case, call for a neurosurgeon. The best diagnostic procedure is a lateral film of the skull to rule out bony involvement.

✓ Because the skin, connective tissue, and aponeurosis are so firmly interconnected, for practical purposes, they form one layer, the surgical zone of the scalp.

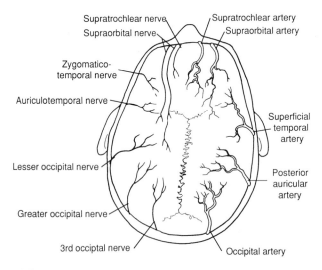

Figure 1.3. Arterial blood supply shown on right. Nerve distribution shown on left. Veins are not shown, but follow the arteries.

Blood Supply (Fig. 1.3)

Arterial

The arteries of the scalp are branches of the external and internal carotid arteries. The internal carotid in this area becomes the supratrochlear and supraorbital arteries, both terminal branches of the ophthalmic artery. The external carotid becomes a large occipital artery and two small arteries, the superficial temporal and the posterior auricular. Abundant anastomosis takes place among all these arteries. All are superficial to the epicranial aponeurosis.

Venous

Veins follow the arteries.

Lymphatic

The lymphatic network of the scalp is located at the deep layer of the dense connective subcutaneous tissue just above the aponeurosis (between the connective tissue and the aponeurosis). The complex network

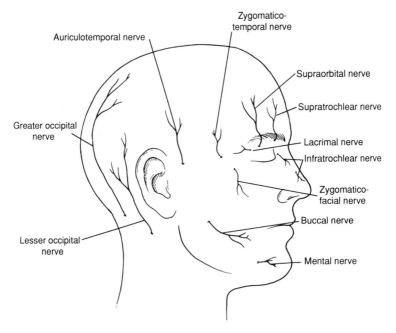

Figure 1.4

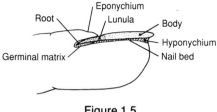

Figure 1.5

has frequent anastomoses. The three principal zones are the frontal, parietal, and occipital.

Nerves (Figs. 1.3 and 1.4)

The following nerves innervate the scalp (their origins are in parentheses):

- lesser occipital (second and third ventral nerves)
- greater occipital (second and third dorsal nerves)
- auriculotemporal (mandibular nerve)
- zygomaticotemporal, zygomaticofacial (zygomatic nerve [maxillary])
- supraorbital (ophthalmic nerve)
- supratrochlear (ophthalmic nerve)

■ THE NAIL

The anatomy of the nail may be appreciated from Figs. 1.5 and 1.6.

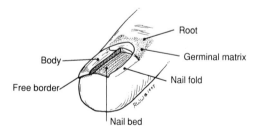

Figure 1.6

TECHNIQUE

■ BENIGN SKIN LESIONS (Figs. 1.7–1.9)

Benign skin lesions fall into several groups. Cystic lesions include epidermal inclusion cysts, sebaceous cysts, pilonidal cysts, and ganglia. Another group includes warts, keratoses, keloids, hemangiomatas, arteriovenous malformations, glomus tumors, and capillary malformations.

A third group includes decubitus ulcers, hidradenitis suppurativae, and burns. Junctional, compound, and intradermal nevi and malignant lentigos compose another group.

Procedure:

Step 1. For a cyst, make an elliptical incision. For a noncystic lesion, be sure to include approximately 0.5 cm of tissue beyond the lesion when making the elliptical incision.

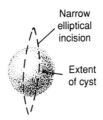

Narrow
elliptical
incision

Extent
of cyst

Figure 1.7

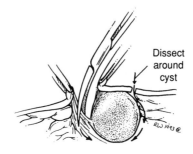

Dissect
around
cyst

Figure 1.8

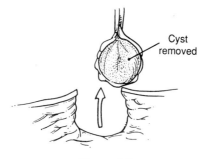

Cyst
removed

Figure 1.9

Step 2. Place the incision along Langer's lines (Kraissl's) and perpendicular to the underlying muscles but seldom parallel to the underlying muscle fibers.

Step 3. Dissect down to the subcutaneous tissue but not to the fascia. Avoid breaking the cyst, if possible.

Step 4. Handle the specimen with care by not crushing the skin or the lesion.

Step 5. Close in two layers. Undermine the skin as required. Remember the dermis is the strongest layer. For the dermis, use absorbable synthetic interrupted suture 4-0 or 5-0 (undyed Vicryl); for the epidermis, use 5-0 Vicryl subcuticular continuous, and reinforce with Steri-strips. It is acceptable to use 6-0 interrupted nonabsorbable sutures very close to the edges of the skin and close to each other.

Step 6. Remove interrupted sutures in 8 to 10 days and again reinforce with Steri-strips, especially if the wound is located close to a joint. A nylon epidermal continuous suture may be left in for 2 weeks without any problems, in most cases.

■ MALIGNANT SKIN LESIONS (Figs. 1.10 and 1.11)

Malignant skin lesions include basal cell carcinoma, squamous cell carcinoma, sweat gland carcinoma, fibrosarcoma, hemangiopericytoma, Kaposi's sarcoma, and dermatofibrosarcoma protuberans.

When removing the lesion, 0.5–1.0 cm of healthy skin around it must also be removed, as well as the subcutaneous layer.

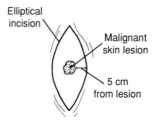

Elliptical incision

Malignant skin lesion

5 cm from lesion

Figure 1.10

Remember:

✓ Send specimen to the lab for frozen section of the lesion and margins.

✓ Explain to the patient prior to surgery about scarring, recurrence, etc.

✓ Remember the medicolegal aspects of the case. If the case involves a large facial lesion, obtain the advice of a plastic surgeon.

Melanoma

Staging of Malignant Melanoma (after Clark)

Level I. Malignant cells are found above the basement membrane.

Level II. Malignant cells infiltrate into the papillary dermis.

Level III. Malignant cells fill the papillary layer and extend to the junction of the papillary and reticular layers but do not enter the reticular layer.

Level IV. Malignant cells extend into the reticular layer of the dermis.

Level V. Malignant cells extend into the subcutaneous tissue.

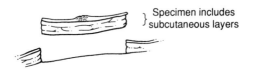

Specimen includes subcutaneous layers

Figure 1.11

Tumor Thickness (after Breslow)

Level I. Tumor thickness less than 0.76 mm

Level II. Tumor thickness 0.76–1.5 mm

Level III. Tumor thickness 1.51–2.25 mm

Level IV. Tumor thickness 2.26–3 mm

Level V. Tumor thickness greater than 3 mm

The Controversy

Surgical oncologists differ in their approach to treatment. Some advocate regional lymphadenectomy when there is clinical adenopathy and no distal metastasis. Others believe in prophylactic lymph node excision.

Remember:

✔ Perform prophylactic lymphadenectomy if the melanoma is located in the neck, axilla, or inguinal area, i.e., when the melanoma is situated just above a lymph node chain. Amputate a digit if melanoma is present. Be sure to consider the size, depth, and topography of the defect. For skin grafts, flaps, etc., refer the case or consult a plastic surgeon.

✔ For all pigmented nevi, ask for a second opinion from another pathologist.

Lesion Thickness and Regional Lymph Node Staging

1. Thin lesion: no lymph node involvement

2. Thick lesion: no lymph node involvement

3. Thin or thick lesion with lymph node involvement

4. Thin or thick lesion with distal metastasis

Cooperation between the surgeon and the pathologist is paramount. The decision regarding curative surgery depends on the thickness of the lesion.

At the present time, the philosophy of surgical treatment of melanoma is:

■ For thickness up to 0.75 mm, remove skin for 0.5 cm around the lesion;

■ For thickness up to 1.5 mm, remove skin for 2 cm around the lesion;

■ For thickness up to 3 mm, remove skin for 4 cm around the lesion.

In-continuity Surgical Treatment

EXAMPLE: Establishment of diagnosis of melanoma with a thickness more than 0.75 mm with some palpable lymph nodes. Primary lesion is on lower third of thigh, anterior.

Procedure:

Step 1. Make a wide excision of the scar with a 5 cm strip of skin and subcutaneous tissue extending upward to the inguinal area.

Step 2. Elevate flaps on each side with a further undercutting of thin skin flaps, producing an additional margin of 5 cm on both sides, thereby removing subcutaneous fat for approximately 10 cm.

Step 3. Remove the superficial inguinal lymph nodes in continuity.

Step 4. If the surgeon is unable to close groin primarily, a skin graft or pedicle graft may be necessary.

Note: Some surgeons advocate removal of the deep inguinal nodes if the superficial nodes have metastases in them.

■ SKIN GRAFTS

Free skin grafts include full-thickness grafts, pinch grafts, split-thickness grafts, and postage-stamp grafts, which are a type of split-thickness graft. Another classification is the pedicle graft. Space permits us to describe only some of them.

Split-Thickness Graft (Epidermis Plus Partial Dermis)

DEFINITION: Large pieces of skin including part of the dermis

INDICATIONS: Noninfected area

CONTRAINDICATIONS: Infection, exposed bone without periosteum, exposed cartilage without perichondrium, exposed tendon without sheath

DONOR AREA: Abdomen, thigh, arm

COMPLICATIONS: Infection, failure to take, contractures

Procedure:

Step 1. Prepare both areas. Skin of donor area must be kept taut by applying hand or board pressure.

Step 2. Remove estimated skin. We use a Zimmer dermatome set at a thickness of 0.03 cm for harvesting of skin. In most cases, we mesh the skin using a 1½-to-1 mesh ratio.

Step 3. Place the graft over the receiving area.

Step 4. Suture the graft to the skin. If the graft was not meshed, perforate it for drainage.

Step 5. Dress using Xeroform gauze covered by moist 4 × 4s or cotton balls. Then cover with roll gauze of appropriate size circumferentially.

Step 6. Change dressing in 3 days.

Alternative procedure: After step 3, do not cut sutures. Instead, tie them above a nonadherent gauze supported by a moist gauze to ensure maximum pressure to the graft.

Full-Thickness Graft

DEFINITION: The skin in toto, but not the subcutaneous tissue

INDICATIONS: Facial defects, fresh wounds, covering of defects after removal of large benign or malignant tumors

CONTRAINDICATIONS: Infections

DONOR AREA: Same as in split thickness grafts; also postauricular, supraclavicular, or nasolabial

TECHNIQUE: Same as in split thickness skin grafts

Meshing

A split-thickness graft may be stretched by a mesher, which produces several parallel openings, thereby permitting coverage of a large area.

Postage-Stamp Graft

In this procedure, multiple grafts are placed 3–5 mm from each other.

Pedicle Graft

We will not describe this procedure. A general surgeon who lacks the proper training should refer such cases to a plastic surgeon. From a medicolegal standpoint, this is best for both the patient and the general surgeon.

■ SCALP SURGERY

Excision of Benign Lesion

Procedure:

Step 1. Cut hair with scissors, then shave hair with razor 1 cm around the lesion.

Step 2. Make longitudinal or elliptical incision, removing small ovoid piece of skin.

Step 3. Elevate flaps.

Step 4. Obtain hemostasis.

Step 5. Remove cyst.

Step 6. Close skin.

Excision of Malignant Lesion (Melanoma, Squamous Cell Epithelioma)

The procedure is similar to that for a benign lesion. For melanoma, make a wide excision depending upon the thickness of the lesion as reported by the pathologist. Scalp melanomas metastasize, and radical neck surgery should be performed: for frontal lesions, include the superficial lobe of the parotid; for temporal and occipital lesions, include the postauricular and occipital nodes. When a posterior scalp melanoma is present, a posterior neck dissection should be done.

See details on malignant skin lesions earlier in this chapter.

For squamous cell epitheliomas, wide excision is the procedure of choice. If the bone is involved, plastic and neurosurgical procedures should follow.

Biopsy of Temporal Artery

Procedure:

Step 1. Shave hair at the point of maximal pulsation at the parietal area over or above the zygomatic process.

Step 2. Make longitudinal incision (Fig. 1.12).

Step 3. Carefully incise the aponeurosis (Fig. 1.13).

Step 4. After proximal and distal ligation with 2-0 silk, remove arterial segment at least 2 cm long (Fig. 1.14).

Step 5. Close in layers.

Remember:

✓ The temporal artery is closely associated with the auriculotemporal nerve, which is behind it, and with the superficial temporal vein, which is also behind it, medially or laterally.

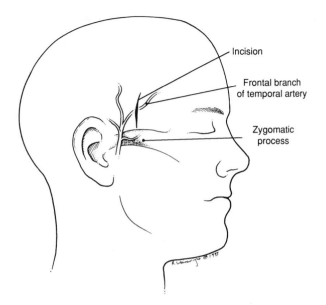

Incision

Frontal branch
of temporal artery

Zygomatic
process

Figure 1.12

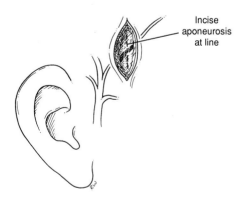

Incise
aponeurosis
at line

Figure 1.13

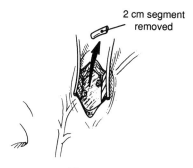

2 cm segment
removed

Figure 1.14

✓ In front of the ear, the temporal artery is subcutaneous and it is crossed by the temporal and zygomatic branches of the facial nerve.

✓ Perform biopsy above the zygomatic process.

■ INGROWN TOENAIL

DEFINITION: Inflammatory process with or without abscess formation secondary to embedment of the lateral or medial edge of the nail into the nail fold.

Conservative Treatment

Good hygiene requires that the nail be cut in transverse, straight fashion without any trimming of the edges (the square nail-cutting technique). Carefully elevate the embedded edge and insert a piece of cotton between the infected nail fold and the nail. Repeat the procedure until the ingrown nail edge grows above and distal to the nail fold.

Surgical Treatment

1. Total excision (avulsion) of nail
2. Partial excision of nail and matrix
3. Radical excision of nail and matrix

Total Excision (Avulsion) of Nail

Procedure:

Step 1. Prepare distal half of foot.

Step 2. Use double rubber band around the proximal phalanx for avascular field. Inject 1 cc of Novocain, 1–2 percent without Adrenalin, at the lateral and medial aspect of the second phalanx.

Step 3. Insert a straight hemostat under the nail at the area of the inflammatory process until the edge of the instrument reaches the lunula.

Step 4. Roll instrument and nail toward the opposite side for the avulsion of the nail.

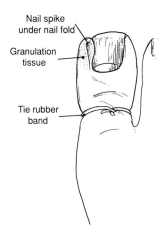

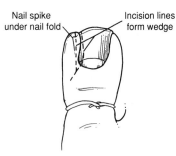

Figure 1.15

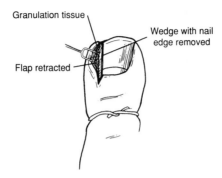

Granulation tissue

Wedge with nail edge removed

Flap retracted

Figure 1.16

Step 5. Occasionally a small fragment of nail remains in situ and should be removed.

Step 6. Excise all granulation tissue.

Step 7. Cover area with antibiotic ointment and apply sterile dressing.

Partial Excision of Nail and Matrix (Figs. 1.15–1.17)

Proceed as in total excision, except in step 4 remove only the involved side of the nail. Remove all granulation tissue, necrotic skin, matrix, and periosteum.

Remember:

✔ The removal of the matrix in the designated area should be complete. Use curette as required. If in doubt, make a small vertical incision at the area for better exposure of the lateral nail and matrix to aid complete removal of these entities.

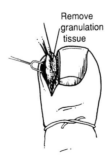

Remove granulation tissue

Figure 1.17

Radical Excision of Nail and Matrix

Include steps 4a–4d in the total excision procedure (above).

Procedure:

Step 4a. Make vertical incisions medially and laterally.

Step 4b. Elevate flaps for exposure of the matrix.

Step 4c. Remove matrix in toto with knife and, as required, with curette.

Step 4d. Loosely approximate the skin.

Note: This procedure is done *only* if there is *no* evidence of inflammatory process.

2

Neck

ANATOMY

■ THE ANTERIOR CERVICAL TRIANGLE (Fig. 2.1)

The boundaries are:

- lateral: sternocleidomastoid muscle
- superior: inferior border of the mandible
- medial: anterior midline of the neck

This large triangle may be subdivided into four more triangles: submandibular, submental, carotid, and muscular.

Submandibular Triangle

The submandibular triangle is demarcated by the inferior border of the mandible above and the anterior and posterior bellies of the digastric muscle below.

The largest structure in the triangle is the submandibular salivary gland. A number of vessels, nerves, and muscles also are found in the triangle.

For the surgeon, the contents of the triangle are best described in four layers, or surgical planes, starting from the skin. It must be noted that severe inflammation of the submandibular gland can destroy all traces of normal anatomy. When this occurs, identifying the essential nerves becomes a great challenge. With this warning, we will describe the structures in the triangle in the four surgical planes.

The Roof of the Submandibular Triangle

It is composed of skin, superficial fascia enclosing platysma muscle and fat, and the mandibular and cervical branches of the facial nerve (VII) (first surgical plane) (Fig. 2.2).

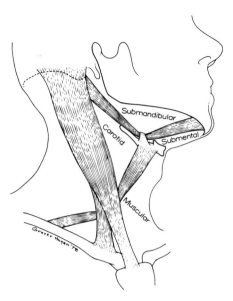

Figure 2.1. The subdivision of the anterior triangle of the neck. (By permission of JE Skandalakis, SW Gray, and JR Rowe, *Am Surg* 45(9):590–596, 1979.)

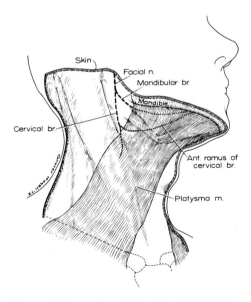

Figure 2.2. The roof of the submandibular triangle (the first surgical plane). The platysma lies over the mandibular and cervical branches of the facial nerve. (By permission of JE Skandalakis, SW Gray, and JR Rowe, *Am Surg* 45(9): 590–596, 1979.)

It is important to remember that (1) the skin should be incised 4 to 5 cm below the mandibular angle; (2) the platysma and fat compose the superficial fascia; and (3) the cervical branch of the facial nerve (VII) lies just below the angle, superficial to the facial artery (Fig. 2.3).

The mandibular, or marginal mandibular, nerve passes approximately 3 cm below the angle of the mandible to supply the muscles of the corner of the mouth and lower lip.

The cervical branch of the facial nerve divides to form descending and anterior branches. The descending branch innervates the platysma and communicates with the anterior cutaneous nerve of the neck. The anterior branch, the ramus colli mandibularis, crosses the mandible superficial to the facial artery and vein and joins the mandibular branch to contribute to the innervation of the muscles of the lower lip.

Injury to the mandibular branch results in severe drooling at the corner of the mouth. Injury to the anterior cervical branch produces minimal drooling that will disappear in 4 to 6 months.

The distance between these two nerves and the lower border of the mandible is shown in Fig. 2.3.

The Contents of the Submandibular Triangle

The structures of the second surgical plane, from superficial to deep, are the anterior and posterior facial vein, part of the facial (external maxillary) artery, the submental branch of the facial artery, the superficial layer of the submaxillary fascia (deep cervical fascia), the lymph nodes, the deep layer of the submaxillary fascia (deep cervical fascia), and the hypoglossal nerve (XII) (Fig. 2.4).

It is necessary to remember that the facial artery pierces the stylomandibular ligament. Therefore, it must be ligated before it is cut to prevent bleeding after retraction. Also, it is important to remember that the lymph nodes lie within the envelope of the submandibular fascia in close relationship with the gland. Differentiation between gland and lymph node may be difficult.

The anterior and posterior facial veins cross the triangle in front of the submandibular gland and unite close to the angle of the mandible to form the common facial vein, which empties into the internal jugular vein near the greater cornu of the hyoid bone. It is wise to identify, isolate, clamp, and ligate both these veins.

The facial artery, a branch of the external carotid artery, enters the submandibular triangle under the posterior belly of the digastric muscle and under the stylohyoid muscle. At its entrance into the triangle, it is under the submandibular gland. After crossing the gland posteriorly, the artery passes over the mandible, lying always under the platysma. It can be ligated easily.

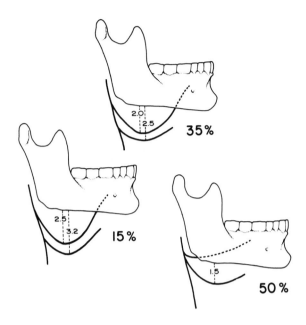

Figure 2.3. The neural "hammocks" formed by the mandibular branch (upper) and the anterior ramus of the cervical branch (lower) of the facial nerve. The distance below the mandible is given in centimeters, and percentages indicate the frequency found in 80 dissections of these nerves. (By permission of JE Skandalakis, SW Gray, and JR Rowe, *Am Surg* 45(9):590–596, 1979.)

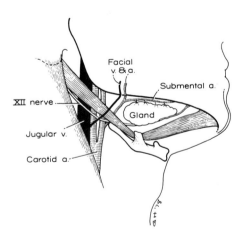

Figure 2.4. The contents of the submandibular triangle (the second surgical plane). Exposure of the superficial portion of the submandibular gland. (By permission of JE Skandalakis, SW Gray, and JR Rowe, *Am Surg* 45(9):590–596, 1979.)

The Floor of the Submandibular Triangle

The structures of the third surgical plane, from superficial to deep, include the mylohyoid muscle with its nerve, the hyoglossus muscle, the middle constrictor muscle covering the lower part of the superior constrictor, and part of the styloglossus muscle (Fig. 2.5).

The mylohyoid muscles are considered to form a true diaphragm of the floor of the mouth. They arise from the mylohyoid line of the inner surface of the mandible and insert on the body of the hyoid bone into the median raphe. The nerve, a branch of the mandibular division of the trigeminal nerve (V), lies on the inferior surface of the muscle. The superior surface is in relationship with the lingual and hypoglossal nerves.

The Basement of the Submandibular Triangle

The structures of the fourth surgical plane, or basement of the triangle, include the deep portion of the submandibular gland, the submandibular (Wharton's) duct, the lingual nerve, the sublingual artery, the sublingual vein, the sublingual gland, the hypoglossal nerve (XII), and the submandibular ganglion (Fig. 2.6).

The submandibular duct lies below the lingual nerve (except where the nerve passes under it) and above the hypoglossal nerve.

The Lymphatic Drainage of the Submandibular Triangle

The submandibular lymph nodes receive afferent channels from the submental nodes, the oral cavity, and the anterior parts of the face. Efferent channels drain primarily into the jugulodigastric, jugulocarotid, and juguloomohyoid nodes of the chain accompanying the internal jugular vein (deep cervical chain). A few channels pass by way of the subparotid nodes to the spinal accessory chain.

Submental Triangle (Fig. 2.1)

The boundaries of this triangle are:

- lateral: anterior belly of digastric muscle
- inferior: hyoid bone
- medial: midline
- floor: mylohyoid muscle
- roof: skin and superficial fascia
- contents: lymph nodes

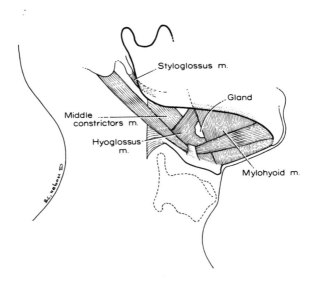

Figure 2.5. The floor of the submandibular triangle (the third surgical plane). Exposure of mylohyoid and hyoglossus muscles. (By permission of JE Skandalakis, SW Gray, and JR Rowe, *Am Surg* 45(9):590–596, 1979.)

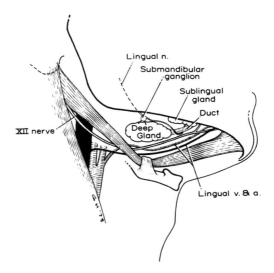

Figure 2.6. The basement of the submandibular triangle (the fourth surgical plane). Exposure of the deep portion of the submandibular gland, the lingual nerve, and the hypoglossal (XII) nerve. (By permission of JE Skandalakis, SW Gray, and JR Rowe, *Am Surg* 45(9):590–596, 1979.)

The lymph nodes of the submental triangle receive lymph from the skin of the chin, the lower lip, the floor of the mouth, and the tip of the tongue. They send lymph to the submandibular and jugular chains of nodes.

Carotid Triangle (Fig. 2.1)

The boundaries are:

- posterior: sternocleidomastoid muscle
- anterior: anterior belly of omohyoid muscle
- superior: posterior belly of digastric muscle
- floor: hyoglossus muscle, inferior constrictor of pharynx, thyrohyoid muscle, longus capitis muscle, and middle constrictor of pharynx
- roof: investing layer of deep cervical fascia
- contents: bifurcation of carotid artery; internal carotid artery (no branches in neck); external carotid artery branches, e.g., superficial temporal artery, internal maxillary artery, occipital artery, ascending pharyngeal artery, sternocleidomastoid artery, lingual artery (occasional), external maxillary artery (occasional); jugular vein tributaries, e.g., superior thyroid vein, occipital vein, common facial vein, pharyngeal vein; and vagus nerve, spinal accessory nerve, hypoglossal nerve, ansa hypoglossi, and sympathetic nerves (partially)

Lymph is received by the jugulodigastric, jugulocarotid, and juguloomohyoid nodes, and by the nodes along the internal jugular vein from submandibular and submental nodes, deep parotid nodes, and posterior deep cervical nodes. Lymph passes to the supraclavicular nodes.

Muscular Triangle (Fig. 2.1)

The boundaries are:

- superior lateral: anterior belly of omohyoid muscle
- inferior lateral: sternocleidomastoid muscle
- medial: midline of neck
- floor: prevertebral fascia and prevertebral muscles
- roof: investing layer of deep fascia, strap muscles, sternohyoid muscle, and cricothyroid muscle
- contents: thyroid and parathyroid glands, trachea, esophagus, and sympathetic nerve trunk

Remember that occasionally the strap muscles must be cut to facilitate thyroid surgery. They should be cut across the upper third of their length to avoid sacrificing their nerve supply.

■ THE POSTERIOR CERVICAL TRIANGLE (Fig. 2.7)

The posterior cervical triangle is sometimes considered to be two triangles, occipital and subclavian, divided by the posterior belly of the omohyoid muscle, or perhaps by the spinal accessory nerve (Fig. 2.7); we will treat it as one.

The boundaries of the posterior triangle are:

- anterior: sternocleidomastoid muscle

- posterior: anterior border of trapezius muscle

- inferior: clavicle

- floor: splenius capitis muscle, levator scapulae muscle, and three scalene muscles

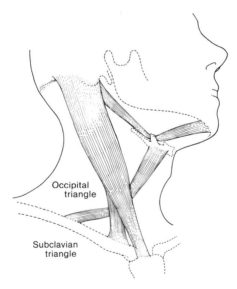

Figure 2.7. The posterior triangle of the neck. The triangle may be divided into two smaller triangles by the omohyoid muscle. (By permission of JE Skandalakis, SW Gray, and JR Rowe, *Am Surg* 45(9):590–596, 1979.)

This muscular floor is covered with investing and prevertebral fascia, between which lie the accessory nerve (XI) and a portion of the external jugular vein.

Deep to the fascia are the cervical nerves, the subclavian vessels, and the motor nerves to the levator scapulae, the rhomboids, the serratus anterior, and the diaphragm.

- roof: investing layer of the deep cervical fascia

- contents: subclavian artery, subclavian vein, cervical nerves, brachial plexus, phrenic nerve, accessory phrenic nerve, spinal accessory nerve, and lymph nodes

The superficial occipital lymph nodes receive lymph from the occipital region of the scalp and the back of the neck. The efferent vessels pass to the deep occipital lymph nodes (usually only one), which drain into the deep cervical nodes along the spinal accessory nerve.

■ FASCIAE OF THE NECK

The following classification of the rather complicated fascial planes of the neck follows the work of several investigators:

1. Superficial fascia
2. Deep fascia
   a. Investing layer (anterior or superficial layer)
   b. Middle, or pretracheal, layer (in front and below hyoid bone only)
   c. Prevertebral layer (posterior or deep layer)

Superficial Fascia

The superficial fascia lies beneath the skin and is composed of loose connective tissue, fat, the platysma muscle, and small unnamed nerves and blood vessels (Fig. 2.8). The surgeon should remember that the cutaneous nerves of the neck and the anterior and external jugular veins are between the platysma and the deep cervical fascia. If these veins are to be cut, they must first be ligated. Because of their attachment to the platysma above and the fascia below, they do not retract; bleeding from them may be serious. For practical purposes, there is no space between this layer and the deep fascia.

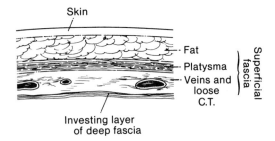

Figure 2.8. The superficial fascia of the neck lies between the skin and the investing layer of the deep cervical fascia. (By permission of JE Skandalakis, SW Gray, and JR Rowe, *Anatomical Complications in General Surgery*, New York: McGraw-Hill, 1983.)

Deep Fascia

Investing Layer (Figs. 2.9 and 2.10)

It envelops two muscles (the trapezius and the sternocleidomastoid), and two glands (the parotid and the submaxillary) and forms two spaces (the

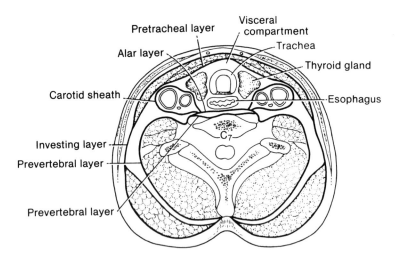

Figure 2.9. Diagrammatic cross section through the neck below the hyoid bone showing the layers of the deep cervical fascia and the structures that they envelop. (By permission of JE Skandalakis, SW Gray, and LJ Skandalakis, In: CG Jamieson (ed), *Surgery of the Esophagus*, Edinburgh: Churchill Livingstone, 19–35, 1988.)

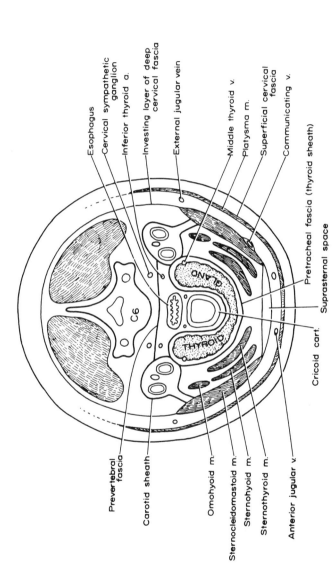

Figure 2.10. Diagrammatic cross section of the neck through the thyroid gland at the level of the 6th cervical vertebra showing the fascial planes, muscles, and vessels that may be encountered in an incision for thyroidectomy. (By permission of JT Akin and JE Skandalakis, *Am Surg* 42(9):648–652, 1976.)

Esophagus
Cervical sympathetic ganglion
Inferior thyroid a.
Investing layer of deep cervical fascia
External jugular vein
Middle thyroid v.
Platysma m.
Superficial cervical fascia
Communicating v.
Pretracheal fascia (thyroid sheath)
Suprasternal space
Cricoid cart.
Anterior jugular v.
Sternothyroid m.
Sternohyoid m.
Sternocleidomastoid m.
Omohyoid m.
Carotid sheath
Prevertebral fascia
C6
GLAND
THYROID

supraclavicular and the suprasternal). It forms the roof of the anterior and posterior cervical triangles and the midline raphe of the strap muscles.

Pretracheal, or Middle, Layer

The middle layer of the deep fascia splits into an anterior portion that envelops the strap muscles and a posterior layer that envelops the thyroid gland, forming the false capsule of the gland.

Prevertebral, or Posterior, Layer

This plane lies in front of the prevertebral muscles. It originates from the posterior surface of the sternocleidomastoid and, together with the pretracheal fascia, forms the carotid sheath. The fascia divides to form a space in front of the vertebral bodies, the anterior layer being the alar fascia and the posterior layer retaining the designation of prevertebral fascia.

Carotid Sheath

Beneath the sternocleidomastoid muscle, the investing fascia, the pretracheal fascia, and the prevertebral fascia contribute to a fascial tube, the carotid sheath. Within this tube lie the common carotid artery, the internal jugular vein, the vagus nerve, and the deep cervical lymph nodes.

Buccopharyngeal Fascia

This layer covers the lateral and posterior surfaces of the pharynx and binds the pharynx to the alar layer of the prevertebral fascia.

Axillary Fascia

This fascia takes its origin from the prevertebral fascia. It is discussed in Chapter 3, "Breast."

■ SPACES OF THE NECK

There are many spaces in the neck defined by the fasciae, but for the general surgeon, the visceral compartment is the most important; be very familiar with its boundaries and contents.

The boundaries of the visceral compartment of the neck are:

■ anterior: pretracheal fascia
■ posterior: prevertebral fascia
■ lateral: carotid sheath

- superior: hyoid bone and thyroid cartilage
- posteroinferior: posterior mediastinum
- anteroinferior: bifurcation of the trachea at the level of the 4th thoracic vertebra
- contents: part of esophagus, larynx, trachea, thyroid gland, and parathyroid glands

■ LYMPHATICS AND THE RIGHT AND LEFT THORACIC LYMPHATIC DUCTS

The overall anatomy of the lymphatics of the head and neck may be appreciated from Table 2.1 and Fig. 2.11.

The thoracic duct originates from the cisterna chyli and terminates in the left subclavian vein (Fig. 2.12). It is approximately 38–45 cm long. The duct begins at about the level of the 2nd lumbar vertebra from the cisterna chyli or, if the cisterna is absent (about 50 percent of cases), from the right and left lumbar lymphatic trunks. It ascends to the right of the midline on the anterior surface of the bodies of the thoracic vertebrae. It crosses the midline between the 7th and 5th thoracic vertebrae to lie on the left side, close to the left esophageal wall. It passes behind the great vessels to the level of the 7th cervical vertebra and descends slightly to enter the left subclavian vein (Fig. 2.12). The duct may have multiple entrances to the vein, and one or more of the contributing lymphatic trunks may enter the subclavian or the jugular vein independently. It may be ligated with impunity.

The thoracic duct collects lymph from the whole of the body below the diaphragm, as well as from the left side of the thorax. Lymph nodes may be present at the caudal end, but there are none along its upward course. Injury to the duct in supraclavicular lymph node dissections results in copious lymphorrhea. Ligation is the answer.

The right lymphatic duct is a variable structure about 1 cm long formed by the right jugular, transverse cervical, internal mammary, and mediastinal lymphatic trunks (Fig. 2.13). If these trunks enter the veins separately, there is no right lymphatic duct. When present, the right lymphatic duct enters the superior surface of the right subclavian vein at its junction with the right internal jugular vein and drains most of the right side of the thorax.

■ ANATOMY OF THE THYROID GLAND

The thyroid gland consists typically of two lobes (right and left), a connecting isthmus, and an ascending pyramidal lobe. One lobe, usually the

Table 2.1 Lymph Nodes and the Lymphatic Drainage of the Head and Neck

		Lymphatics	
	Location	From	To
Superior horizontal chain: Submental nodes	Submental triangle	Skin of chin, lip, floor of mouth, tip of tongue	Submandibular nodes or jugular chain
Submandibular nodes	Submandibular triangle	Submental nodes, oral cavity, face, except forehead and part of lower lip	Intermediate jugular nodes, deep posterior cervical nodes
Preauricular (parotid) nodes	In front of tragus	Lateral surface of pinna, side of scalp	Deep cervical nodes
Postauricular (mastoid) nodes	Mastoid process	Temporal scalp, medial surface of pinna, external auditory meatus	Deep cervical nodes
Occipital node	Between mastoid process and external occipital protuberance	Back of scalp	Deep cervical nodes
Vertical chain: Posterior cervical (posterior triangle) nodes		Subparotid nodes, jugular chain, occipital, and mastoid area	Supraclavicular and deep cervical nodes
Superficial	Along exterior jugular vein		
Deep	Along spinal accessory nerve		

Node	Location	Afferents from	Efferents to
Intermediate (jugular) nodes		All other nodes of neck	Lymphatic trunks to left and right thoracic ducts
Juguloparotid (subparotid) nodes	Angle of mandible, near parotid nodes		
Jugulodigastric (subdigastric) nodes	Junction of common facial and internal jugular veins	Palatine tonsils	
Jugulocarotid (bifurcation) nodes	Bifurcation of common carotid artery close to carotid body	Tongue, except tip	
Juguloomohyoid (omohyoid) nodes	Crossing of omohyoid and internal jugular vein	Tip of tongue	
Anterior (visceral) nodes			
Parapharyngeal nodes	Lateral and posterior wall of pharynx	Deep face and esophagus	Intermediate nodes
Paralaryngeal nodes	Lateral wall of larynx	Larynx and thyroid gland	Deep cervical nodes
Paratracheal nodes	Lateral wall of trachea	Thyroid gland, trachea, esophagus	Deep cervical and mediastinal nodes
Prelaryngeal (Delphian) nodes	Cricothyroid ligament	Thyroid gland, pharynx	Deep cervical nodes
Pretracheal nodes	Anterior wall of trachea below isthmus of thyroid gland	Thyroid gland, trachea, esophagus	Deep cervical and mediastinal nodes
Inferior horizontal chain: Supraclavicular and scalene nodes	Subclavian triangle	Axilla, thorax, vertical chain	Jugular or subclavian trunks to right lymphatic duct and thoracic duct

(By permission of JE Skandalakis, SW Gray, and JR Rowe, *Anatomical Complications in General Surgery*, New York: McGraw-Hill, 1983.)

33

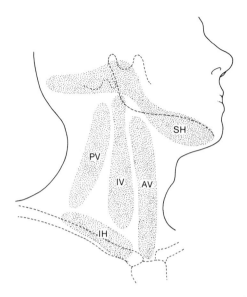

Figure 2.11. The lymph nodes of the neck. SH = superior horizontal chain; IH = inferior horizontal chain; PV = posterior vertical chain; IV = intermediate vertical chain; AV = anterior vertical chain. (By permission of JE Skandalakis, SW Gray, and JR Rowe, *Anatomical Complications in General Surgery*, New York: McGraw-Hill, 1983.)

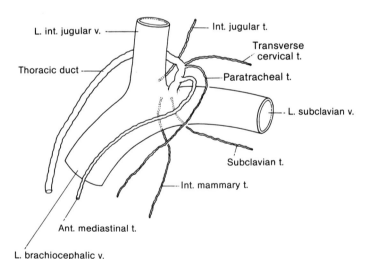

Figure 2.12. The thoracic duct and main left lymphatic trunks. Trunks are variable and may enter the veins with the thoracic duct or separately. (By permission of JE Skandalakis, SW Gray, and JR Rowe, *Anatomical Complications in General Surgery*, New York: McGraw-Hill, 1983.)

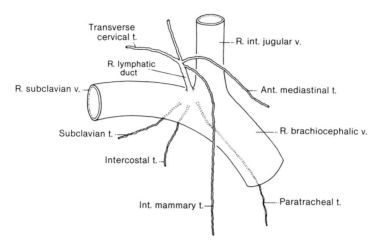

Transverse
cervical t.

R. int. jugular v.

R. lymphatic
duct

R. subclavian v.

Ant. mediastinal t.

Subclavian t.

R. brachiocephalic v.

Intercostal t.

Int. mammary t.

Paratracheal t.

Figure 2.13. The right lymphatic duct is formed by the junction of several lymphatic trunks. If they enter the veins separately, there may be no right lymphatic duct. (By permission of JE Skandalakis, SW Gray, and JR Rowe, *Anatomical Complications in General Surgery*, New York: McGraw-Hill, 1983.)

right, may be smaller than the other (7 percent of cases) or completely absent (1.7 percent). The isthmus is absent in about 10 percent of thyroid glands, and the pyramidal lobe is absent in about 50 percent (Fig. 2.14). A minute epithelial tube or fibrous cord, the thyroglossal duct, almost always extends between the thyroid gland and the foramen cecum of the tongue.

The thyroid gland normally extends from the level of the 5th cervical vertebra to that of the 1st thoracic vertebra. It may lie higher (lingual thyroid) but rarely lower than normal.

The Capsule of the Thyroid Gland

The thyroid gland has a connective tissue capsule continuous with the septa that make up the stroma of the organ. This is the *true* capsule of the thyroid.

External to the true capsule is a more or less well-developed layer of fascia derived from the pretracheal fascia. This is the *false* capsule, *perithyroid sheath*, or *surgical capsule*. The false capsule, or fascia, is not removed with the gland at thyroidectomy.

The sternohyoid muscle is most superficial and the sternothyroid and thyrohyoid muscles are underneath. For all practical purposes, the thyrohyoid is an upward continuation of the sternothyroid.

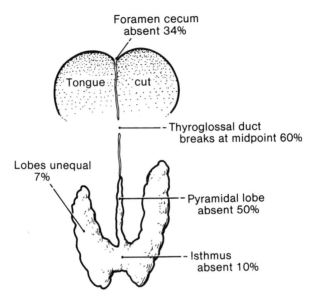

Figure 2.14. Normal vestiges of thyroid gland development. None are of clinical significance, but their presence may be of concern to the surgeon. (By permission of JE Skandalakis, SW Gray, and JR Rowe, *Anatomical Complications in General Surgery*, New York: McGraw-Hill, 1983.)

The superior parathyroid glands normally lie between the true capsule of the thyroid and the fascial false capsule. The inferior parathyroids may be between the true and the false capsules, within the thyroid parenchyma, or lying on the outer surface of the fascia.

Arterial Supply of the Thyroid and Parathyroid Glands

Two paired arteries, the superior and inferior thyroid arteries, and an inconstant midline vessel, the thyroid ima artery, supply the thyroid (Fig. 2.15).

The superior thyroid artery arises from the external carotid artery just above, at, or just below the bifurcation of the common carotid artery. It passes downward and anteriorly to reach the superior pole of the thyroid gland. In part of its course, the artery parallels the superior laryngeal nerve. At the superior pole the artery divides into anterior and posterior branches. From the posterior branch, a small parathyroid artery passes to the superior parathyroid gland.

The inferior thyroid artery usually arises from the thyrocervical trunk,

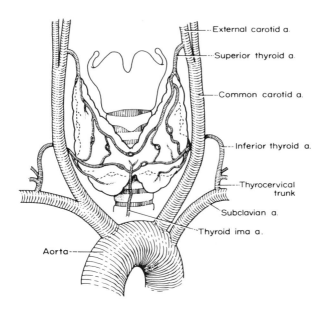

Figure 2.15. The arterial supply to the thyroid gland. The thyroid ima artery is only occasionally present. (By permission of S Tzinas, C Droulias, N Harlaftis, et al., *Am Surg* 42(9):639–644, 1976.)

or from the subclavian artery. It ascends behind the carotid artery and the jugular vein, passing medially and posteriorly on the anterior surface of the longus colli muscle. After piercing the prevertebral fascia, the artery divides into two or more branches as it crosses the ascending recurrent laryngeal nerve. The nerve may pass anterior or posterior to the artery, or between its branches (Fig. 2.16). The lowest branch sends a twig to the inferior parathyroid gland. On the right, the inferior thyroid artery is absent in about 2 percent of individuals. On the left, it is absent in about 5 percent. The artery is occasionally double.

The arteria thyroidea ima is unpaired and inconstant. It arises from the brachiocephalic artery, the right common carotid artery, or the aortic arch. Its position anterior to the trachea makes it important for tracheostomy.

Venous Drainage

The veins of the thyroid gland form a plexus of vessels lying in the substance and on the surface of the gland. The plexus is drained by three pairs of veins (Fig. 2.17):

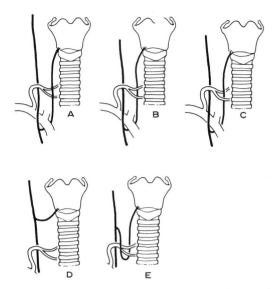

Figure 2.16. Relations at the crossing of the recurrent laryngeal nerve and the inferior thyroid artery. (A–C) Common variations. Their frequencies are given in Table 2.2. (D) A nonrecurrent nerve is not related to the inferior thyroid artery. (E) The nerve loops beneath the artery. (By permission S Tzinas, C Droulias, N Harlaftis, et al., *Am Surg* 42(9):639–644, 1976.)

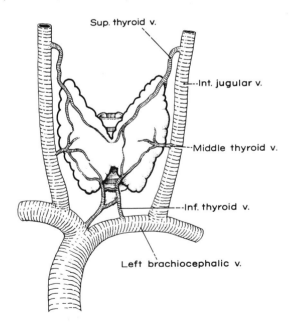

Figure 2.17. The venous drainage of the thyroid gland. The inferior thyroid veins are quite variable. (By permission S Tzinas, C Droulias, N Harlaftis, et al., *Am Surg* 42(9):639–644, 1976.)

1. The superior thyroid vein accompanies the superior thyroid artery.

2. The middle thyroid vein arises on the lateral surface of the gland at about two-thirds of its anteroposterior extent. No artery accompanies it. This vein may be absent and occasionally is double.

3. The inferior thyroid vein is the largest and most variable.

Thyroid Gland and Recurrent Laryngeal Nerves
(Figs. 2.18A and B, and 2.16)

The right recurrent laryngeal nerve crosses anterior to the right subclavian artery, loops around the artery from anterior to posterior, and ascends in or near the tracheoesophageal groove, passing posterior to the right lobe of the thyroid gland to enter the larynx behind the cricothyroid articulation and the inferior corner of the thyroid cartilage.

The left recurrent laryngeal nerve loops under the aorta and ascends in the same manner as the right nerve. Both nerves cross the inferior thyroid arteries near the lower border of the middle third of the gland.

In about 1 percent of patients, the right recurrent nerve arises normally from the vagus but passes medially almost directly from its origin to the larynx without looping under the subclavian artery. In these cases, the right subclavian artery arises from the descending aorta and passes to the right behind the esophagus. This anomaly is asymptomatic, and the thyroid surgeon will rarely be aware of it prior to operation. Even less common is a nonrecurrent left nerve in the presence of a right aortic arch and a retroesophageal left subclavian artery.

In the lower third of its course, the recurrent laryngeal nerve ascends behind the pretracheal fascia at a slight angle to the tracheoesophageal groove. In the middle third of its course, the nerve may lie in the groove or within the substance of the thyroid gland.

The vulnerability of the recurrent laryngeal nerve may be appreciated from Table 2.2.

Exposure of the Laryngeal Nerves

The recurrent laryngeal nerve forms the medial border of a triangle bounded superiorly by the inferior thyroid artery and laterally by the carotid artery. The nerve may be identified where it enters the larynx just posterior to the inferior cornu of the thyroid cartilage. If the nerve is not found, a nonrecurrent nerve should be suspected, especially on the right.

In the lower portion of its course, the nerve may be palpated as a tight strand over the tracheal surface. There is more connective tissue between the nerve and the trachea on the right than on the left. Visual identifica-

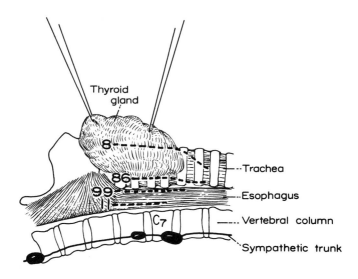

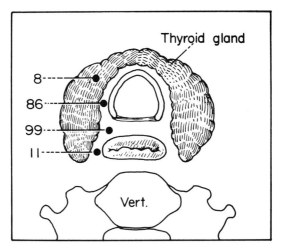

Figure 2.18. The course of the recurrent laryngeal nerve at the level of the thyroid gland in 102 cadavers. In about one-half of the cases, the nerve lay in the groove between the trachea and the esophagus. (Top) Lateral view. (Bottom) Cross-sectional view. (By permission of JE Skandalakis, C Droulias, N Harlaftis, et al., *Am Surg* 42(9):629–634, 1976.)

Table 2.2 Recurrent Laryngeal Nerve Vulnerability

Cause of vulnerability	Percent encountered
Lateral and anterior location	1.5–3.0
Tunnelling through thyroid tissue	2.5–15.0
Fascial fixation	2.0–3.0
Arterial fixation	5.0–12.5
Close proximity to inferior thyroid vein	1.5–2.0 +

Data from Chang-Chien Y. Surgical anatomy and vulnerability of the recurrent laryngeal nerve. *Int Surg* 1980; 65: 23.

tion, with avoidance of traction, compression, or stripping the connective tissue, is all that is necessary.

The superior laryngeal nerve passes inferiorly, medial to the carotid artery. At the level of the superior cornu of the hyoid bone, it divides into a large, sensory, internal laryngeal branch and a smaller, motor, external laryngeal branch, serving only the cricothyroid muscle. The bifurcation is usually within the bifurcation of the carotid artery (Fig. 2.19).

The internal laryngeal branch is rarely identified by the surgeon (Fig. 2.20).

The external laryngeal branch, together with the superior thyroid vein and artery, passes under the sternothyroid muscles and continues inferiorly and innervates the cricothyroid muscle.

Remember:

✓ The results of injury to the recurrent laryngeal and the external branch of the superior laryngeal nerves have been outlined:

  1. *Unilateral recurrent nerve injury.* The affected vocal cord is paramedian owing to adduction by the cricothyroid muscle. Voice is preserved (not unchanged).

  2. *Unilateral recurrent and superior laryngeal nerve injury.* The affected cord is in an intermediate position, resulting in hoarseness and inability to cough. The affected cord will move toward the midline with time. Voice improves, but improvement is followed by narrowing of the airway. Tracheostomy becomes necessary.

Postoperative hoarseness is not always the result of operative injury to laryngeal nerves. From 1 to 2 percent of patients have a paralyzed vocal cord prior to thyroid operations. Researchers at the Mayo Clinic examined 202 cases of vocal cord paralysis, of which 153 (76 percent) followed

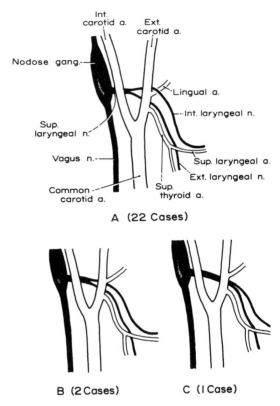

Figure 2.19. Branching of the superior laryngeal nerve and the carotid arteries. (A) The internal branch crosses the external carotid artery above the origin of the lingual artery. (B) The internal branch crosses below the origin of the lingual artery. (C) The nerve divides medial to the external carotid artery. (By permission of C Droulias, S Tzinas, N Harlaftis, et al., *Am Surg* 42(9):635–638, 1976.)

thyroidectomy, 36 (18 percent) were of various known etiologies, and 13 (6 percent) were of idiopathic origin. We strongly advise the general surgeon to perform a mirror laryngoscopy prior to thyroidectomy.

We believe that the patient should be told that in spite of all precautions, there is a possibility of some vocal disability following thyroidectomy.

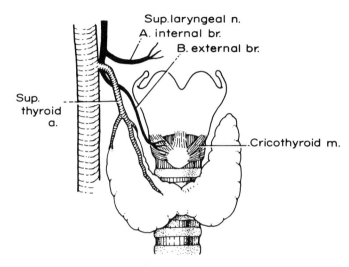

Figure 2.20. Relations of the internal and external branches of the superior laryngeal nerve to the superior thyroid artery and the upper pole of the thyroid gland. (By permission of C Droulias, S Tzinas, N Harlaftis, et al., *Am Surg* 42(9):635–638, 1976.)

A sympathetic ganglion may be confused with a lymph node and removed when the surgeon operates for metastatic papillary carcinoma of the thyroid. In one of our patients, the inferior cervical and first thoracic ganglia were fused to form a nodelike structure that was removed. The surgeon must identify any apparent lymph node related to the vertebral artery and fixed in front of the transverse process of the seventh cervical vertebra.

Injury to the cervical sympathetic nerve results in Horner's syndrome: (1) constriction of the pupil, (2) ptosis of the upper eyelid, (3) apparent enophthalmos, and (4) dilatation of the retinal vessels.

Persistent Remnants of the Thyroglossal Duct

The foramen cecum of the tongue and the pyramidal lobe of the thyroid gland are normal remnants of the thyroglossal duct. Between these structures is a very small epithelial tube, usually broken in several places. Occasionally these epithelial fragments hypertrophy, secrete fluid, and form cysts. Drainage or aspiration of these cysts is futile and often results in formation of a fistula, usually infected.

All fragments of the duct, the foramen cecum, and the midportion of the hyoid bone should be removed (Sistrunk procedure). Recurrence of the cyst is the result of failure to remove the entire duct or the central portion of the hyoid bone.

■ ANATOMY OF THE PARATHYROID GLANDS

The parathyroid glands are usually found on the posterior surface of the thyroid gland, each with its own capsule of connective tissue. They are occasionally included in the thyroid capsule, or one of them may even follow a blood vessel deep into a sulcus of the thyroid.

Extreme locations are very rare, although glands have been found as high as the bifurcation of the carotid artery and as low as the mediastinum. In practice, the surgeon should start at the point at which the inferior thyroid artery enters the thyroid gland. The superior parathyroid glands will *probably* lie about 1.27 cm (½ inch) above it, and the inferior parathyroid glands will *probably* lie 1.27 cm (½ inch) below it. If the inferior gland is not found, it is more likely to be lower than higher.

It is not uncommon to have more or fewer than four parathyroid glands.

Blood Supply

The inferior thyroid artery is responsible in most cases for the blood supply of both the upper and the lower parathyroid glands.

■ ANATOMY OF THE TRACHEA

The trachea, together with the esophagus and the thyroid gland, lies in the visceral compartment of the neck. The anterior wall of the compartment comprises sternothyroid and sternohyoid muscles covered anteriorly by the investing layer of the deep cervical fascia and posteriorly by the prevertebral fascia (Fig. 2.9). The trachea begins at the level of the 6th cervical vertebra and its bifurcation is at the level of the 6th thoracic vertebra in the erect position or the 4th to the 5th thoracic vertebrae when supine.

Arterial Supply

The chief source of arterial blood to the trachea is the inferior thyroid arteries. At the bifurcation, these descending branches anastomose with ascending branches of the bronchial arteries.

Venous Drainage

Small tracheal veins join the laryngeal vein or empty directly into the left inferior thyroid vein.

Lymphatic Drainage

The pretracheal and paratracheal lymph nodes receive the lymphatic vessels from the trachea.

Nerve Supply

The trachealis muscle and the tracheal mucosa receive fibers from the vagus, the recurrent laryngeal nerves, and the sympathetic trunks. Small autonomic ganglia are numerous in the tracheal wall.

Anatomical Landmarks

The usual site of a tracheostomy is between the 2nd and the 4th tracheal rings. The structures encountered are as follows:

Skin and Superficial Fascia

The platysma lies in the superficial fascia and is absent in the midline. The anterior jugular veins may lie close to the midline, and more importantly, they may be united by a jugular venous arch at the level of the 7th to the 8th tracheal rings.

Investing Layer of Deep Cervical Fascia

The sternohyoid muscle lies between the investing layer and the pretracheal fascia on either side of the midline.

Visceral Compartment under the Pretracheal Fascia

The inferior thyroid veins, the isthmus of the thyroid gland, and the possibility of an arteria thyroidea ima should not be forgotten.

■ THE PAROTID GLAND (Fig. 2.21)

Relations of the Parotid Gland

The parotid gland lies beneath the skin in front of and below the ear. It is contained within the investing layer of the deep fascia of the neck,

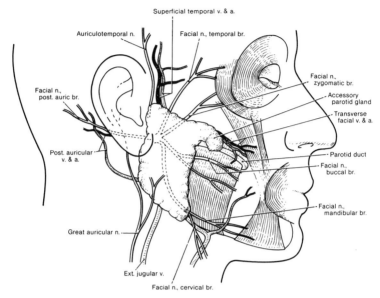

Figure 2.21. Relations of the parotid gland to the facial nerve and its branches. (By permission of JE Skandalakis, SW Gray, and JR Rowe, *Anatomical Complications in General Surgery*, New York: McGraw-Hill, 1983.)

called locally the parotid fascia, and the gland can be felt only under pathological conditions.

The boundaries are:

- anterior: masseter muscle, ramus of mandible, and internal pterygoid muscle
- posterior: mastoid process and sternocleidomastoid muscle
- superior: external auditory meatus and temporomandibular joint
- inferior: sternocleidomastoid muscle and posterior belly of digastric muscle
- lateral: investing layer of deep cervical fascia, skin, and platysma muscle
- medial: investing layer of deep cervical fascia, styloid process, internal jugular vein, internal carotid artery, and pharyngeal wall

From the anterolateral edge of the gland, the parotid duct (Stensen's) passes lateral to the masseter muscle and turns medial at the anterior margin of the muscle to pierce the buccinator muscle and enters the oral cavity at the level of the upper 2nd molar tooth.

Structures Traversing the Parotid Gland

Facial Nerve

There is a superficial lobe and a deep lobe of the gland; the branches of the facial nerve run between them. In contrast, some anatomists visualize the gland as essentially unilobular, with the branches of the facial nerve enmeshed within the gland tissue with no cleavage plane between nerve and gland. The view that one may accept does not change the actual surgical procedure.

The main trunk of the facial nerve enters the posterior surface of the parotid gland about 1 cm from its emergence from the skull through the stylomastoid foramen about midway between the angle of the mandible and the cartilaginous ear canal (Fig. 2.21). At birth the child has no mastoid process and the stylomastoid foramen is subcutaneous.

About 1 cm from its entrance into the gland, the facial nerve divides to form five branches: temporal, zygomatic, buccal, mandibular, and cervical. In most individuals, an initial bifurcation forms an upper temporofacial and a lower cervicofacial division, but six major patterns of branching (from simple to complex) have been distinguished.

Arteries

The external carotid artery enters the inferior surface of the gland and divides into the maxillary and superficial temporal arteries. The latter gives rise to the transverse facial artery. Each of these branches emerges separately from the superior or anterior surface of the parotid gland (Fig. 2.22).

Veins

The superficial temporal vein enters the superior surface of the parotid gland and receives the middle temporal vein to become the posterior facial vein. Still within the gland, the posterior facial vein divides; the posterior branch joins the posterior auricular vein to form the external jugular vein, while the anterior branch emerges from the gland to enter the common facial vein (Fig. 2.23). Remember, the nerve is superficial, the artery is deep, and the vein lies between them.

Lymphatics

The preauricular lymph nodes in the superficial fascia drain the temporal area of the scalp, the upper face, and the anterior pinna. Parotid nodes within the gland drain the gland itself, as well as the nasopharynx, nose, palate, middle ear, and external auditory meatus. These nodes, in turn,

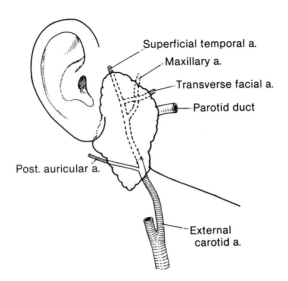

Figure 2.22. Relations of the parotid gland to branches of the external carotid artery. (By permission of JE Skandalakis, SW Gray, and JR Rowe, *Anatomical Complications in General Surgery*, New York: McGraw-Hill, 1983.)

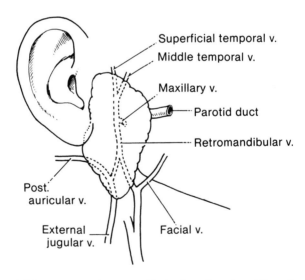

Figure 2.23. Relations of the parotid gland to tributaries of the external and internal jugular veins. (By permission of JE Skandalakis, SW Gray, and JR Rowe, *Anatomical Complications in General Surgery*, New York: McGraw-Hill, 1983.)

send lymph to the subparotid nodes and eventually to the nodes of the internal jugular and spinal accessory chains (Table 2.1).

Great Auricular Nerve

The great auricular nerve reaches the posterior border of the sternocleidomastoid muscle and, on the surface of the parotid gland, follows the course of the external jugular vein. It is sacrificed at parotidectomy. Numbness in the preauricular region, the lower auricle, and the lobe of the ear results from injury to this nerve, but it disappears after 4 to 6 months.

Auriculotemporal Nerve

The auriculotemporal nerve, a branch of the mandibular nerve (V_3), traverses the upper part of the parotid gland and emerges with the superficial temporal blood vessels from the superior surface of the gland. Within the gland, the auriculotemporal nerve communicates with the facial nerve.

Usually, the order of the structures from the tragus anteriorly is: auriculotemporal nerve, superficial temporal artery and vein, and temporal branch of the facial nerve. The auriculotemporal nerve carries sensory fibers from the trigeminal nerve and motor (secretory) fibers from the glossopharyngeal nerve.

Injury to the auriculotemporal nerve produces Frey's syndrome, in which the skin anterior to the ear sweats during eating ("gustatory sweating").

The Parotid Bed

Complete removal of the parotid gland reveals the following structures (the acronym VANS may be helpful in remembering them):

- one **V**ein: internal jugular
- two **A**rteries: external and internal carotid
- four **N**erves: glossopharyngeal (IX), vagus (X), spinal accessory (XI), and hypoglossal (XII) (Fig. 2.24);
- four anatomical entities starting with "**S**": one styloid process and three muscles: styloglossus, stylopharyngeus, and stylohyoid

■ IDENTIFICATION OF THE FACIAL NERVE

The main trunk of the facial nerve is within a triangle bounded by the mastoid process, the external auditory meatus, and the angle of the man-

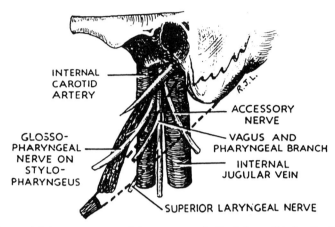

INTERNAL
CAROTID
ARTERY

ACCESSORY
NERVE

GLOSSO-
PHARYNGEAL
NERVE ON
STYLO-
PHARYNGEUS

VAGUS AND
PHARYNGEAL BRANCH

INTERNAL
JUGULAR VEIN

SUPERIOR LARYNGEAL NERVE

Figure 2.24. Lateral view of the structures in the left carotid sheath at the base of the skull. The posterior belly of the digastric is shown in dotted outline. The hypoglossal nerve (not shown) hooks around the vagus and appears between the artery and the vein below the lower border of the digastric. (By permission of RJ Last, *Anatomy: Regional and Applied*. Baltimore: Williams & Wilkins, 1972.)

dible. The lower tip of the mastoid process is palpated and a fingertip is placed on the lateral surface pointing forward. The trunk of the facial nerve will be found deep and anterior to the center of the fingertip.

Remember:

✓ The stem of the nerve lies between the parotid gland and its fascia, deep in front of the mastoid, and medially at the midpoint between the mandibular angle and the cartilaginous ear canal. The stylomastoid foramen and the facial nerve are subcutaneous.

The facial nerve and its branches are in danger during parotidectomy. The facial trunk is large enough for anastomosis of the cut ends, should this be necessary.

■ BRANCHIAL CLEFT SINUSES AND CYSTS

Anatomy of Branchial Remnants

Fistulas

Fistulas are patent ductlike structures that have both external and internal orifices.

Cervicoaural fistulas extend from the skin at the angle of the jaw and may open into the external auditory canal. These fistulas lie anterior or, occasionally, posterior, to the facial nerve. They are remnants of the ventral portion of the 1st branchial cleft (Fig. 2.25).

Lateral cervical fistulas are almost always from the ventral portion of the 2nd branchial cleft and pouch. They originate on the lower third of the neck on the anterior border of the sternocleidomastoid muscle. The path is upward through the platysma muscle and deep fascia. Above the hyoid bone the track turns medially to pass beneath the stylohyoid and the posterior belly of the digastric muscle, in front of the hypoglossal nerve, and between the external and internal carotid arteries. It enters the pharynx on the anterior surface of the upper half of the posterior pillar of the fauces (Fig. 2.26A). It may open into the supratonsillar fossa or even the tonsil itself.

Sinuses

External sinuses are blindly ending spaces that extend inward from openings in the skin. *Internal sinuses* are blindly ending spaces that extend outward from openings in the pharynx.

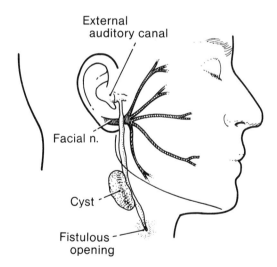

Figure 2.25. Congenital cervicoaural fistula or cyst. This is a persistent remnant of the ventral portion of the 1st branchial cleft. The tract may or may not open into the external auditory canal. (Modified by permission of AH Bill and JL Vadheim, *Ann Surg* 142:904, 1955.)

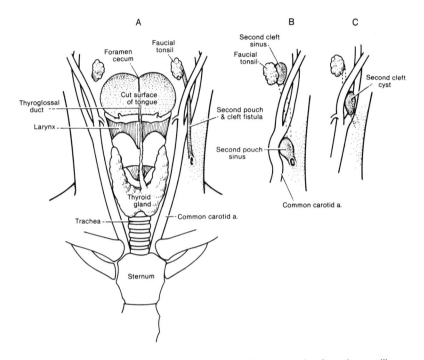

Figure 2.26. Track of a 2nd-pouch and -cleft fistula passing from the tonsillar fossa of the palatine (faucial) tonsils to the neck. (A) Complete fistula. (B) External (cervical) and internal (pharyngeal) sinuses. (C) Cyst of branchial cleft origin lying in the carotid notch. (By permission of JE Skandalakis, SW Gray, and JR Rowe, *Anatomical Complications in General Surgery*, New York: McGraw-Hill, 1983.)

Internal sinuses are usually asymptomatic and hence undetected. External sinuses usually arise at the anterior border of the sternocleidomastoid muscle and end in a cystic dilatation (Fig. 2.26B).

Cysts

Cysts lie in the track of a branchial pouch or cleft and have no communication with the pharynx or skin.

Superficial cysts lie at the edge of the sternocleidomastoid muscle. Deeper cysts lie on the jugular vein or in the bifurcation of the carotid artery (Fig. 2.26C). These are of branchial cleft origin and are lined with stratified squamous epithelium. Cysts on the pharyngeal wall deep to the carotid arteries are usually of branchial cleft origin and are lined with ciliated epithelium unless inflammatory or pressure changes have occurred (Fig. 2.27).

The external and internal carotid arteries just above the bifurcation of the common carotid artery are especially exposed to injury, because a 2nd-cleft cyst or the path of a 2nd-cleft fistula will lie in the crotch of the bifurcation.

Remember:

✓ A 1st-cleft sinus or cyst passes over or under the facial nerve below and anterior to the ear. The cyst may displace the nerve either upward or downward. While removing the cyst, the surgeon must take care to protect the nerve.

✓ Several nerves will be found above the pathway of a 2nd-cleft or -pouch branchial fistula:

    1. The mandibular and cervical branches of the facial nerve

    2. The spinal accessory nerve, which may be injured when trying to free a cyst or fistulous tract from the sternocleidomastoid muscle

    3. The ansa hypoglossis, which may be cut with impunity

    4. The hypoglossal nerve (Above the bifurcation of the common carotid artery the fistula crosses the nerve.)

    5. The superior laryngeal nerves

    6. The vagus nerve, which lies parallel to the carotid artery (The fistula crosses the nerve near the level of the carotid bifurcation.)

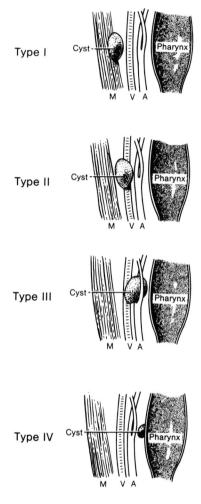

Type I

Type II

Type III

Type IV

Figure 2.27. Incomplete closure of the 2nd branchial cleft or pouch may leave cysts. Type I, superficial, at the border of the sternocleidomastoid muscle. Type II, between the muscle and the jugular vein. Type III, in the bifurcation of the carotid artery. Type IV, in the pharyngeal wall. Types I, II, and III are of 2nd-cleft origin; Type IV is from the second pouch. M = sternocleidomastoid muscle; V = jugular vein; A = carotid artery. (By permission of JE Skandalakis, SW Gray, and JR Rowe, *Anatomical Complications in General Surgery*, New York: McGraw-Hill, 1983.)

TECHNIQUE

■ MASSES OF THE NECK

Diagnosis of nonthyroid neck masses follows a well-marked pathway. With a little rounding of the figures, an easily remembered rule is apparent:

Rule of 80

- 80 percent of nonthyroid neck masses are neoplastic.

- 80 percent of neoplastic neck masses are in males.

- 80 percent of neoplastic neck masses are malignant.

- 80 percent of malignant neck masses are metastatic.

- 80 percent of metastatic neck masses are from primary sites above the clavicle.

In addition, the probable diagnosis may be based on the average duration of the patient's symptoms:

Rule of 7

- Mass from inflammation has existed for 7 days.

- Mass from a neoplasm has existed for 7 months.

- Mass from a congenital defect has existed for 7 years.

However, the plague of AIDS perhaps changes these rules a little.

■ PAROTIDECTOMY

Position and prepare the skin as in thyroid surgery, but uncover the lateral angle of the eye and the labial commissure. Sterilize the external auditory canal. Use intravenous antibiotic of choice.

Procedure:

Step 1. Incision: Inverted T or modified Y (Figs. 2.28 and 2.29)

Inverted T: Make a vertical preauricular incision about 3 mm in front of the ear with downward curved extension at the posterior angle of the mandible. Make a transverse curved incision 3 cm below the mandible with posterior extension close to the mastoid.

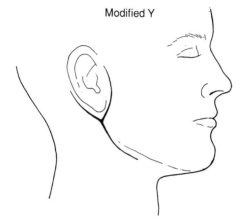

Figure 2.28

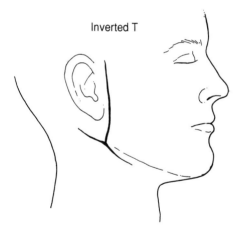

Figure 2.29

Modified Y: Make vertical pre- and postauricular incisions which unite approximately at the angle of the mandible, forming a Y which again meets a transverse incision 3 cm below the mandible.

Make a deep incision into the superficial cervical fascia (anteriorly: fat and platysma; posteriorly: fat only).

Step 2. Formation of flaps (Fig. 2.30)
Carefully elevate skin and fat using knife, scissors, and blunt dissection upward, medially, laterally, downward, and posteriorly.
For the upper flap, provide traction upward and medially on the dissected skin, and laterally toward the external auditory canal. Form the lower flap by dissection of the skin downward and posteriorly toward the mastoid process.

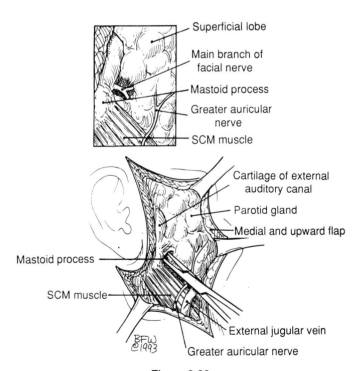

Figure 2.30

Remember:
✓ Sacrifice the great auricular nerve and the posterior facial vein, both very close and topographicoanatomically situated in the vicinity of the lower flap and the lower parotid border.

Step 3. Facial nerve identification (Fig. 2.31)

    a. Place the distal phalanx of the left index finger on the mastoid, pointing to the eye of the patient.

    b. Carefully incise the parotid fascia and further mobilize the superficial part of the parotid.

    c. Insert a hemostat between the mastoid and the gland and bluntly spread the gland medially.

    d. The stem of the nerve will always be found at a depth of less than 0.5 cm. If there is any doubt about identifying the nerve, use electrical stimulation.

    e. Exert upward traction on the superficial lobe and, with a curved hemostat, begin dissection over the nerve.

    f. Identify all five branches.

Step 4. Resection of the superficial lobe (Fig. 2.32)
With gentle traction of the gland and further anterior nerve dissection toward the periphery of the gland, totally mobilize

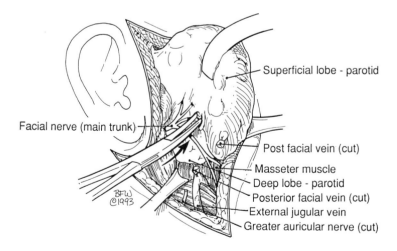

Figure 2.31

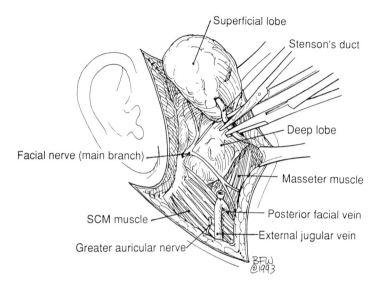

Superficial lobe

Stenson's duct

Deep lobe

Facial nerve (main branch)

Masseter muscle

Posterior facial vein

SCM muscle

External jugular vein

Greater auricular nerve

Figure 2.32

and resect the superficial lobe. As the dissection is carried toward the ends of the branches of the facial nerve, Stensen's duct will be encountered and should be ligated and divided.

Step 5. Resection of the deep lobe (Fig. 2.33)
The following anatomical entities should be kept in mind:

a. pterygoid venous plexus

b. external carotid artery

c. maxillary nerve

d. superficial temporal nerve

e. posterior facial vein

All the above should be ligated using fine chromic catgut. Pterygoid venous plexus bleeding may be stopped by compression. Do not go deep: remember VANS (see p. 49). Remove the deep lobe carefully, working under the facial nerve by the piecemeal dissection technique. Obtain good hemostasis.

Radical Parotidectomy (Fig. 2.34)

Excise the parotid in toto, as well as the facial nerve and the regional lymph nodes; also perform ipsilateral radical neck dissection, if necessary.

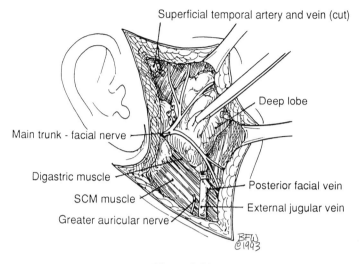

Superficial temporal artery and vein (cut)

Deep lobe

Main trunk - facial nerve

Digastric muscle

SCM muscle

Greater auricular nerve

Posterior facial vein

External jugular vein

BFW
©1993

Figure 2.33

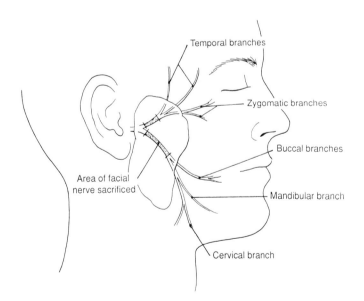

Temporal branches

Zygomatic branches

Buccal branches

Area of facial
nerve sacrificed

Mandibular branch

Cervical branch

Figure 2.34

In such an operation, the authors strongly recommend the presence of a plastic surgeon as a member of the team to avoid medicolegal problems. Autologous graft microanastomosis should be considered for reconstruction of the facial nerve.

The greater and lesser occipital nerves can serve as donors.

Remember:

✓ Try to save zygomatic marginal branches if possible. If not, use microanastomosis end-to-end proximal and distal with 10-0 silk.

Insert a Jackson–Pratt drain through a lower stab wound. To close the wound, use interrupted 4-0 catgut for platysma and fat, and interrupted 6-0 nylon for skin.

■ RESECTION OF SUBMAXILLARY GLAND (Figs. 2.1 to 2.6)

POSITION AND PREPARATION: As in parotidectomy. The upper half of the face should be covered, but the labial commissure should be uncovered.

INCISION: Make a transverse incision 3 cm below the lower border of the mandible. Incise the superficial fascia from the anterior border of the sternocleidomastoid muscle to 2–3 cm from the midline (Fig. 2.35).

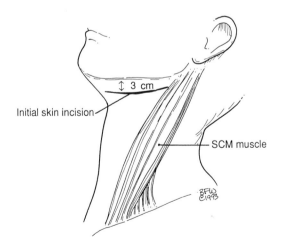

↕ 3 cm

Initial skin incision

SCM muscle

BFW
©1993

Figure 2.35

Remember:

✓ The two branches of the facial nerve (mandibular and cervical) are under the platysma and the deep fascia of the gland. Identify and protect them. Apply retractors carefully.

SURGICAL FIELD IN VIEW:

- superior: inferior border of mandible
- inferior: digastric and stylohyoid muscles
- medially: mylohyoid muscle
- laterally: sternocleidomastoid muscle
- center: deep cervical fascia covering the gland

The common facial vein, its anterior vein, or its posterior vein is now in view close to the sternocleidomastoid muscle. Continue to observe the marginal branch of the facial nerve, which is superficial to the facial vessels (occasionally at a lower level).

Remember:

✓ There are lymph nodes outside the capsule close to the vessels. With benign disease, removal of these is not necessary.

Procedure:

Step 1. Ligate the facial vessels (Fig. 2.36).

Step 2. With curved hemostat, separate inferiorly the gland from the digastric muscle (Fig. 2.37).

> **Remember:**
>
> ✓ The hypoglossal nerve is located very close to the digastric tendon and is accompanied by the lingual vein and, deeper, by the external maxillary artery. Both vessels should be ligated carefully. Elevate the mylohyoid muscle to expose the deep part of the submaxillary gland. Separate the gland slowly. Just under the gland and cephalad to it, the following anatomical entities are in view: lingual nerve, chorda tympani, submaxillary ganglion, and Wharton's duct.

Step 3. Ligate and cut Wharton's duct. Protect the lingual nerve (Fig. 2.38). Continue blunt dissection.

Step 4. Insert Jackson–Pratt drain and close in layers.

Caution: The three points of danger are the mandibular, hypoglossal, and lingual nerves.

■ EXCISION OF STONE FROM WHARTON'S DUCT

If possible, dilate the opening of the duct (Fig. 2.39). Make an incision over the duct. Remove the stone (Fig. 2.40). Do not close the incision.

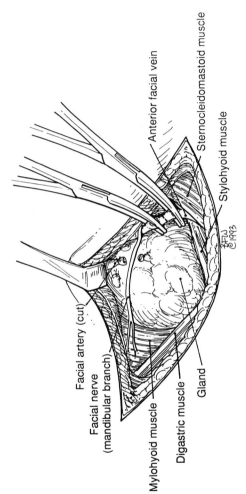

Facial artery (cut)

Facial nerve
(mandibular branch)

Mylohyoid muscle

Digastric muscle

Gland

Anterior facial vein

Sternocleidomastoid muscle

Stylohyoid muscle

Figure 2.36

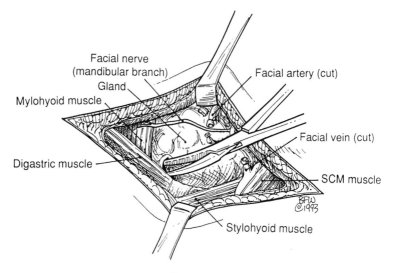

Facial nerve
(mandibular branch)
Gland
Mylohyoid muscle

Facial artery (cut)

Facial vein (cut)

Digastric muscle

SCM muscle

Stylohyoid muscle

Figure 2.37

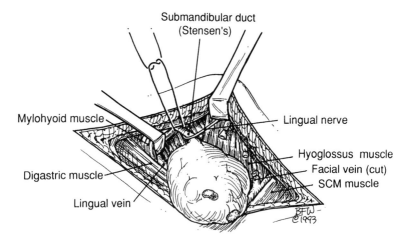

Submandibular duct
(Stensen's)

Mylohyoid muscle

Lingual nerve

Digastric muscle

Hyoglossus muscle
Facial vein (cut)
SCM muscle

Lingual vein

Figure 2.38

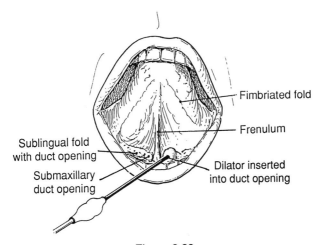

Fimbriated fold

Frenulum

Sublingual fold
with duct opening

Submaxillary
duct opening

Dilator inserted
into duct opening

Figure 2.39

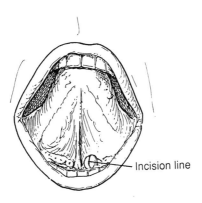

Incision line

Figure 2.40

■ THYROIDECTOMY AND PARATHYROIDECTOMY

Procedure:

Step 1. Position

    a. Put the patient in semi-Fowler position.

    b. Patient's neck should be hyperextended.

    c. Place small pillow at the area of the upper thoracic spine, beneath the shoulders.

    d. Place a doughnut support under the head.

Step 2. Preparation of skin

    a. Use Betadine or any other solution of the surgeon's choice.

    b. Be sure the chin and long axis of the body are aligned at the midline.

    c. With 2-0 silk, mark the location of the incision, two finger breadths above the sternal notch.

    d. Use a knife to mark very superficially the middle and edges of the previously marked location of the incision.

Step 3. Incise the low collar symmetrical mark of the skin, carrying out the incision through the superficial fascia (subcutaneous fat and platysma). Establish good hemostasis by electrocoagulation or ligation using silk (Figs. 2.41 and 2.42).

Step 4. Formation of flaps (Fig. 2.43)
By blunt dissection, elevate the upper flap to the notch of the thyroid cartilage and the lower flap to the jugular (sternal) notch. Use Mahorner's, Murphy's, or other self-retaining retractors.

Step 5. Opening of the deep fascia (Figs. 2.44 and 2.45)
The opening is accomplished by a longitudinal midline incision along the raphe of the strap muscles, which is actually the deep fascia.

Step 6. Elevation of the strap muscles (Figs. 2.46–2.48)
The sternohyoid muscles are easily elevated, but the thyrohyoid and sternothyroid muscles are attached to the false thyroid capsule and should be separated carefully to avoid injuring the gland and causing bleeding. In extremely rare cases, when the thyroid gland is huge, section of the strap muscles becomes necessary. Divide them at the proximal (upper) one-

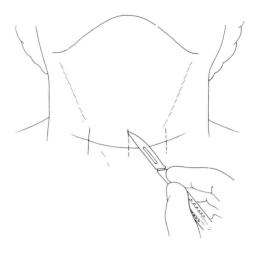

Figure 2.41

third to avoid paralysis due to injury of the ansa hypoglossi
(C_1, C_2, C_3 and XII).

The sternohyoid muscles are the most superficial, and the
sternothyroid and thyrohyoid are underneath. For practical
purposes, the thyrohyoid is an upward continuation of the
sternothyroid.

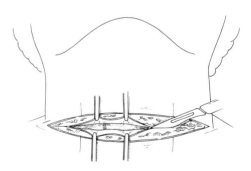

Figure 2.42

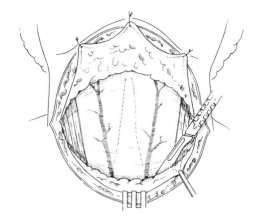

Figure 2.43

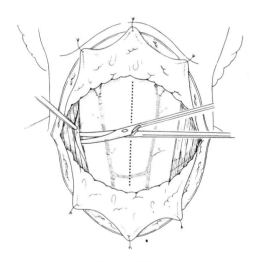

Figure 2.44

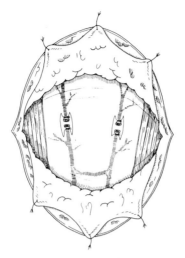

Figure 2.45

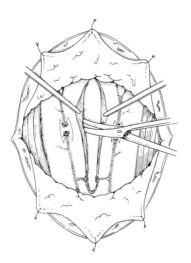

Figure 2.46

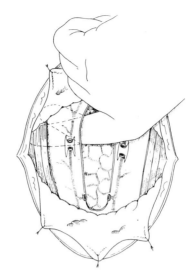

Figure 2.47

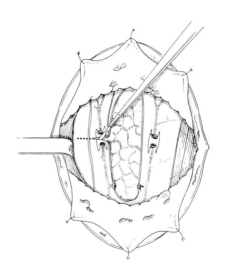

Figure 2.48

Step 7. Exposure and mobilization of the gland

With all strap muscles elevated and retracted, the index finger of the surgeon is gently inserted between the thyroid and the muscles. A lateral elevation is also taking place, occasionally using all the fingers except the thumb. It not only breaks the remaining muscular or pathological attachments, but enables the surgeon to appreciate the gross pathology of the gland in toto. Occasionally the strap muscles should be divided.

The surgeon now decides whether to perform a total or a partial (subtotal) lobectomy (Figs. 2.47–2.49).

The anatomy of the normal and the abnormal must be studied carefully regarding size, extension, consistency, and fixation of the gland. Is a pyramidal lobe present? How thick is the isthmus? Are a Delphian node or other lymph nodes present? If so, excision of the Delphian node and perhaps of one or two of the other palpable lymph nodes is in order. Frozen section should follow.

Step 8. Total lobectomy (Figs. 2.50–2.52)

    a. Retract the lobe medially and anteriorly by special clamps or deep sutures outside the lesion.

    b. Ligate the middle thyroid vein.

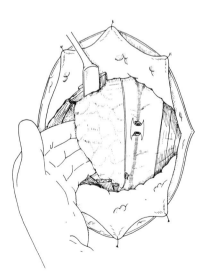

Figure 2.49

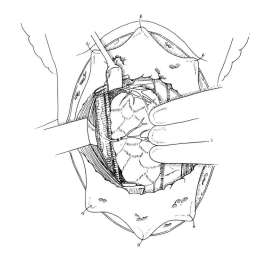

Figure 2.50

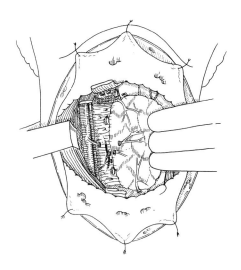

Figure 2.51

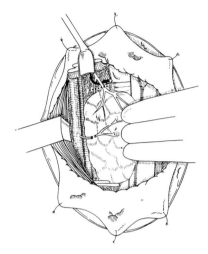

Figure 2.52

c. Identify the recurrent laryngeal nerve by blunt dissection into the tracheoesophageal groove.

d. Identify and protect the parathyroids.

e. Ligate the inferior thyroid artery.

f. Ligate the lower pole vessels.

g. Carefully ligate the upper pole. Perform en masse ligation, thereby ligating the superior thyroid artery, or, if possible, prepare the artery above the pole and ligate.

h. Dissect the lobe from the trachea by dividing the gland between straight mosquitoes. Suture ligate the tissue that is clamped over the trachea with 3-0 silk.

i. If the pyramidal lobe is present, ligate its most distal part and remove it together with the lobe. Send the specimen to the lab for frozen section.

j. Ligate the isthmus, if present.

k. Obtain meticulous hemostasis.

Step 9. Partial (subtotal) thyroidectomy.
Apply multiple hemostats at the thyroid parenchyma and partially transect the gland. Use 4-0 silk suture ligature for su-

ture ligation of the thyroid parenchyma and surface veins. If possible, approximate the segment to the trachea. Both upper pole remnants or the tracheoesophageal remnant should weigh approximately 5-6 g.

Step 10. Strategy for finding parathyroid glands.
The following steps are suggested for abnormal parathyroid location.

  a. Explore the superior surface of the thyroid gland. Ligate the middle thyroid veins, retract the lobe medially and anteriorly, and expose the recurrent laryngeal nerve.

  b. Dissect the superior anterior mediastinum as far as possible, with special attention to the thymus or its remnant behind the manubrium.

  c. Explore the region above the upper pole of the thyroid gland as far as the hyoid bone.

  d. Explore the retroesophageal and retropharyngeal spaces.

  e. Perform subtotal thyroidectomy.

  f. Further explore the mediastinum at a second operation. This should be done only after the pathology report on thymus and thyroid tissue has been received and no parathyroid tissue is reported.

Remember:

✔ The best anatomical landmark is the inferior thyroid artery.

✔ The most useful instrument for palpation is the distal phalanx of the index finger.

Step 11. In a patient with hyperplasia, remove 3½ glands. The remaining ½ gland can be left in situ or implanted into the sternocleidomastoid muscle. In any case, cryopreserve a parathyroid for reimplantation in case the patient becomes hypothyroid. When a patient is explored for a suspected adenoma, the healthy glands will be smaller than normal. Try to identify all the glands, and do not stop after having removed the adenoma, because in a small percentage of cases multiple adenomas are found. Always send adenomas for frozen section. If the gland is determined to be malignant, the surrounding tissue should be removed.

Step 12. Reconstruction

Insert a Penrose or a Jackson–Pratt drain. Close the midline and the superficial fascia, approximating the marked points and avoiding dog-ears. Closure of the skin is up to the surgeon: Use subcuticular sutures with Steri-strips, interrupted 6-0 nylon, or clips. Remember to check the vocal cords as soon as the endotracheal tube has been removed.

■ THYROID REOPERATION

Procedure:

Step 1. Carefully read the previous operating report.

Step 2. Inspect vocal cords.

Step 3. Incise through the previous scar, but add 1–2 cm on each side laterally.

Step 4. Make flaps as in thyroidectomy.

Step 5. Identify the sternocleidomastoid; incise, dissect, and elevate its medial border.

Step 6. Carefully elevate the strap muscles.

Step 7. There are two ways to reexplore the thyroid: from the periphery (this anatomically intact area has less scar tissue) to the center, and from the midline/isthmic area to the periphery.

    a. From the periphery to the center

Most likely, the virgin area after thyroid surgery is the area corresponding to the medial border of the sternocleidomastoid. The best anatomical landmark is the proximal part of the inferior thyroid artery, since the distal was probably ligated. Any white, thin, cordlike structure should be protected, since this is probably the recurrent laryngeal nerve. If in doubt, stop the dissection in this area and try to find the nerve at the cricothyroid area above, or at the supraclavicular area below. The most virgin area is just above the clavicle, and the least virgin (if total lobectomy was done previously) is the cricothyroid area. The parathyroids will be found above and below the inferior thyroid artery.

The remnants of the thyroid glands will be found in the tracheoesophageal groove or in the area of the upper thyroid pole.

b. From the midline/isthmic area to the periphery
The anatomical area to be explored with this procedure is the tracheoesophageal groove, in the hope that the recurrent laryngeal nerve is somewhere in the vicinity. Small curved mosquito or Mixter clamps may be used for elevation of the thyroid remnants, location of the nerve, and location of the parathyroids.

If reexploration was done for malignant disease, then a modified radical neck dissection is in order. The recurrent nerve should be saved; only if it is fixed to the tumor should it be sacrificed.

■ PARATHYROID REOPERATION

Procedure:

Step 1. Read about normal and abnormal locations.

Step 2. Carefully read the previous operating report and pay special attention to:

    a. Number of parathyroids removed

    b. Sites (right or left)

    c. Together with the radiologist, study all possible results of techniques for localization (ultrasonography, CT scan, MRI, thallium 201, technetium 99m subtraction scan, selective venous catheterization with parathyroid hormone immunoassay evaluation, digital subtraction angiography)

Step 3. Reexplore the neck as in thyroidectomy.

Step 4. Locate and mark the inferior thyroid artery.

Step 5. Protect the recurrent laryngeal nerve.

Step 6. Palpate the "certain" location and all possible locations of parathyroid glands, such as: tracheoesophageal groove, retropharyngeal, retroesophageal, retrocarotid, anterior mediastinum (thymus), posterior mediastinum, middle mediastinum (pericardium) within the carotid sheath, suprathyroid, infrathyroid, intrathyroid, and posterior triangle.

Step 7. Remove the tumor. A patient diagnosed with hyperplasia probably has one gland or only ½ of the fourth gland (if the patient has only four glands) with hyperplasia or adenomatous changes. Remove 50 percent of this remnant and be sure it has a good blood supply. If uncertain, perform a total parathyroidectomy and transplant multiple pieces (1 mm in diameter) of the adenoma or the hyperplastic gland into the biceps muscle, being sure to mark the location. If there is an adenoma that was not found previously, remove it. If the frozen section is determined to be malignant, the surrounding tissue should be removed.

■ THYROGLOSSAL DUCT CYSTECTOMY (Fig. 2.53)

Position and prepare as for thyroidectomy.

Procedure:

Step 1. Make a transverse incision over the cyst. Incise the superficial fascia (fat and platysma) and mark the skin at the midline to facilitate good closure. Formation of flaps: The upward elevation reaches the hyoid bone and extends cephalad 1–2 cm. Elevate the lower flap almost to the isthmus of the thyroid gland. One self-retaining retractor is enough to keep the field open. Open the deep fascia in a longitudinal fashion.

Step 2. Dissect the cyst and isolate it with a small hemostat and plastic scissors (Fig. 2.54). The involved anatomical entities depend upon the location of the cyst (Fig. 2.55): suprahyoid (rare), hyoid (common), infrahyoid or suprasternal (rare). (Embryology plays a great role here.)

Remember:

✓ The embryologic path of descent of the thyroid gland (from the foramen cecum to the manubrium sterni).

✓ The thyroglossal duct (a midline cordlike formation) travels, in most cases, through the hyoid bone.

✓ The anatomical entities involved in most of the cases are:
  - foramen cecum
  - thyroid membrane
  - mylohyoid muscle
  - geniohyoid muscle
  - genioglossus muscle
  - sternohyoid muscle
  - anterior belly of digastric muscle

✓ The mylohyoid is fixed to the hyoid bone above and the sternohyoid is fixed to the hyoid bone below.

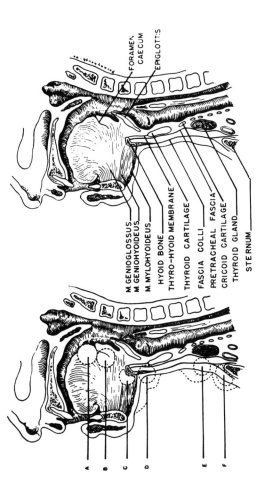

FORAMEN CAECUM

EPIGLOTTIS

M. GENIOGLOSSUS
M. GENIOHYOIDEUS
M. MYLOHYOIDEUS
HYOID BONE
THYRO-HYOID MEMBRANE
THYROID CARTILAGE
FASCIA COLLI
PRETRACHEAL FASCIA
CRICOID CARTILAGE
THYROID GLAND
STERNUM

Figure 2.53. Various locations of thyroglossal duct cysts. (A) In front of the foramen cecum. (B) At the foramen cecum. (C) Above the hyoid bone. (D) Below the hyoid bone. (E) In the region of the thyroid gland. (F) At the suprasternal notch. About 50 percent of the cysts are located at D, below the hyoid bone. (By permission of GE Ward, JW Hendrick, and RG Chambers, *Surg Obstet Gynecol* 89:728, 1949.)

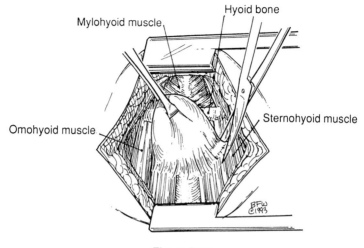

Figure 2.54

✓ The anterior belly of the digastric muscle occasionally may partially cover the hyoid bone laterally.

✓ The geniohyoid is between the thyroid membrane and the mylohyoid.

Step 3. Take special care of the hyoid bone and tract. Clean the central part of the hyoid bone. Leave some cuffs of sternohyoid and mylohyoid attached to the bone, as well as some cuffs of the underlying geniohyoid and genioglossus attached to the cephalad tract. Insert a curved hemostat under the central part of the hyoid bone. With heavy scissors or small bone cutter, cut the bone on both sides. Continue upward dissection bilaterally to the midline where the tract is located as advised above. The thyrohyoid membrane is now exposed (Figs. 2.56 and 2.57).

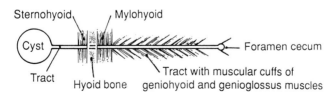

Figure 2.55

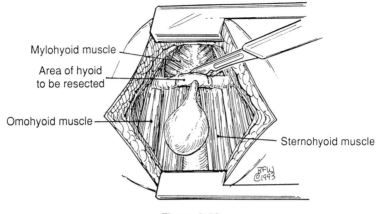

Mylohyoid muscle

Area of hyoid
to be resected

Omohyoid muscle

Sternohyoid muscle

Figure 2.56

Step 4. The foramen cecum also requires special attention. The anesthesiologist's index finger is inserted into the patient's mouth, elevating the foramen cecum. With continuous cephalad dissection, the surgeon reaches the foramen cecum by palpating the finger of the anesthesiologist just under the thyrohyoid membrane. Excise the foramen cecum in continuity and close the defect with figure-of-eight 4–0 chromic catgut or any other

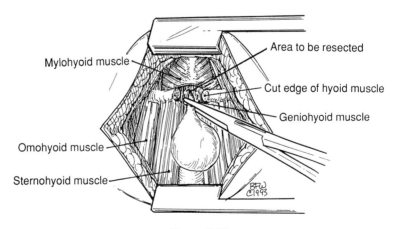

Area to be resected

Mylohyoid muscle

Cut edge of hyoid muscle

Geniohyoid muscle

Omohyoid muscle

Sternohyoid muscle

Figure 2.57

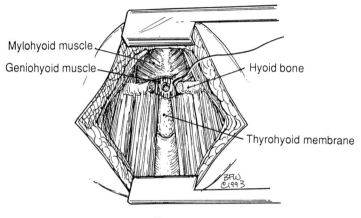

Mylohyoid muscle

Geniohyoid muscle

Hyoid bone

Thyrohyoid membrane

BRW
©1993

Figure 2.58

absorbable suture. Drainage is up to the surgeon. Establish good hemostasis. Irrigate with normal saline (Fig. 2.58).

Step 5. Reconstruction. Perform midline approximation of the mylohyoid and sternohyoid with interrupted sutures as for thyroid operation.

Note: In the case of a sinus without cyst, follow the same steps.

■ EXCISION OF BRANCHIAL CLEFT CYST OR FISTULA

Procedure:

Step 1. Above a cyst, make a small transverse incision; around a sinus, make an elliptical incision. Multiple incisions will be necessary if the cyst or sinus is low (Fig. 2.59).

Step 2. Separate and elevate the sternocleidomastoid muscle, always using the medial border (Fig. 2.60).

Step 3. Visualize the carotid sheath and hypoglossal nerve (Fig. 2.61).

Step 4. Continue dissection of the cyst or sinus cephalad toward the pharyngeal wall.

Step 5. Excise the minute pharyngeal wall if pathology exists.

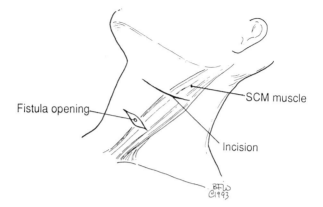

Figure 2.59

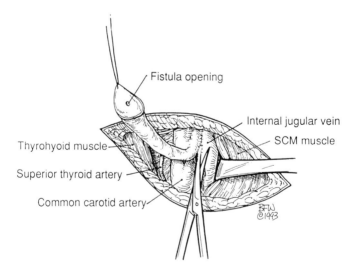

Figure 2.60

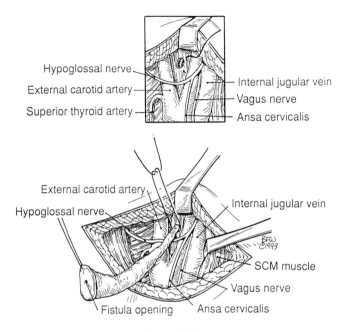

Figure 2.61

■ RADICAL NECK DISSECTION

Definition

A radical neck dissection must be planned as a curative procedure. It involves complete excision of the primary lesion, together with all nonessential structures and their lymph nodes, collecting lymph trunks, fascia, and fat. The bed of a radical neck dissection is bounded superiorly by the inferior border of the mandible, inferiorly by the clavicle, posteriorly by the anterior border of the trapezius muscle, and anteriorly by the midline.

Lymphatic tissue must be removed as completely as possible. Nonlymphatic tissue falls into three categories: (1) structures that can be sacrificed with impunity, (2) structures whose sacrifice is controversial, especially for cosmetic reasons, and (3) structures that must be preserved unless directly invaded by cancer. Structures in these categories are listed in Table 2.3.

Table 2.3 Synopsis of Radical Neck Procedures

Structures	May be sacrificed	Controversial	Must be preserved[a]
Organs	Submaxillary gland, lower pole of parotid gland	None	Thyroid gland, parathyroid glands
Muscles	Omohyoid, sternocleidomastoid	Platysma, digastric, stylohyoid	All other muscles
Vessels	External jugular vein, facial artery and vein, superior thyroid artery, lingual artery	Internal jugular vein	External carotid artery, internal carotid artery, subclavian artery and vein, thoracic duct
Nerves	Anterior cutaneous C_2–C_3, supraclavicular C_3–C_4, ansa hypoglossi, great auricular nerve	Spinal accessory nerve	Mandibular branch of facial nerve, superior laryngeal nerve, recurrent laryngeal nerve, facial nerve, lingual nerve, hypoglossal nerve, phrenic nerve, vagus nerve, cervical sympathetic nerve, carotid sinus nerves, brachial plexus, nerves to rhomboid and serratus muscles

[a]Unless invaded by cancer.
(By permission of JE Skandalakis, SW Gray, and JR Rowe, *Anatomical Complications in General Surgery*, New York: McGraw-Hill, 1983.)

Anatomical Elements

Superficial cervical fascia

The anterior cutaneous nerves and the supraclavicular nerves must be sacrificed. The platysma muscle should be preserved.

Deep cervical fascia

The deep cervical fascia must be removed as completely as possible, since lymph nodes and lymphatic vessels are largely distributed in the connective tissue between the layers of the fascia. The carotid sheath and the internal jugular vein also should be sacrificed.

Anterior triangle

1. Submental triangle: Remove the entire contents.

2. Submandibular triangle: Remove the submaxillary gland and lymph nodes.

3. Carotid triangle: Remove the internal jugular vein. High ligation of the vein is facilitated by removal of the lower pole of the parotid gland. The great auricular nerve and all superficial branches of the cervical nerves should be cut. All lymph nodes along the internal jugular vein must be removed. The final result is shown in Fig. 2.62.

Posterior triangle

Remove all tissue above the spinal accessory nerve without injury to the nerve. With blunt dissection, free the nerve from the underlying tissue. Ligate the external jugular vein close to the subclavian vein, and transect the sternocleidomastoid and omohyoid muscles.

The area beneath the spinal accessory nerve is the "danger zone" of Beahrs and contains a number of structures that must be saved: the nerves to rhomboid and serratus muscles, the brachial plexus, the subclavian artery and vein with the anterior scalene muscle between, and the phrenic nerve. All these should be preserved if possible. The object of dissection in this area is to remove completely the transverse cervical (inferior horizontal) and spinal accessory chains of lymph nodes (see Fig. 2.11).

Deep to the sternocleidomastoid muscle and posterolateral to the internal jugular vein, the thoracic duct on the left and the right lymphatic duct on the right lie in a mass of areolar connective tissue. They should be preserved if possible; if they have been injured, ligate.

Between the jugular vein and the carotid artery lies the ansa cervicalis, which innervates the strap muscles of the neck. This nerve is on or in the carotid sheath medial to the internal jugular vein. It may be cut with impunity.

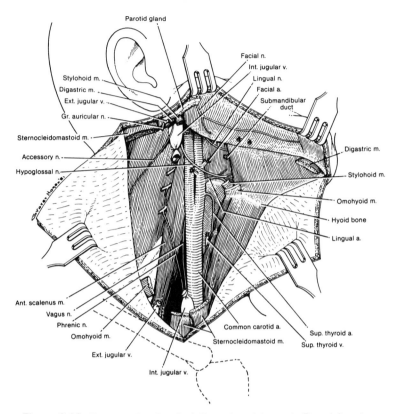

Figure 2.62. The completed radical dissection of the neck. Remaining structures may be removed if they are involved in malignant growth. (Modified by permission of OH Beahrs, *Surg Clin NA* 57:477–493, 1977.)

Procedure:

Position and prepare as in parotidectomy.

Step 1. Incision (Figs. 2.63–2.65)

Make a T-incision with the horizontal part extending from the midline to the submastoid area approximately 3 cm below the inferior border of the mandible and the vertical part extending from the midpoint of the horizontal down to 1 cm above the clavicle. Alternative incisions are the H type, the I type, or one shaped like an H lying on its side (⊥).

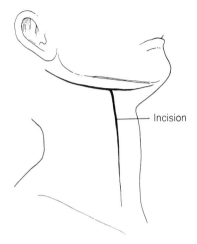

Figure 2.63

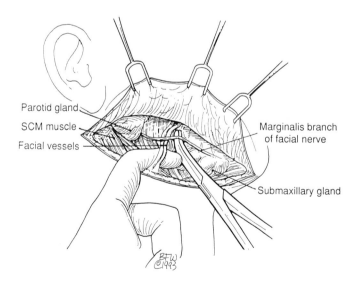

Figure 2.64

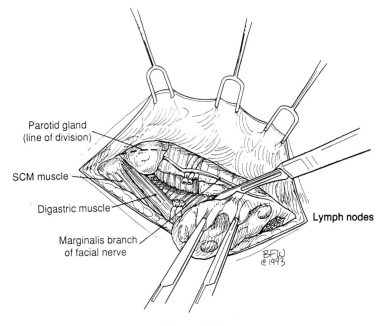

Parotid gland
(line of division)

SCM muscle

Digastric muscle

Lymph nodes

Marginalis branch
of facial nerve

Figure 2.65

The upper flap of the horizontal part. Incise the superficial fascia (fat and platysma) by deepening the skin incision and elevate the upper flap. The anterior facial vessels are located at the upper part of the flap snaking in front of the mandible. The mandibular and cervical branches of the facial nerves are located superficially to these vessels. Protect both nerves, especially the marginal branch, by careful dissection and isolation. The cervical branch may be cut, if necessary. Elevate the anterior facial vessels, then clamp, divide, and ligate them.

Detach the deep cervical fascia from the mandible and push it downward bluntly, including the submental area and the submaxillary gland, fat, and lymph nodes. Occasionally, the lower pole of the parotid is removed below the disappearing point of the marginal branch. Then, in this procedure, the contents of the submental and submandibular triangles are dissected as well as the lower pole of the parotid.

Vertical incision and formation of flaps. To form flaps, deepen the existing skin incision. Prepare the anterior neck triangle and elevate the anterior flap to the midline and the posterior flap to the anterior border of the trapezius muscle. The sternocleidomastoid muscle is practically in the middle of the surgical field.

Step 2. Exploration of the posterior triangle (Fig. 2.66)
The following anatomical entities should be identified:

    a. spinal accessory nerve

    b. external jugular vein

    c. cervical nerves (not shown)

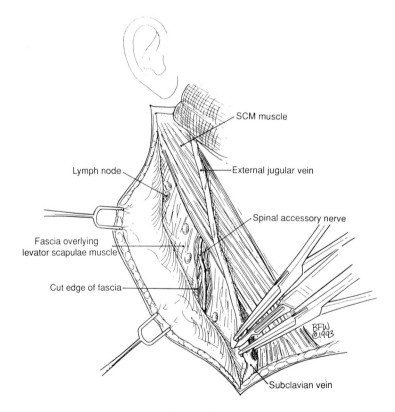

Figure 2.66

    d. brachial plexus (between anterior and middle scalene) (not shown)

    e. phrenic nerve (resting on the anterior scalene) (not shown)

All but the spinal accessory nerve are under the carpet of the floor of the posterior triangle, which is the splitting of the deep fascia.

Carefully ligate the external jugular vein close to the subclavian vein while protecting the other four entities listed above. The upper part of the posterior triangle is cleaned by blunt dissection, pushing fibrofatty tissue and lymph nodes cephalad.

Step 3. After elevating and protecting the anatomical entities of the carotid sheath, carefully transect the clavicular and sternal insertions of the sternocleidomastoid muscle.

The next step is a low division of the omohyoid behind the sternocleidomastoid muscle. Continue to clean up the floor of the posterior triangle (Figs. 2.67 and 2.68).

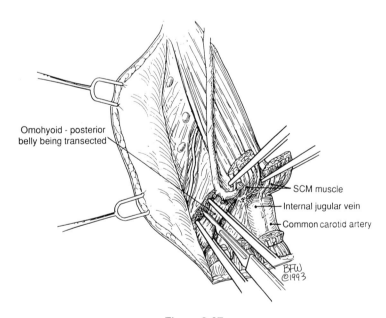

Omohyoid - posterior belly being transected

SCM muscle

Internal jugular vein

Common carotid artery

BFW
©1993

Figure 2.67

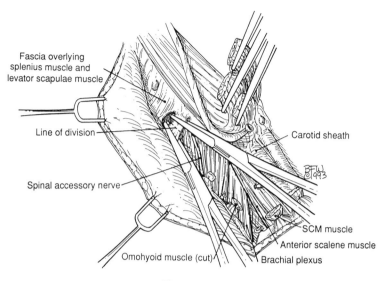

Fascia overlying
splenius muscle and
levator scapulae muscle

Line of division

Spinal accessory nerve

Omohyoid muscle (cut)

Carotid sheath

SCM muscle

Anterior scalene muscle

Brachial plexus

Figure 2.68

Step 4. Open the anterior wall of the carotid sheath, ligate the internal jugular vein close to the clavicle, and remove the sheath together with the vein and all fibrofatty tissue in the vicinity. Protect the phrenic nerve, and ligate the transverse scapular and transverse cervical arteries and the right or left thoracic ducts as required. Proceeding upward, remember: The posterior belly of the digastric muscle is an excellent anatomical landmark. Just underneath are internal and external carotid arteries; the internal jugular vein, which should be ligated; cranial nerves (X, XI, XII); and the sympathetic chain (Fig. 2.69).

Step 5. Working now at the anterior triangle, avoid cutting the external branch of the superior laryngeal nerve. Ligate the branches of the external carotid artery. Protect and save the hypoglossal nerve. Continue to work on both the submental and the submandibular triangles. Ligate the submaxillary duct, but protect and save its fellow traveler, the lingual nerve. Spare the submaxillary ganglion. Establish good hemostasis (Fig. 2.70).

Step 6. Remove the specimen en bloc (Fig. 2.71). Fig. 2.62 shows the surgical field after removal of the specimen.

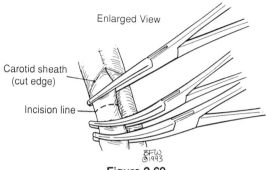

Enlarged View

Carotid sheath
(cut edge)

Incision line —

BFW
©1993

Figure 2.69

In the beautiful book *An Atlas of the Surgical Techniques of Oliver H. Beahrs* (Beahrs OH, Kiernan PD, Hubert JP Jr, Philadelphia: W.B. Saunders Co., 1985), Dr. Beahrs gives an excellent description of the technique of radical neck, one of the most complicated surgeries of the human body. We strongly advise the reader to consult his book and article in Surgical Clinics of North America, August 1977; 57(4):663–700) (W.B. Saunders, Philadelphia).

■ TRACHEOSTOMY

Procedure

Step 1. Position:

    a. semi-Fowler position

    b. hyperextension of neck

    c. small pillow at the area of the upper thoracic spine beneath the shoulders

    d. doughnut support under the head

Step 2. Preparation of skin:

    a. Use Betadine or any other solution of surgeon's choice.

    b. Be sure that chin and long axis of the body are aligned at the midline.

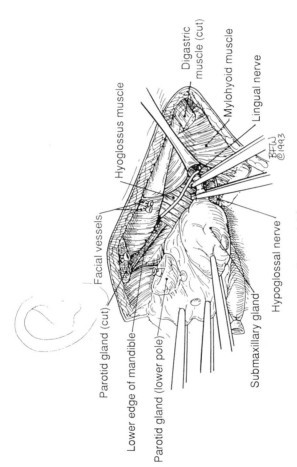

Facial vessels

Parotid gland (cut)

Lower edge of mandible

Parotid gland (lower pole)

Hyoglossus muscle

Digastric muscle (cut)

Mylohyoid muscle

Lingual nerve

Submaxillary gland

Hypoglossal nerve

BFW
©1993

Figure 2.70

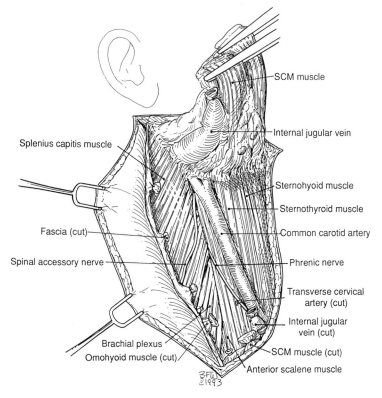

Figure 2.71

    c. Mark the location of the incision with 2–0 silk, two finger
breadths above the sternal notch.

    d. With a knife, mark very superficially the middle and
edges of the previously marked location of the incision.
Using an endotracheal tube is a wise step.

Step 3. In children, make a vertical incision to avoid injury of the
arteries and veins located under the anterior border of the
sternocleidomastoid muscle.

    In adults, use vertical or transverse incision and proceed as in
thyroid surgery (Fig. 2.72).

Step 4. Locate the thyroid isthmus. The inferior thyroid vein and thyroid ima artery should be ligated (Fig. 2.73).

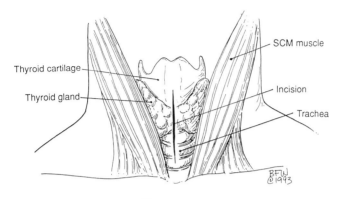

Figure 2.72

Step 5. Clean the anterior wall of the trachea below the isthmus.

Remember:

✓ Dissection too deep toward the superior mediastinum will injure the jugular venous arch, and too lateral dissection will injure the vessels of the carotid sheath. The thyroid isthmus should be retracted or cut between clamps for more tracheal room.

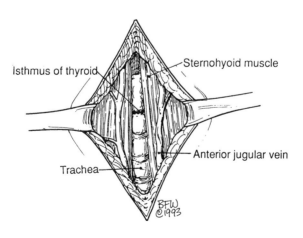

Figure 2.73

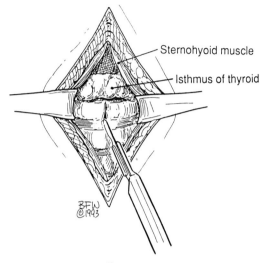

Sternohyoid muscle

Isthmus of thyroid

Figure 2.74

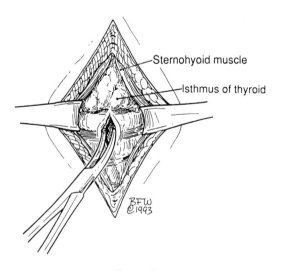

Sternohyoid muscle

Isthmus of thyroid

Figure 2.75

Step 6. Immobilize and elevate the anterior tracheal wall using a hook at the lower border of the cricoid cartilage.

Step 7. Make a vertical incision through the 2–3 tracheal ring or form a window at the anterior tracheal wall by removing the anterior central segment of the two rings (Fig. 2.74).

> **Remember:**
>
> Be careful when you incise the trachea. The posterior wall of the trachea is not protected, so the danger of esophageal injury is obvious.
>
> Protect the cricoid cartilage and 1st tracheal ring to avoid postoperative tracheal stenosis.

Step 8. Spread the tracheal opening with a tracheal spreader. Insert a Hardy–Shiley tracheostomy tube as the endotracheal tube is slowly backed out (Fig. 2.75).

Step 9. With umbilical tape, secure the tube around the patient's neck. Pack iodoform in the subcutaneous tissue around the tracheostomy tube.

3

Breast

ANATOMY

■ GENERAL DESCRIPTION OF THE BREAST

The adult female breast is located within the superficial fascia of the anterior chest wall. The base of the breast extends from the 2nd rib above to the 6th or 7th rib below, and from the sternal border medially to the midaxillary line laterally. Two-thirds of the base of the breast lies anterior to the pectoralis major muscle; the remainder lies anterior to the serratus anterior muscle. A small part may lie over the aponeurosis of the external oblique muscle.

In about 95 percent of women, there is a prolongation of the upper lateral quadrant toward the axilla. This tail (of Spence) of breast tissue enters a hiatus (of Langer) in the deep fascia of the medial axillary wall. This is the only breast tissue found beneath the deep fascia.

■ DEEP FASCIA

The deep pectoral fascia envelops the pectoralis, and the clavipectoral fascia envelops the pectoralis minor and part of the subclavius muscles. The axillary fascia lying across the base of the axillary pyramidal space is an extension of the pectoralis major fascia and continues as the fascia of the latissimus dorsi. It forms the dome of the axilla (Fig. 3.1A).

Where the axillary vessels and the nerves to the arm pass through it, they take with them a tubular fascial sleeve, the axillary sheath.

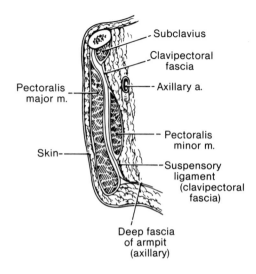

A   Anterior Wall

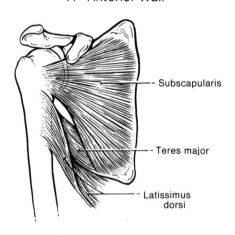

B   Posterior Wall

Figure 3.1. Diagram of the walls of the axilla. (Modified by permission of JV Basmajian and CE Slonecker, *Grant's Method of Anatomy*, 11th ed. Baltimore: Williams & Wilkins, 1989.)

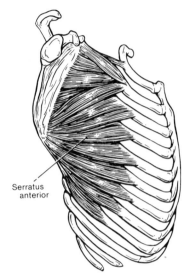

C   Medial Wall

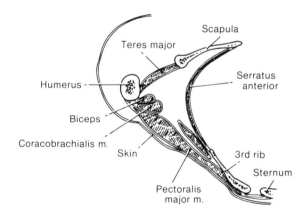

D   Lateral Wall

The clavipectoral fascia is thus formed of four parts (Fig. 3.1A):

1. The attachment to the clavicle and the envelope of the subclavian muscle
2. The costocoracoid ligament between the subclavius and pectoralis minor muscles
3. The pectoralis minor envelope
4. The suspensory ligament of the axilla attaching to the axillary fascia

■ AXILLA

The axilla is defined as a pyramidal space having an apex, a base, and four walls. The apex is at the junction of the clavicle, the upper border of the scapula, and the 1st rib. The base consists of the axillary fascia beneath the skin of the axillary fossa. The anterior wall is composed of three muscles, the pectoralis major, the pectoralis minor, and the subclavius, and the clavipectoral fascia, which envelops the muscles and fills the spaces between them. The posterior wall is formed by the scapula and three muscles, the subscapularis, the latissimus dorsi, and the teres major. The medial wall consists of the lateral chest wall, which contains the 2nd to the 6th ribs and the serratus anterior muscle. The lateral wall is the narrowest of the walls, being formed by the bicipital groove of the humerus (Fig. 3.1D).

The axilla contains lymph nodes, about which more will be said; the axillary sheath, which covers blood vessels and nerves; and the tendons of the long and short heads of the biceps and of the coracobrachialis muscles (Fig. 3.2).

■ MUSCLES

The muscles and nerves with which the surgeon must be familiar are listed in Table 3.1.

■ MORPHOLOGY OF THE BREAST

Between the superficial and the deep fasciae is the submammary space, which is rich in lymphatics (Fig. 3.3).

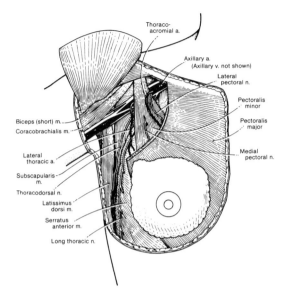

Figure 3.2. Topography of the axilla. Anterior view. (By permission of JE Skandalakis, SW Gray, and JR Rowe, *Anatomical Complications in General Surgery*, New York: McGraw-Hill, 1983.)

Each lobe has a duct terminating at the nipple. These lobes, together with their ducts, are anatomical but not surgical units. A breast biopsy is not a lobectomy; in the latter, parts of one or more lobes are removed.

In the fat-free area under the areola, the ducts dilate to form the lactiferous sinuses. These sinuses are the only sites of actual milk storage. Intraductal papillomas may develop here.

The suspensory ligaments of Cooper form a network of strong connective tissue fibers passing between the lobes of parenchyma and connecting the dermis of the skin with the deep layer of the superficial fascia. With malignant invasion, portions of this ligament may contract, producing a characteristic fixation and retraction of the skin. This must not be confused with the retraction called *peau d'orange* secondary to lymphatic obstruction. Occasionally the superficial fascia is fixed to the skin in such a way that ideal subcutaneous total mastectomy is impossible.

Table 3.1 Muscles and Nerves Involved in Mastectomy

Muscle	Origin	Insertion	Nerve supply	Comments
Pectoralis major	Medial half of clavicle, lateral half of sternum, 2nd to 6th costal cartilages, aponeurosis of external oblique muscle	Greater tubercle of humerus	Lateral anterior thoracic nerve	Clavicular portion of pectoralis forms upper extent of radical mastectomy; lateral border forms medial boundary of modified radical mastectomy; both nerves should be preserved in modified radical procedure
Pectoralis minor	2nd to 5th ribs	Coracoid process of scapula	Medial anterior thoracic nerve	
Deltoid	Lateral half of clavicle, lateral border of acromion process, spine of scapula	Deltoid tuberosity of humerus	Axillary nerve	
Serratus anterior (3 parts)	1. 1st and 2nd ribs	Costal surface of scapula at superior angle	Long thoracic nerve	Injury produces "winged scapula"
	2. 2nd to 4th ribs	Vertebral border of scapula		
	3. 4th to 8th ribs	Costal surface of scapula at inferior angle		

Muscle	Origin	Insertion	Nerve	Comment
Latissimus dorsi	Back, to crest of ilium	Crest of lesser tubercle and intertubercular groove of humerus	Thoracodorsal nerve	Anterior border forms lateral extent of radical mastectomy; injury results in weakness of rotation and abduction of arm
Subclavius	Junction of 1st rib and its cartilage	Groove of lower surface of clavicle	Subclavian nerve	
Subscapularis	Costal surface of scapula	Lesser tubercle of humerus	Subscapular nerve	Subscapular nerve should be spared
External oblique aponeurosis	External oblique muscle	Rectus sheath and linea alba, crest of ilium		Remember the interdigitation with serratus anterior and pectoralis muscles
Rectus abdominis	Ventral surface of 5th to 7th costal cartilages and xiphoid process	Crest and superior ramus of pubis	Branches of 7th to 12th thoracic nerves	Rectus sheath is lower limit of radical mastectomy

(By permission of JE Skandalakis, SW Gray, and JR Rowe, *Anatomical Complications in General Surgery*, New York: McGraw-Hill, 1983.)

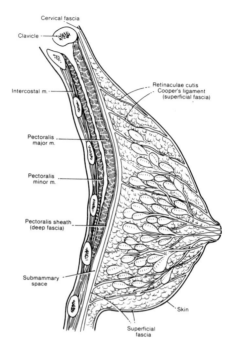

Figure 3.3. Diagrammatic sagittal section through the nonlactating female breast and anterior thoracic wall. (By permission of JE Skandalakis, SW Gray, and JR Rowe, *Anatomical Complications in General Surgery*, New York: McGraw-Hill, 1983.)

■ BLOOD SUPPLY OF THE BREAST

Arterial Supply

The breast is supplied with blood from three sources, with considerable variation (Figs. 3.2 and 3.4).

Internal Thoracic Artery

The internal thoracic artery is a branch of the subclavian artery that parallels the lateral border of the sternum behind the internal intercostal muscles.

Branches of the Axillary Artery

Three branches of the axillary artery may supply the breast. They are, in order: (1) the supreme thoracic, (2) the pectoral branch of the thoracoacromial, and (3) the lateral thoracic arteries.

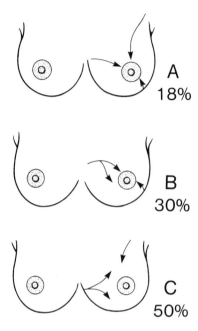

Figure 3.4. (A) The breast may be supplied with blood from the internal thoracic, axillary, and intercostal arteries in 18 percent of individuals. (B) In 30 percent, the contribution from the axillary artery is negligible. (C) In 50 percent, the intercostal arteries contribute little or no blood to the breast. In the remaining 2 percent, other variations may be found. (By permission of JE Skandalakis, SW Gray, and JR Rowe, *Anatomical Complications in General Surgery*, New York: McGraw-Hill, 1983.)

Intercostal Arteries

The lateral half of the breast may receive branches of the 3rd, 4th, and 5th intercostal arteries.

Venous Drainage

The axillary, the internal thoracic, and the 3rd to 5th intercostal veins drain the mammary gland. These veins follow the arteries.

Lymphatic Drainage (as Reported by Haagensen) (Fig. 3.5)

Lymph nodes occur in inconstant groups of varying numbers, and many nodes are very small. The following is a useful grouping, including the average number of nodes in each group.

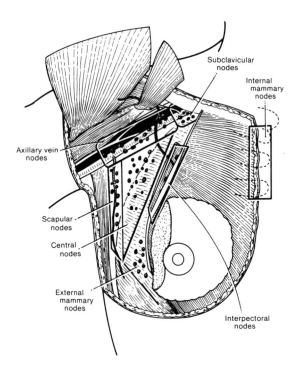

Figure 3.5. Lymph nodes of the breast and axilla. Classification of Haage-nsen and coworkers. (By permission of CD Haagensen. Lymphatics of the breast. In: Haagensen CD, Feind CR, Herter FP, Slanetz CA Jr, Weinberg JA, *The Lymphatics In Cancer*. Philadelphia: W.B. Saunders, 1972, pp. 300–398.)

Axillary Drainage (35.3 nodes)

Group 1. External mammary nodes (1.7 nodes). These lie beneath the lateral edge of the pectoralis major, along the medial side of the axilla, following the course of the lateral thoracic artery on the chest wall from the 2nd to the 6th rib.

Group 2. Scapular nodes (5.8 nodes). These lie on the subscapular vessels and their thoracodorsal branches.

Group 3. Central nodes (12.1 nodes). This is the largest group of lymph nodes and the nodes most easily palpated in the ax-illa. They are embedded in fat in the center of the axilla.

Group 4. Interpectoral nodes (Rotter's nodes) (1.4 nodes). These lie between the pectoralis major and minor muscles. Often there is a single node. They are the smallest group of the axillary nodes and will not be found unless the pectoralis major is removed.

Group 5. Axillary vein nodes (10.7 nodes). This is the second largest group of lymph nodes in the axilla. They lie on the caudal and ventral surfaces of the lateral part of the axillary vein.

Group 6. Subclavicular nodes (3.5 nodes). These lie on the caudal and ventral surfaces of the medial part of the axillary vein. Haagensen and co-workers consider them to be inaccessible unless the pectoralis minor muscle is divided.

Internal Thoracic (Mammary) Drainage (8.5 nodes)

The nodes, about four or five on each side, are small and are usually in the fat and connective tissue of the intercostal spaces. The internal thoracic trunks empty into the thoracic duct or the right lymphatic duct. This route to the venous system is shorter than the axillary route.

Some authors have stated that regional lymph nodes are primary indicators and not instigators of distal disease, and they advise that lower axillary dissection is more than adequate to fulfill the aims of the operation. These authors believe that with removal of a few lymph nodes, the qualitative axillary nodal status (positive or negative) can be determined with accuracy.

■ SURGICAL ANATOMY OF MASTECTOMY

Anatomy of the Triangular Bed of Modified Radical Mastectomy

The medial side of the surgical field is the upward and medially retracted axillary margin of the pectoralis major. The lateral side is the medial border of the latissimus dorsi muscle and the superior side is the axillary vein. The floor of the triangular bed is formed by the serratus anterior and the subscapularis muscles. This results in a smaller triangle than would be used for a radical mastectomy, but one that is adequate for good dissection (Fig. 3.6).

After the breast and the underlying fascia are removed, a good dissection consists of (1) removing remnants of the pectoralis major fascia at its axillary border, (2) entering the axilla by incising and stripping the axillary fascia, (3) further stripping the fascia of the pectoralis minor (lower clavipectoral fascia), (4) exposing the axillary vein, (5) downward dissection of axillary fat and lymph nodes after ligating tributaries of the axillary vein from the thoracic wall, and (6) continuing the dissection

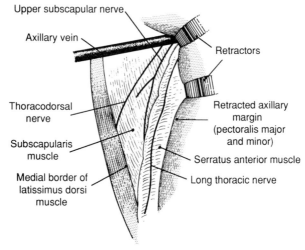

Upper subscapular nerve

Axillary vein

Retractors

Thoracodorsal nerve

Retracted axillary margin (pectoralis major and minor)

Subscapularis muscle

Serratus anterior muscle

Medial border of latissimus dorsi muscle

Long thoracic nerve

Figure 3.6. The triangular bed of a modified radical mastectomy. The pectoralis muscles are retracted, rather than removed. (By permission of LJ Skandalakis, MD Vohman, and JE Skandalakis, et al., *Am Surg* 45(9):552–555, 1979.)

downward, partially removing the fasciae of the serratus anterior, the subscapularis, and the medial border of the latissimus dorsi muscles.

Remember:

✓ The *thoracodorsal nerve* lies on the subscapularis muscle and innervates the latissimus dorsi muscle (Fig. 3.6). If it is cut, internal rotation and abduction will be weakened, although there is no deformity. The nerve and its associated vessels can be found near the medial border of the latissimus dorsi about 5 cm above a plane passing through the 3rd sternochondral junction. Once located, the neurovascular bundle should be marked with an umbilical tape. If there is obvious involvement of lymph nodes around the nerve, it must be sacrificed.

✓ The *long thoracic nerve* innervates the serratus anterior muscle and lies on it (Fig. 3.6). Section of the nerve results in the "winged scapula" deformity. Unless actually invaded by cancer, this nerve should be spared. The landmark for locating the nerve is the point at which the axillary vein passes over the 2nd rib. Careful dissection of this area will reveal the nerve descending on the 2nd rib posterior to the axillary vein.

✓ The *medial anterior thoracic nerve* is superficial to the axillary vein and lateral to the pectoralis minor muscle. The *lateral anterior thoracic nerve*, which is the nerve supply of the clavicular as well as of the sternal portions of the pectoralis major muscle, also is superficial to the axillary vein and lies at the medial edge of the pectoralis minor.

✓ If branches of one or both anterior thoracic nerves are injured, the result will be atrophy of the pectoralis major and minor muscles. If the few lymph nodes of the interpectoral group are involved and are fixed to the nerves, these nerves should be sacrificed.

TECHNIQUE

■ BREAST BIOPSY

Excisional Breast Biopsy

Procedure:

Step 1. Make a circumareolar or curved incision directly over the lesion along Langer's lines (Fig. 3.7).

Step 2. Raise skin flaps to approach the lesion (Fig. 3.8).

Step 3. Excise the lesion with a margin of normal breast tissue.

Step 4. Establish good hemostasis with electrocautery. Approximate the mammary tissue with 2-0 Vicryl. Some surgeons prefer not to approximate the breast defect, reasoning that if hemostasis is good, in time the formed seroma will form fibrous tissue and no skin depression will result. We prefer to place a few superficial sutures, approximating the edges of the defect and leaving the cavity in situ. Use subcutaneous interrupted sutures with 4-0 Vicryl and close the skin with running 4-0 Vicryl subcuticular sutures (Fig. 3.9).

Step 5. Apply an ice bag to the breast for 24 hours.

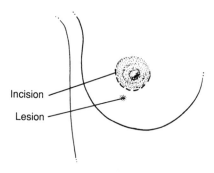

Incision

Lesion

Figure 3.7

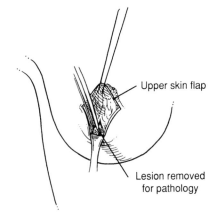

Figure 3.8

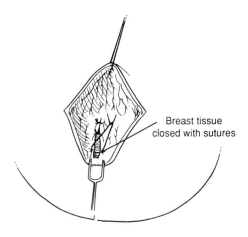

Figure 3.9

Radiologic Breast Evaluation with Needle

Procedure:

Step 1. Perform mammography.

Step 2. Insert needle and localize into the previously radiologically described lesion.

Step 3. Take the patient into the operating room very carefully with the needle in situ.

Step 4. Perform biopsy. X-ray the specimen and obtain frozen section.

Step 5. If benign, close the wound. If malignant, continue procedure of your choice.

■ MODIFIED RADICAL MASTECTOMY

Procedure:

Step 1. Mark the contour of the breast to determine its edges, especially when the patient is obese. This minimizes unnecessary dissection (Figs. 3.10A and B).

Step 2. Use the incision of your choice and allow 4–5 cm around the lesion, if it has been found by aspiration biopsy to be malignant. Use the same procedure when previous biopsy was done and an incision or scar is present.

Step 3. Use electrocautery for the formation of the upper and lower flaps (medial or lateral as per incision) (Fig. 3.11).

Step 4. Begin the dissection of the breast medially. Elevate it sharply off the pectoralis fascia. There are many arterial perforators entering the breast in this area that will require ligation with 2-0 Vicryl.

Step 5. As the breast is elevated and the axilla is approached, the clavipectoral fascia is encountered. When this is opened, one will have access to the axilla (Figs. 3.12A and B). Protect the pectoralis major and minor. Occasionally, however, the pectoralis minor should be cut for a more complete axillary dissection (Fig. 3.13).

Step 6. Locate the axillary vein and its tributaries. Ligate in continuity with 3-0 or 4-0 silk all the tributaries toward the breast. Protect the brachial plexus and axillary artery (Fig. 3.14).

Step 7. Using a scalpel or Metzenbaum scissors, gently evacuate the axillary contents of fat and lymph nodes, pushing them towards the breast in continuity (Fig. 3.15).

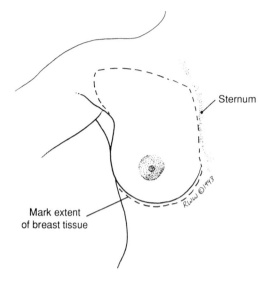

Sternum

Mark extent
of breast tissue

Figure 3.10A

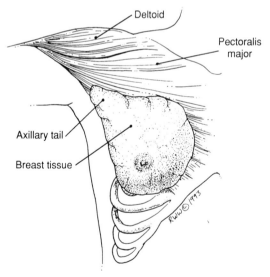

Deltoid

Pectoralis
major

Axillary tail

Breast tissue

Figure 3.10B

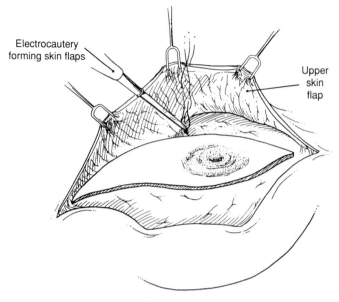

Electrocautery forming skin flaps

Upper skin flap

Figure 3.11

Step 8. Five nerves should be identified and protected if possible (Figs. 3.2 and 3.16):

   a. long thoracic, where the axillary vein passes over the 2nd rib

   b. thoracodorsal, at the medial border of the latissimus dorsi

   c. medial anterior thoracic (pectoral), superficial to the axillary vein and lateral to the pectoralis minor muscle

   d. lateral anterior thoracic (pectoral), at the medial edge of of the pectoralis minor and superficial to the axillary vein

   e. subscapular, at the vicinity of the subscapular artery and vein.

Step 9. Place two Jackson–Pratt drains: the first to drain the inferior skin flap and the axilla, and the second to drain the superior skin flap. Close the subcutaneous tissue with interrupted 3-0 Vicryl and close the skin with the stapler (Fig. 3.17).

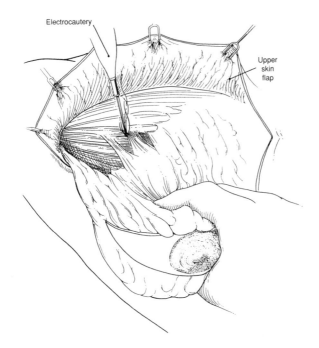

Electrocautery

Upper skin flap

Figure 3.12A

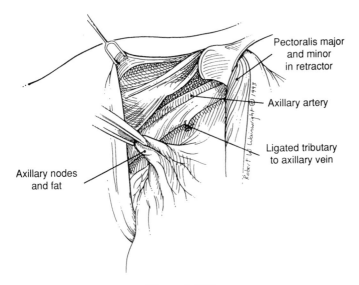

Pectoralis major and minor in retractor

Axillary artery

Ligated tributary to axillary vein

Axillary nodes and fat

Figure 3.12B

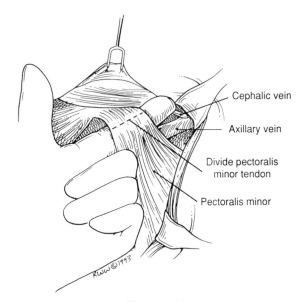

Figure 3.13

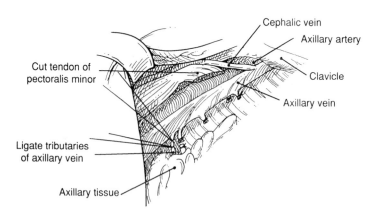

Figure 3.14

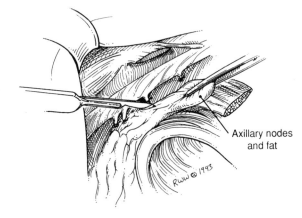

Axillary nodes
and fat

Figure 3.15

■ LUMPECTOMY WITH AXILLARY DISSECTION

A lumpectomy is the removal of a lesion with an adequate margin of mammary tissue determined by frozen section to be free of tumor. The surgeon must present the pathologist with a well-oriented specimen and demand that the pathologist use the newest techniques for establishing and diagnosing tumor-free margins. The surgeon emphasizes to the pathologist the importance of obtaining hormone receptor assays. The specimen should be submitted as soon as it is removed. We use five sutures (superior, medial, lateral, inferior, and center). Or, if the overlying skin is present, we use four sutures, omitting the center.

Procedure:

Step 1. Make a cosmetic incision. Remove the tumor and healthy mammary tissue and send it to the lab for frozen section. (See the previous technique for excisional breast biopsy, p. 112).

Step 2. We prefer to make a transverse incision at the lower axilla. Try to avoid making skin flaps, but if absolutely necessary, make only an upper flap. Retract both pectoral muscles. Locate the axillary vein at the medial area of the pectoralis minor and begin ligating its tributaries. Remember that the anterior border of the latissimus dorsi is located at the lateral wall of the axilla. Carefully proceed towards the medial axillary wall. Be sure to protect the thoracodorsal nerve, which is close to

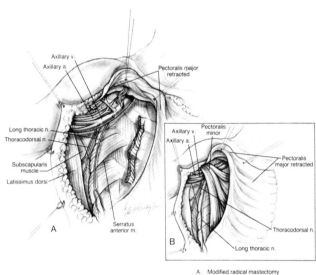

Figure 3.16. (By permission of SW Gray, JE Skandalakis, and DA McClusky, *Atlas of Surgical Anatomy for General Surgeons*, Baltimore: Williams and Wilkins, 1985.)

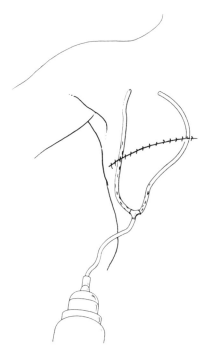

Figure 3.17

the anterior margin of the latissimus dorsi muscle, and the long thoracic nerve, which is under the fascia of the serratus anterior muscle. Complete the dissection and separate the specimen from the axillary vein. Remove the specimen and mark its upper portion with a silk suture. Drain the axillary cavity with two Jackson-Pratt drains. For more information, read about axillary dissection described in the technique for modified radical mastectomy, pp. 114–118.

Step 3. Close the wound in two layers.

4

Abdominal Wall and Hernias

ANATOMY

■ GENERAL DESCRIPTION OF THE ANTERIOR ABDOMINAL WALL

The anterior abdominal wall may be considered to have two parts: an anterolateral portion composed of the external oblique, internal oblique, and transversus abdominis muscles; and a midline portion composed of the rectus abdominis and pyramidalis muscles.

Anterolateral Portion

The three flat muscles mentioned above are arranged so that their fibers are roughly parallel as they approach their insertion on the rectus sheath.

Midline Portion

When present, the insertion of the pyramidalis into the linea alba is a landmark for an accurate midline incision.

The rectus muscle is enclosed in a stout sheath formed by the bilaminar aponeuroses of the abdominal muscles, which pass anteriorly and posteriorly around the muscle and attach medially to the linea alba (Fig. 4.1), which is formed by decussation.

In the lower ¼ of the abdominal wall, the aponeuroses of the internal oblique and transversus abdominis muscles pass anterior to the muscle, which is bounded posteriorly by the transversalis fascia only (Fig. 4.1).

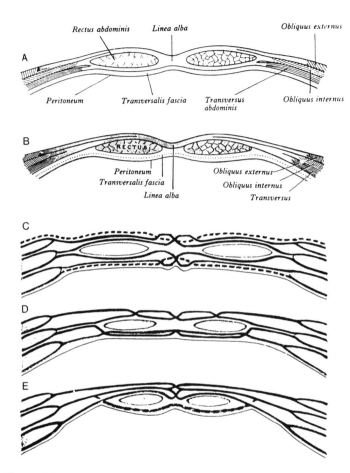

Figure 4.1. Transverse sections through the anterior abdominal wall. Traditional view: (A) Immediately above the umbilicus. (B) Below the arcuate line. Schematic transverse section through the ventral abdominal wall showing bilaminar aponeuroses, external oblique, transversus abdominis, and sites of linear decussation that, compacted, form the linea alba. (C–E) Tenuous layers are dotted or omitted. (By permission of PL Williams, R Warwick, M Dyson, et al. (eds) *Gray's Anatomy*, 37th ed. Edinburgh: Churchill Livingstone, 1989.)

The dividing line is the linea semicircularis of Douglas, which marks the level at which the rectus sheath loses its posterior wall. The line is well marked if the change is abrupt; it is less definite if the change is gradual.

The following array shows some comparisons between the structures of the upper ¾ and the lower ¼ of the abdominal wall:

Upper Abdominal Wall	**Lower Abdominal Wall**
1. Linea alba well developed	Linea alba not well developed
2. Right and left recti well separated	Right and left recti very close together
3. External oblique fascia and aponeurosis weak or absent	External oblique fascia strong and well developed
4. Both layers of rectus sheath present	Only anterior layer of rectus sheath present

■ UMBILICAL REGION

Variations of the Umbilical Ring and the Umbilical Fascia

The anatomy of the umbilical region may be appreciated from the drawing presenting the relations of the umbilical ring to the linea alba, round ligament, urachus (median umbilical ligament), and umbilical fascia (Fig. 4.2)

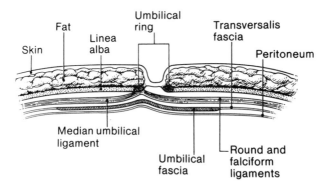

Figure 4.2. Diagrammatic sagittal section through a normal umbilicus showing the relation of the umbilical ring to the linea alba, the round ligament, the urachus, and the umbilical and transversalis fasciae. Note the absence of subcutaneous fat over the umbilical ring. (By permission of JE Skandalakis, SW Gray, AR Mansberger, et al, *Hernia: Surgical Anatomy and Technique,* New York: McGraw-Hill, 1989.)

Figs. 4.3 and 4.4 present variations of the umbilical fascia in relation to several anatomical entities. Note that in Fig. 4.4A, the fascia covers the umbilical ring in toto.

■ BLOOD SUPPLY TO THE ANTERIOR ABDOMINAL WALL

Arterial Supply

Where there have been no previous incisions, the blood supply to the abdominal wall creates no problem. Where scars are present, the surgeon should be familiar with the blood supply to avoid necrosis from ischemia to specific areas. Proceed through the same scar if possible.

The lower anterolateral abdominal wall is supplied by three branches of the femoral artery. They are, from above downward, the superficial circumflex iliac artery, the superficial epigastric artery, and the superficial external pudendal artery. These arteries travel toward the umbilicus

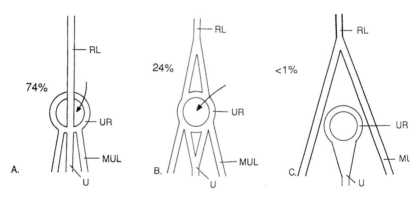

Figure 4.3. Variations in the disposition of the umbilical ligaments as seen from the posterior (peritoneal) surface of the body wall. Arrows indicate: (A) Usual relations (74 percent) of the umbilical ring (UR), the round ligament (RL), the urachus (U), and the medial umbilical ligaments (MUL). The round ligament crosses the umbilical ring to insert on its inferior margin. (B) Less common configuration (24 percent). The round ligament splits and is attached to the superior margin of the umbilical ring. (C) Rare configuration (less than 1 percent). The round ligament branches before reaching the umbilical ring. Each branch continues with the medial umbilical ligament without attaching to the umbilical ring. (Modified by permission of R Orda and H Nathan, *Int Surg* 58(7):454–464, 1973.)

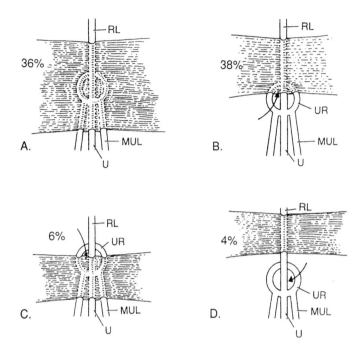

Figure 4.4. Variations in the presence and form of the insertion of the umbilical fascia as seen from the posterior (peritoneal) surface of the body wall. (A) The thickened transversalis fascia forms the umbilical fascia covering the umbilical ring (36 percent). Arrows indicate: (B) the umbilical fascia covers only the superior portion of the umbilical ring (38 percent); (C) the umbilical fascia covers only the inferior portion of the umbilical ring (6 percent); (D) though present, the umbilical fascia does not underlie the umbilical ring (4 percent). (E) (Not shown.) The fascia is entirely absent in 16 percent. (Modified by permission of R Orda and H Nathan, *Int Surg* 58(7):454–464, 1973.)

in the subcutaneous connective tissue. The superficial epigastric artery anastomoses with the contralateral artery, and all three arteries have anastomoses with the deep arteries.

The deep arteries lie between the transversus abdominis and the internal oblique muscles. They are the posterior intercostal arteries 10 and 11, the anterior branch of the subcostal artery, the anterior branches of the four lumbar arteries, and the deep circumflex iliac artery.

The rectus sheath is supplied by the superior epigastric artery, which arises from the internal thoracic artery, and the inferior epigastric artery, which arises from the external iliac artery just above the inguinal ligament.

The superior epigastric artery enters the upper end of the rectus sheath deep to the rectus muscle. Musculocutaneous branches pierce the anterior rectus sheath to supply the overlying skin. The perforating arteries are closer to the lateral border of the rectus than to the linea alba. An incision too far lateral will result in bleeding from the several perforating arteries and muscle paralysis from the cut musculocutaneous nerves.

The inferior epigastric artery lies first in the preperitoneal connective tissue and enters the sheath at or above the level of the linea semilunaris, passing between the rectus muscle and the posterior layer of the sheath.

Venous Drainage

The veins follow the arteries.

■ NERVE SUPPLY TO THE ANTERIOR ABDOMINAL WALL

Both the anterolateral portion of the abdominal wall and the rectus abdominis muscle are supplied by anterior rami of the 7th to the 12th thoracic and the 1st lumbar nerves. A branch, the lateral cutaneous ramus, arises from each anterior ramus and pierces the outer two flat muscles, innervating the external oblique and forming the lateral cutaneous nerve. The anterior rami of the last six thoracic nerves enter the posterior layer of the rectus sheath, innervating the rectus muscle and sending perforating branches through the anterior layer of the sheath to form the anterior cutaneous nerves. The 1st lumbar nerve forms an anterior cutaneous nerve without passing through the sheath. These relationships are shown diagrammatically in Fig. 4.5. Rectus paralysis with weakening of the abdominal wall will result from section of more than one of these nerves.

■ THE ANATOMICAL ENTITIES OF THE GROIN

Superficial Fascia (Fig. 4.6)

This fascia (described here only for the male) is divided into a superficial part (Camper's) and a deep part (Scarpa's). The superficial part extends upward on the abdominal wall and downward over the penis, scrotum,

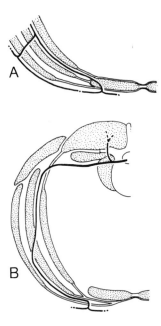

Figure 4.5. The course of the anterior ramus of segmental nerves in the anterior body wall. (A) 7th to 12th thoracic nerves. (B) 1st lumbar nerve. (By permission of JE Skandalakis, SW Gray, and JR Rowe, *Anatomical Complications in General Surgery*, New York: McGraw-Hill, 1983.)

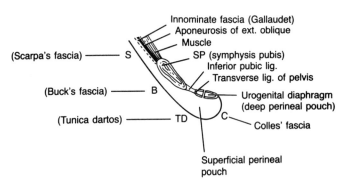

Figure 4.6. Diagram of the relations of the superficial fasciae of the inguinal area showing the formation of the superficial perineal pouch. (By permission of JE Skandalakis, SW Gray, AR Mansberger, et al, *Hernia: Surgical Anatomy and Technique*, New York: McGraw-Hill, 1989.)

perineum, thigh, and buttocks. The deep part extends from the abdominal wall to the penis (Buck's fascia), the scrotum (dartos), and the perineum (Colles' fascia).

Perhaps two spaces are formed: the superficial perineal cleft and the superficial perineal pouch. The cleft is situated between Colles' fascia and the muscle fascia that covers the muscles of the superficial perineal pouch. The pouch is defined by the perineal membrane, the external perineal fascia (Gallaudet), and the ischiopubic rami.

Aponeurosis of the External Oblique Muscle

Below the arcuate line (Douglas'), this aponeurosis joins with the aponeuroses of the internal oblique and transversus abdominis muscles to form the anterior layer of the rectus sheath. This aponeurosis forms or contributes to three anatomical entities in the inguinal canal:

- inguinal ligament (Poupart's)
- lacunar ligament (Gimbernat's)
- reflected inguinal ligament (Colles')
  (Included sometimes is the pectineal ligament [Cooper's], which is also formed from tendinous fibers of the internal oblique, transversus, and pectineus muscles)

Inguinal Ligament (Poupart's) (Fig. 4.7)

This is the thickened lower part of the external oblique aponeurosis from the anterosuperior iliac spine laterally to the superior ramus of the pubis. The middle ⅓ has a free edge. The lateral ⅔ is attached strongly to the underlying iliopsoas fascia.

Lacunar Ligament (Gimbernat's) (Fig. 4.8)

This is the most inferior portion of the inguinal ligament and is formed from external oblique tendon fibers arising at the anterior superior iliac spine. Its fibers recurve through an angle of less than 45 degrees before attaching to the pectineal ligament. Occasionally it forms the medial border of the femoral canal.

Pectineal Ligament (Cooper's) (Fig. 4.8)

This is a thick, strong tendinous band formed principally by tendinous fibers of the lacunar ligament and aponeurotic fibers of the internal

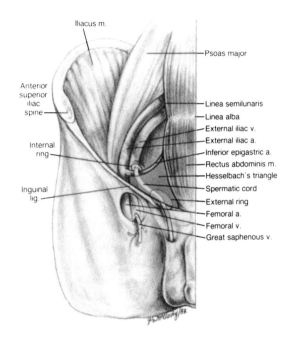

Figure 4.7. (By permission of SW Gray, JE Skandalakis, and DA McClusky, *Atlas of Surgical Anatomy for General Surgeons*, Baltimore: Williams and Wilkins, 1985.)

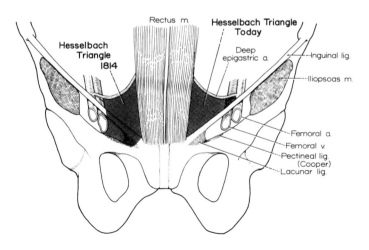

Figure 4.8. (By permission of JE Skandalakis, SW Gray, and JR Rowe, *Anatomical Complications in General Surgery*, New York: McGraw-Hill, 1983.)

oblique, transversus abdominis, and pectineus muscles, and, with variation, the inguinal falx. It is fixed to the periosteum of the superior pubic
ramus and, laterally, the periosteum of the ilium. The tendinous fibers
are lined internally by transversalis fascia.

Conjoined Area (Fig. 4.9)

By definition, this is the fusion of fibers of the internal oblique aponeurosis with similar fibers from the aponeurosis of the transversus abdominis
muscle just as they insert on the pubic tubercle, the pectineal ligament,
and the superior ramus of the pubis.

The above configuration is rarely encountered; published data suggest
that it will be found in 5 percent of individuals or fewer. We have proposed the term *conjoined area*. This has obvious practical application to
the region containing the falx inguinalis (Henle's ligament), the transversus abdominis aponeurosis, the inferomedial fibers of the internal
oblique muscle or aponeurosis, the reflected inguinal ligament, and the
lateral border of the rectus sheath.

Arch of the Transversus Abdominis

The inferior portion of the transversus abdominis, the transversus arch,
becomes increasingly less muscular and more aponeurotic as it approaches the rectus sheath. Close to the internal ring, it is covered by the

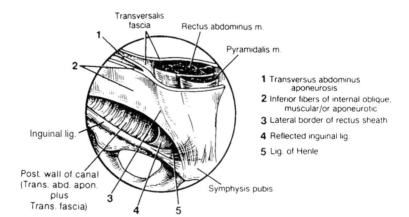

Figure 4.9. The "conjoined area." (By permission of JE Skandalakis, GL Colborn, SW Gray, et al., *Contemp Surg* 38(1):20–34, 1991.)

much more muscular arch of the internal oblique muscle. Remember, in the vicinity of the internal ring, the internal oblique is muscular and the transversus abdominis is aponeurotic.

Falx Inguinalis (Henle's Ligament) (Fig. 4.9)

Henle's ligament is the lateral, vertical expansion of the rectus sheath that inserts on the pecten of the pubis. It is present in 30–50 percent of individuals and is fused with the transversus abdominis aponeurosis and transversalis fascia.

Interfoveolar Ligament (Hesselbach's)

This is not a true ligament. It is a thickening of the transversalis fascia at the medial side of the internal ring. It lies anterior to the inferior epigastric vessels.

Reflected Inguinal Ligament (Colles') (Fig. 4.9)

This is formed by aponeurotic fibers from the inferior crus of the external ring which pass superomedially to the linea alba.

Iliopubic Tract (Fig. 4.10)

This is an aponeurotic band extending from the iliopectineal arch to the superior ramus of the pubis. It forms part of the deep musculoaponeurotic layer together with the transversus abdominis muscle and aponeurosis and the transversalis fascia.

The tract passes medially, contributing to the inferior border of the internal ring. It crosses the femoral vessels to form the anterior margin of the femoral sheath, together with the transversalis fascia. The tract curves around the medial surface of the femoral sheath to attach to the pectineal ligament. It can be confused with the inguinal ligament.

Transversalis Fascia (Fig. 4.11)

Although the name transversalis fascia may be restricted to the internal fascia lining the transversus abdominis muscle, it is often applied to the entire connective tissue sheet lining the abdominal cavity. In the latter sense, it is a fascial layer covering muscles, aponeuroses, ligaments, and bones. In the inguinal area the transversalis fascia is bilaminar, enveloping the inferior epigastric vessels.

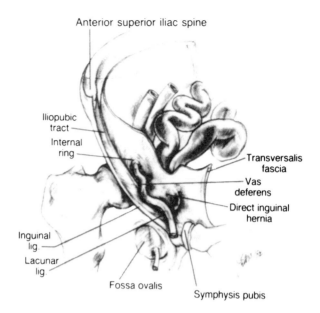

Figure 4.10. (By permission of SW Gray, JE Skandalakis, and DA McClusky, *Atlas of Surgical Anatomy for General Surgeons*, Baltimore: Williams and Wilkins, 1985.)

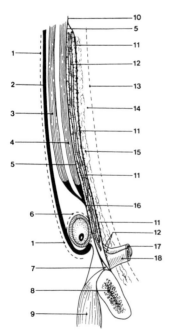

Figure 4.11. The space of Bogros. 1 = innominate fascia; 2 = external oblique aponeurosis; 3 = internal oblique muscle; 4 = transversus abdominis muscle; 5 = transversalis fascia anterior; 6 = external spermatic fascia; 7 = Cooper's ligament; 8 = pubic bone; 9 = pectineus muscle; 10 = transversalis fascia; 11 = transversalis fascia posterior lamina; 12 = vessels; 13 = peritoneum; 14 = home (space) of the prosthesis; space of Bogros; 15 = preperitoneal fat; 16 = transversus abdominis aponeurosis and anterior lamina of transversalis fascia; 17 = femoral artery; 18 = femoral vein. (By permission of JE Skandalakis, GL Colborn, JA Androulakis, et al., *Surg Clin NA* 73(4):799–836, 1993.)

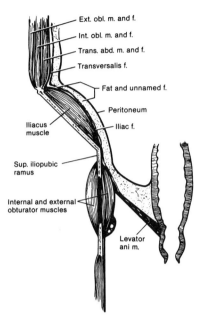

Ext. obl. m. and f.

Int. obl. m. and f.

Trans. abd. m. and f.

Transversalis f.

Fat and unnamed f.

Peritoneum

Iliacus muscle

Iliac f.

Sup. iliopubic ramus

Internal and external obturator muscles

Levator ani m.

Figure 4.12. Diagram of the normal relations of the transversalis fascia in the lateral and lower parts of the abdominal wall. (By permission of EW Lampe. Transversalis fascia. In: Nyhus LM, Condon RL. *Hernia*, 3rd ed. Philadelphia, JB Lippincott, 1989.)

Related to the transversalis fascia is the space of Bogros, which is, for all practical purposes, a lateral extension of the retropubic space of Retzius. It is located just beneath the posterior lamina of the transversalis fascia out in front of the peritoneum (Fig. 4.11). The space of Bogros is used for the location of prostheses during the repair of inguinal hernias.

Fig. 4.12 shows normal relations of the transversalis fascia in the lateral and lower parts of the abdominal wall.

Iliopectineal Arch

This is a medial thickening of the iliopsoas fascia deep to the inguinal ligament. The surgeon does not directly use this arch, but it is important as the junction of a number of structures of the groin. These are:

1. Insertions of fibers of the external oblique aponeurosis and fibers of the inguinal ligament

2. The origin of part of the internal oblique muscle and a part of the transversus abdominis muscle

3. The lateral attachment of the iliopubic tract

Hesselbach's Triangle (Fig. 4.8)

As described by Hesselbach in 1814, the base of the triangle was formed by the pubic pecten and the pectineal ligament. The boundaries of this triangle as usually described today are:

- superolateral: the inferior (deep) epigastric vessels
- medial: the rectus sheath (lateral border)
- inferior (or, the base): the inguinal ligament

This is smaller than that described by Hesselbach in 1814. Most direct inguinal hernias occur in this area.

The Inguinal Canal

The inguinal canal in the adult is an oblique rift measuring approximately 4 cm in length. It is located 2–4 cm above the inguinal ligament between the internal (deep inguinal) ring and the external (superficial inguinal) ring opening. The subcutaneous inguinal ring is on the opening of the aponeurosis of the external oblique lateral and above the pubic crest, and the deep inguinal ring is an opening of the transversalis fascia corresponding to the middle of the inguinal ligament. The canal contains either the spermatic cord or the round ligament of the uterus (Fig. 4.13).

The anterior wall is formed by the aponeurosis of the external oblique muscle and laterally by participation of the internal oblique muscle. The superior wall ("roof") is formed by the internal oblique and transversus abdominis muscles and their aponeuroses. The inferior wall ("floor") is formed by the inguinal and lacunar ligaments.

The posterior wall is the fusion of the aponeurosis of the transversus abdominis muscles and the transversalis fascia. In 77 percent of cases, the wall is strong; in 23 percent, it is weak (Figs. 4.14 and 4.15).

Fruchaud viewed hernias not by their clinical presentation but rather by their origin within the groin. He termed this area the myopectineal orifice (Fig. 4.16). This area in the groin is bounded superiorly by the arch of the internal oblique muscle and the transversus abdominis muscle, laterally by the iliopsoas muscle, medially by the lateral border of the rectus muscle and its anterior lamina, and inferiorly by the pubic pecten. The inguinal ligament spans and divides this framework.

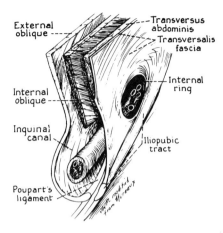

Figure 4.13. (By permission of LM Nyhus. The preperitoneal approach and iliopubic tract repair of inguinal hernia. In: Nyhus LM, Condon RL. *Hernia*, 3rd ed. Philadelphia: JB Lippincott, 1989.)

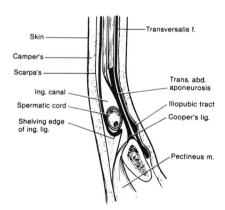

Figure 4.14. Diagrammatic cross section of a "strong" posterior inguinal canal wall. Notice the thickness and extent of the aponeurosis of the transversus abdominis muscle. (By permission of EW Lampe. Transversalis fascia. In: Nyhus LM, Condon RL. *Hernia*, 3rd ed. Philadelphia: JB Lippincott, 1989.)

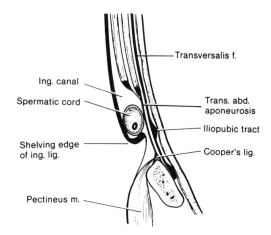

Figure 4.15. Diagrammatic cross section of a "weak" posterior inguinal canal wall. Compare with Figure 4.14. (By permission of EW Lampe. Transversalis fascia. In: Nyhus LM, Condon RL. *Hernia*, 3rd ed. Philadelphia: JB Lippincott, 1989.)

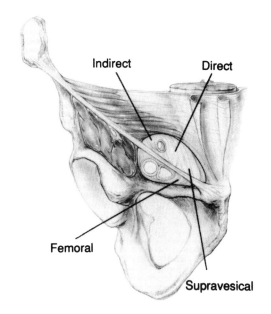

Figure 4.16. Anterior view of Fruchaud's myopectineal orifice. (Modified by permission of GE Wantz. *Atlas of Hernia Surgery*. New York: Raven Press, 1991.)

Blood Supply and Nerves

The blood supply of the lower abdominal wall may be appreciated from Fig. 4.17. The nerves of the area are illustrated in Fig. 4.18.

The Surgical Ellipse (Fig. 4.19)

With the patient in the supine position, the surgeon is dealing with the following anatomical areas and entities of the inguinal region which are incorporated into an elliptical area: floor of the inguinal canal; superior medial edge (above); inferior lateral edge (below); medial apex; lateral apex.

The *floor* (posterior wall) of the ellipse is formed by the transversus abdominis aponeurosis and the transversalis fascia.

Remember:

✔ The transversalis fascia and transversus abdominis aponeurosis together are "good stuff" for repair of inguinofemoral herniation.

If the posterior wall is intact, none of the four types of inguinal hernia (indirect, direct, external supravesical, femoral) will develop.

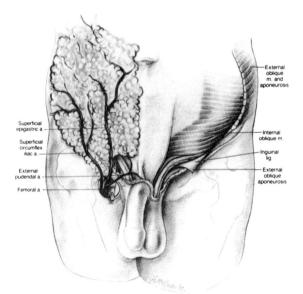

Figure 4.17. The skin of the lower abdominal wall has been removed to show the superficial branches of the femoral artery. (By permission of SW Gray, JE Skandalakis, and DA McClusky, *Atlas of Surgical Anatomy for General Surgeons*, Baltimore: Williams and Wilkins, 1985.)

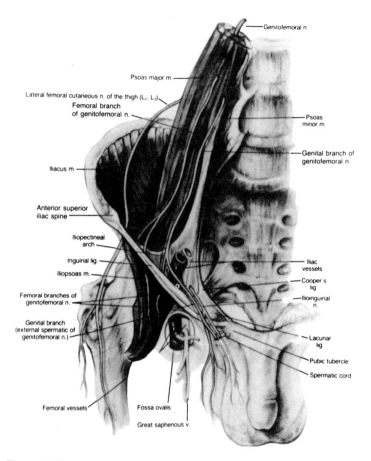

Figure 4.18. Nerves of the inguinal region with which the surgeon should be familiar. (By permission of SW Gray, JE Skandalakis, and DA McClusky, *Atlas of Surgical Anatomy for General Surgeons*, Baltimore: Williams and Wilkins, 1985.)

The transversus abdominis layer is the most important of the three strata. Its integrity prevents herniation (Figs. 4.14 and 4.15).

The *superior medial edge* (above) of the ellipse is formed by the conjoined area and the arch (internal oblique muscle and transversus abdominis muscle with their aponeuroses).

The *inferior lateral edge* (below) is formed by the inguinal ligament, iliopubic tract, femoral sheath, and Cooper's ligament. The iliopubic

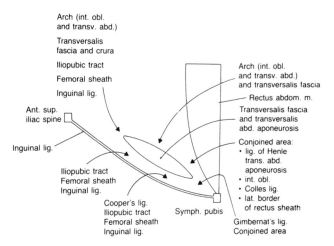

Arch (int. obl.
and transv. abd.)

Transversalis
fascia and crura

Iliopubic tract

Femoral sheath

Inguinal lig.

Ant. sup.
iliac spine

Inguinal lig.

Iliopubic tract
Femoral sheath
Inguinal lig.

Cooper's lig.
Iliopubic tract
Femoral sheath
Inguinal lig.

Symph. pubis

Arch (int. obl.
and transv. abd.)
and transversalis fascia

Rectus abdom. m.

Transversalis fascia
and transversalis
abd. aponeurosis

Conjoined area:
• lig. of Henle
  trans. abd.
  aponeurosis
• int. obl.
• Colles lig.
• lat. border
  of rectus sheath

Gimbernat's lig.
Conjoined area

Figure 4.19. (By permission of JE Skandalakis, SW Gray, AR Mansberger, et al, *Hernia: Surgical Anatomy and Technique*, New York: McGraw-Hill, 1989.)

tract, femoral sheath, Cooper's ligament, and occasionally the inguinal ligament are used for repair.

The *medial apex*, close to the symphysis pubis, is formed by Gimbernat's ligament below and the conjoined area above.

The *lateral apex*, at the internal ring, is formed by the arch (internal oblique and transversus abdominis muscles and aponeuroses), transversalis fascia and crura, iliopubic tract, femoral sheath, and inguinal ligament.

TECHNIQUE

■ INCISIONS OF THE ANTERIOR ABDOMINAL WALL

Principles

There are three requirements for a proper abdominal incision: (1) accessibility, (2) extensibility, and (3) security.

A surgeon must plan the incision, taking personal preferences into account. The following rules should be observed where they apply:

✓ The incision should be long enough for a good exposure and for room to work, but short enough to avoid unnecessary complications.

✓ Where possible, skin incisions should follow Langer's lines.

✓ Excise existing scars and proceed, rather than making incisions parallel to the scars.

✓ Split muscles in the direction of their fibers, rather than transecting them. The rectus muscle is an exception, because it has a segmental nerve supply and therefore no risk of denervation.

✓ Do not superimpose the openings formed through different layers of the abdominal wall.

✓ Wherever possible, avoid cutting nerves.

✓ Retract muscles and abdominal organs toward, not away from, their neurovascular supply.

✓ Insert drainage tubes in separate small incisions. Insertion in the main incision may weaken the wound.

✓ Pay close attention to cosmetic considerations, but not at the expense of the requirements of accessibility, extensibility, and security, as noted previously.

✓ Be sure closure follows anatomical topography.

Surgical Anatomy of Specific Incisions

Abdominal incisions are legion. Some have descriptive names; others are eponymous. For practical purposes, we will describe only the major types of incisions without discussing their many variations (Fig. 4.20).

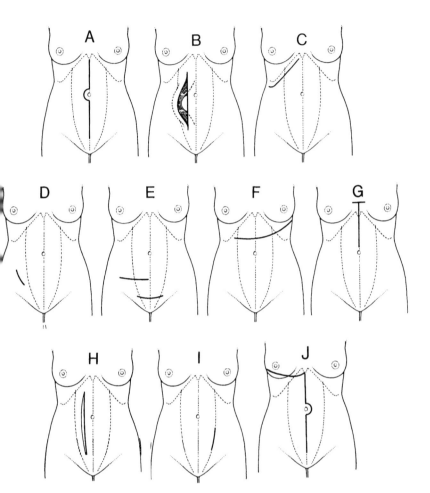

Figure 4.20. Varieties of abdominal incisions. (A) Midline (linea alba) incision. (B) Paramedian (rectus) incision with muscle retraction. (C) Subcostal incision. (D) McBurney incision. (E) Transverse abdominal incision. (F and G) Two types of thoracoabdominal incisions. (H) Paramedian (rectus) incision with muscle splitting. (I) Pararectus incision. (J) "Hockey stick" (thoracoabdominal) incision. (By permission of JE Skandalakis, SW Gray, and JR Rowe, *Anatomical Complications in General Surgery*, New York: McGraw-Hill, 1983.)

Vertical Incisions

Upper Midline Incision

Incisions of the linea alba and the transversalis fascia may reveal abundant and well-vascularized fat in the upper midline (Fig. 4.21A). We suggest that the incisions of the peritoneum be made slightly to the left of the midline to avoid the ligamentum teres in the edge of the falciform ligament. If it is encountered, it may be ligated and divided. As soon as the linea alba is incised, mark the opposite sides of the incision with a stitch of 0 silk. This will ensure alignment during closure. Close the linea alba from above downward. Alternatively, closing from caudal to cranial may be easier and cause less evisceration as you approach the costal margin.

A *thoracic extension* of a midline abdominal incision may be made through the 8th intercostal space as far as the scapula. In this procedure, the midline incision is exploratory, and the need for the thoracic extension depends on the pathology revealed by the exploration.

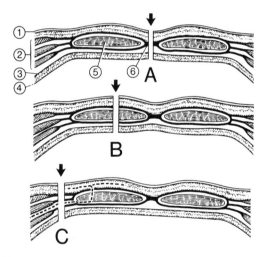

Figure 4.21. Vertical incisions. (A) Incision through the linea alba. (B) Incision through the rectus muscle (paramedian) splitting the muscle. (C) Incision lateral to the rectus sheath (pararectus). Segmental nerves to the rectus muscle (broken line) will be cut. (1) Skin, (2) three flat muscles and their aponeuroses, (3) transversalis fascia, (4) peritoneum, (5) rectus abdominis muscle, (6) linea alba. (By permission of JE Skandalakis, SW Gray, and JR Rowe, *Anatomical Complications in General Surgery*, New York: McGraw-Hill, 1983.)

Sternal splitting may be used to continue the midline incision superiorly.

A *lateral extension* to one or even both sides may be L- or T-shaped.

A *downward continuation* of an upper midline incision is always an available option.

Lower Midline Incision

There are some anatomical differences in the midline above and below the umbilicus. The linea alba is narrow and more difficult to identify below. Remember that the bladder always must be decompressed.

An *upward extension* of a lower midline incision is always available to the surgeon. The incision should go around the umbilicus to the left to avoid the ligamentum teres and an unclean umbilicus.

Lateral extensions are the same as those of upper midline extensions.

Occasionally the anatomy of the umbilicus permits a *transumbilical extension*. The surgeon must be sure the umbilical folds are clean.

Rectus (Paramedian) Incision

This incision is preferred by the surgeon who wishes to close the abdominal wall in layers (Fig. 4.21B). It does not destroy muscle tissue or nerves. Retract the rectus muscle laterally to prevent tension on vessels and nerves (Fig. 4.22).

Feasible extensions may be made as described for midline incisions.

Pararectus Incision

The incision is made along the lateral border of the rectus sheath. It is undesirable because it cuts across the nerve supply to the rectus muscle (Fig. 4.21C). The blood supply from the inferior epigastric artery also may be compromised.

Extensions will further injure nerves and blood vessels.

Transverse Incisions

In this type of incision, both rectus sheath and muscle are cut.

Upper Abdomen

The rectus muscle and the flat muscles may be cut in the line of the skin incision.

Lower Abdomen (Pfannenstiel Incision)

This incision is made horizontally just above the pubis. The anterior rectus sheaths and the linea alba are transected and reflected upward 8–10 cm. The rectus muscles are retracted laterally, and the transversalis fascia and the peritoneum may be cut in the midline. The iliohypogastric nerve must be identified and protected (Fig. 4.23).

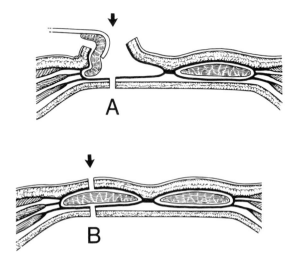

Figure 4.22. Incision through the rectus sheath without muscle splitting. (A) Lateral retraction of the rectus muscle following incision of the anterior layer of the sheath. (B) Release of traction allows intact muscle to bridge the incision through the sheath (compare with Figure 4.21B). (By permission of JE Skandalakis, SW Gray, and JR Rowe, *Anatomical Complications in General Surgery*, New York: McGraw-Hill, 1983.)

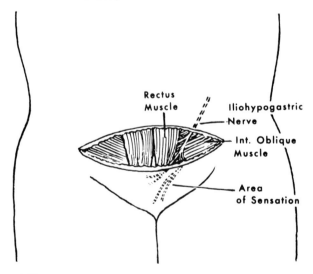

Figure 4.23. Pfannenstiel transverse abdominal incision showing the iliohypogastric nerve between the internal oblique muscle and the external oblique aponeurosis just lateral to the border of the rectus muscle. (By permission of CR Grosz, *Am J Surg* 142:628, 1981.)

All the transverse incisions may be extended in the midline. The lower abdominal incision may be extended laterally by dividing the tendinous attachment of the rectus muscle to the pubis. Lateral extension also may be attained by leaving the rectus muscle attached, but retracting it medially and splitting the muscles of the anterolateral wall. This usually requires ligation of the inferior epigastric vessels. Extension too far laterally may jeopardize the iliohypogastric and ilioinguinal nerves (Fig. 4.24).

Oblique Incisions

Subcostal Incision

The rectus sheath is incised transversely. The rectus muscle is cut and the external oblique muscle is split and retracted. The incision should extend laterally no further than necessary in order to avoid cutting intercostal nerves. The operator usually sees the small 8th and the larger 9th nerves. The latter should be retracted and preserved.

The external oblique, internal oblique, and transversus abdominis

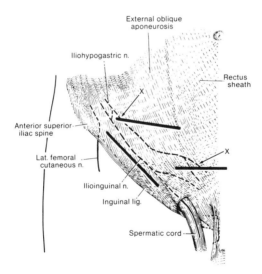

Figure 4.24. The courses of the iliohypogastric and ilioinguinal nerves. Transverse incisions carried too far laterally may cut the iliohypogastric nerve. Inguinal incisions may injure the ilioinguinal nerve directly or it may be inadvertently included in a suture during closure of the incision. (By permission of JE Skandalakis, SW Gray, and JR Rowe, *Anatomical Complications in General Surgery*, New York: McGraw-Hill, 1983.)

muscles usually can be split. Occasionally, the external oblique fibers must be cut laterally and downward.

A subcostal incision two finger breadths below and parallel to the right costal margin is the incision most frequently used.

An oblique incision can be extended laterally to the contralateral side of the body or to the same side by following the costal arch and avoiding the nerves. It may be extended upward or downward on the linea alba. It may be extended obliquely upward through the costal arch if it is necessary to convert it to a thoracoabdominal incision.

McBurney Incision

The skin is incised for about 8 cm starting 4 cm medial to the right anterosuperior spine and extending downward on a line from the spine to the umbilicus. The aponeurosis of the external oblique muscle and the internal oblique and transversus abdominis muscles are split in the direction of their fibers. The iliohypogastric nerve, deep to the internal oblique muscle, must be identified and preserved.

A McBurney incision may be extended upward and laterally for several centimeters without cutting muscles. Medial extension requires transecting the rectus sheath and muscle. In some instances, it is easier to close the incision and make a new one.

Thoracoabdominal Incisions

A wide variety of incisions to expose lesions in the upper abdomen and lower thorax have been reported.

Thoracic incisions have been made through intercostal spaces 5 through 9 or by resection of ribs 7 to 9. The abdominal portion of the incision has been either a midline or a transverse continuation of the thoracic incisions. It may or may not extend into the rectus abdominis.

Use this incision only if it is absolutely necessary.

Dehiscence of the Incision

Obesity, prolonged ileus or bowel obstruction, and wound infection are important factors of dehiscence. Dehiscence is caused by poor quality of the tissue or suturing with bites that are too small, placed too far apart, or tied too tightly. Because wounds in patients with hypoproteinemia heal slowly, hyperalimentation is recommended for those whose protein intake is at all questionable.

In contaminated cases, secondary closure of the skin 4–5 days later is a mature surgical decision. The sutures at the initial closure may be placed, but not tied until later. Good hemostasis, debridement, irrigation, good approximation of skin, absence of tension, and avoidance of dead spaces all contribute to good healing without wound dehiscence, postoperative incisional hernia, or a disfiguring scar.

■ MYOAPONEUROTIC INCISIONAL HERNIAS

Location

These hernias may be located in any part of the abdominal wall, since they are the result of incisions made for some type of surgery. The usual sites are as follows:

- upper midline
- umbilical
- lower midline
- lateral upper quadrant
- lateral lower quadrant
- suprapubic, transverse
- lumbar

Overall Etiology and Pathogenesis

- surgery: dehiscence, infection, poor anatomical knowledge or technique
- obesity
- pregnancy
- straining or severe cough
- abdominal distention
- collagen synthesis (enzymatic lysis)
- diabetes
- malnutrition
- ascites
- concomitant steroid therapy

Preoperative Evaluation and Care

- gastrointestinal and small bowel series, if indicated
- barium enema, if indicated
- bowel prep, if indicated
- erythromycin base 500 mg and neomycin 500 mg four times daily for 1 day prior to surgery, if involvement of large bowel is suspected

■ cleansing of the abdominal wall with Hibiclens or PhisoHex 12 hours and 1 hour prior to surgery

■ shaving the abdominal wall in the operating room

■ intravenous antibiotics in the operating room prior to making the incision and for the first 24 hours postoperatively

Operating Room Strategy

The closure for the defect depends upon its size. We recommend the following:

■ Very small or small (1–3 cm): Close defect in two layers anatomically.

■ Larger than 4 cm: Close defect with prosthesis.

Very Small or Small Defects (1–3 cm)
Procedure:

Step 1. Remove scar by elliptical incision (Fig. 4.25).

Step 2. Dissect skin flaps and subcutaneous tissue on both sides of defect down to the aponeurotic area, approximately 3–4 cm around the defect (Fig. 4.26).

Step 3. If possible, avoid opening the sac. If this is not possible, remove sac and carefully palpate the defect or defects. Remove all scars and attenuated tissues.

Step 4. Close the posterior and anterior laminae, vertically or trans-

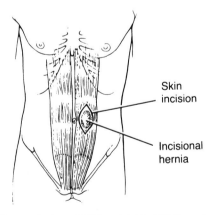

Skin incision

Incisional hernia

Figure 4.25. (By permission of JE Skandalakis, SW Gray, AR Mansberger, et al, *Hernia: Surgical Anatomy and Technique*, New York: McGraw-Hill, 1989.)

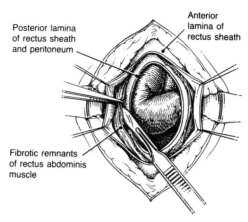

Posterior lamina
of rectus sheath
and peritoneum

Anterior
lamina of
rectus sheath

Fibrotic remnants
of rectus abdominis
muscle

Figure 4.26. (By permission of JE Skandalakis, SW Gray, AR Mansberger, et al, *Hernia: Surgical Anatomy and Technique*, New York: McGraw-Hill, 1989.)

versely, with continuous or interrupted No. 1 Prolene (the authors prefer interrupted), with bites 2–2.5 cm from the ring (Fig. 4.27). Alternatively, the defect may be closed by imbrication in a side-to-side closure (Fig. 4.28).

Step 5. Use Jackson-Pratt or Snyder drain, if required, and close in layers (Fig. 4.29).

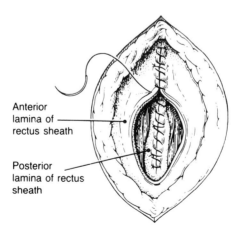

Anterior
lamina of
rectus sheath

Posterior
lamina of rectus
sheath

Figure 4.27. (By permission of JE Skandalakis, SW Gray, AR Mansberger, et al, *Hernia: Surgical Anatomy and Technique*, New York: McGraw-Hill, 1989.)

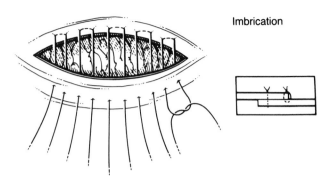

Imbrication

Figure 4.28. (By permission of JE Skandalakis, SW Gray, AR Mansberger, et al, *Hernia: Surgical Anatomy and Technique*, New York: McGraw-Hill, 1989.)

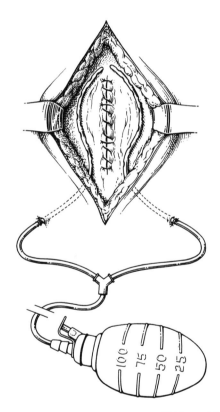

Figure 4.29. (By permission of JE Skandalakis, SW Gray, AR Mansberger, et al, *Hernia: Surgical Anatomy and Technique*, New York: McGraw-Hill, 1989.)

Defects Larger than 4 cm

For defects larger than 4 cm, the Stoppa procedure is highly recommended: it consists of implanting a large prosthesis deep between the
muscles of the abdominal wall and the peritoneum (Figs. 4.30A-C).
Stoppa does not use sutures; however, in practically all our cases we have
used sutures.

An alternative procedure follows.

Step 1. With Mersilene, Prolene, or Marlex prosthesis, use the Usher
repair with two layers. Suture one layer to the posterior surface of the transversalis fascia.

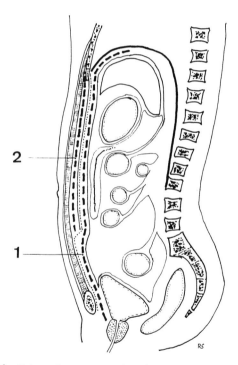

Figure 4.30A. Schematic representation of a paramedial sagittal cross section of the trunk showing the two retroparietal cleavable spaces used for prosthetic repair of large hernias. Broken line 1 = the retrofascial preperitoneal
space used at the lower part of the wall. Broken line 2 = the retrorectal space
used at the supraumbilical part of the wall. (Modified by permission of Odimba
BFK, Stoppa R, Laude M, Henry X, Verhaeghe P. *J Chir (Paris)* 117(11):621–
627; 1980).

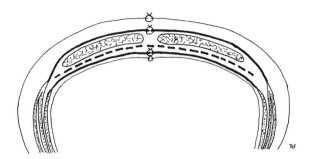

Figure 4.30B. Schematic representation of a horizontal cross section of the wall at its upper level, with a mesh prosthesis (broken line) in the retrorectal cleavable space. (Courtesy Dr. Rene F. Stoppa)

Step 2. Using interrupted 0 or 00 polypropylene monofilament sutures, attach a second layer to the anterior surface of the fascia (Fig. 4.31).

Step 3. Jackson–Pratt or Snyder drains should be used, by separate stab wounds. Secure the catheter with skin sutures.

Remember:

✓ The lines of mesh should match with the oblique aponeurotic pattern of Askar.

✓ Though there are surgeons who believe that abdominal pressure alone keeps a large prosthesis in place, the authors prefer fixation. The anatomical fixation of a large prosthesis is *only approximately* as follows:

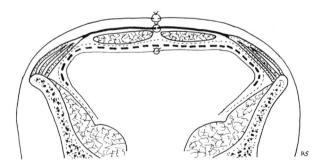

Figure 4.30C. Schematic representation of a horizontal cross section of the wall at its lower level, with a mesh prosthesis (broken line) in the retrofascial preperitoneal cleavable space. (Courtesy Dr. Rene F. Stoppa)

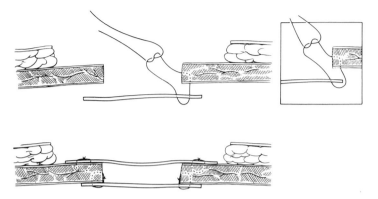

Figure 4.31. (By permission of JE Skandalakis, SW Gray, AR Mansberger, et al, *Hernia: Surgical Anatomy and Technique*, New York: McGraw-Hill, 1989.)

- **a.** Upper midline: costal arch, lateral flat muscles, or rectus sheath.

- **b.** Umbilical: lower costal arch; superior-anterior iliac spine, if possible; lateral flat muscles; or rectus sheath.

- **c.** Lower midline: linea semicircularis, pectineal ligament, space of Retzius, rectus sheath, or lateral flat muscles.

- **d.** Lateral upper: costal arch; superior-anterior iliac spine, if possible; rectus sheath; opposite myoaponeurotic flat muscles; or lateral flat muscles.

- **e.** Spigelian: anatomical closure of defect. **Remember:** the sac is under the aponeurosis of the external oblique.

- **f.** Lateral lower: iliac crest, right and left ligaments of Cooper, rectus sheath, or lateral flat muscles.

- **g.** Lumbar (both): external oblique, latissimus dorsi, or iliac crest. You may need double prosthesis.

■ EPIGASTRIC HERNIA (HERNIA THROUGH THE LINEA ALBA)

An epigastric hernia (or hernia through the linea alba) is a protrusion of preperitoneal fat or a peritoneal sac with or without an incarcerated viscus. It occurs in the midline between the xiphoid process and the umbilicus.

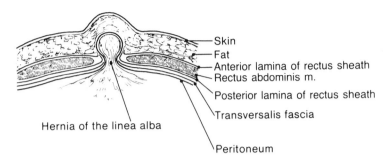

Skin
Fat
Anterior lamina of rectus sheath
Rectus abdominis m.
Posterior lamina of rectus sheath
Transversalis fascia
Hernia of the linea alba
Peritoneum

Figure 4.32. (By permission of JE Skandalakis, SW Gray, AR Mansberger, et al, *Hernia: Surgical Anatomy and Technique*, New York: McGraw-Hill, 1989.)

In Fig. 4.32, a peritoneal sac containing omentum has formed through a defect in the rectus sheath. The sac is covered only with skin and fat.

Procedure:

Step 1. Make a vertical or transverse incision over the mass.

Step 2. Dissect the fat down to the linea alba superiorly and inferiorly and to the anterior lamina of the rectus sheath laterally (Fig. 4.33).

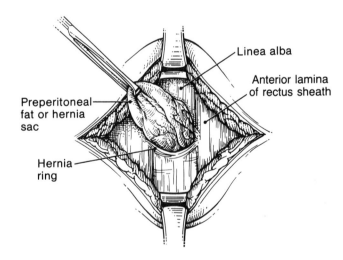

Linea alba

Anterior lamina of rectus sheath

Preperitoneal fat or hernia sac

Hernia ring

Figure 4.33. (By permission of JE Skandalakis, SW Gray, AR Mansberger, et al, *Hernia: Surgical Anatomy and Technique*, New York: McGraw-Hill, 1989.)

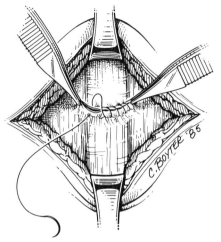

Figure 4.34. (By permission of JE Skandalakis, SW Gray, AR Mansberger, et al, *Hernia: Surgical Anatomy and Technique*, New York: McGraw-Hill, 1989.)

Step 3. Close the small defect in the linea alba transversely with interrupted 0 Surgilon suture. A running suture can be used (Fig. 4.34).

Step 4. Imbrication may be used, but not at the risk of overstretching the aponeurosis. Close subcutaneous tissue and skin.

■ UMBILICAL HERNIA

Small Umbilical Hernia (Figs. 4.35A–G)
Procedure:

Step 1. Make an infraumbilical incision from the 3 to the 9 o'clock position.

Step 2. Dissect the sac circumferentially free of the surrounding subcutaneous tissue.

Step 3. Divide the sac and excise the excess sac down to the ring.

Step 4. Use an interrupted 0 Surgilon to close the ring.

Step 5. Close the skin.

Large Umbilical Hernia
Umbilical hernias in adults may be the result of large, untreated infantile hernias that failed to close spontaneously. Umbilical hernias in the adult do not close spontaneously.

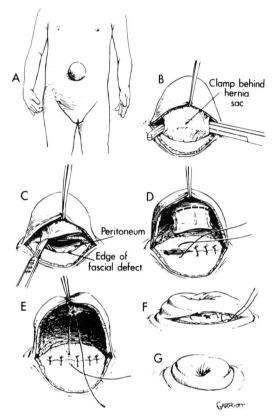

Figs. 4-35A–G. (By permission of RP Harmel, Umbilical hernia. In: Nyhus LM, Condon RL. *Hernia*, 3rd ed. Philadelphia: JB Lippincott, 1989.)

Repair of Umbilical Hernia in Adults

Procedures:

Step 1. If the skin is degenerated and if the patient is old, the umbilicus need not be preserved. However, try to save the umbilicus in all other cases. If possible, make an incision from the 9 to the 3 o'clock position above or below the umbilicus (Fig. 4.36).

Step 2. Separate the sac from the fat with knife or scissors and, after satisfactory isolation and elevation, open it.

Incision

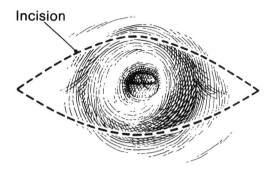

Figure 4.36. (By permission of JE Skandalakis, SW Gray, AR Mansberger, et al, *Hernia: Surgical Anatomy and Technique*, New York: McGraw-Hill, 1989.)

Step 3. Trim the sac down to the ring or just above the ring if the sac is to be closed separately. Ligate all bleeding points. We ligate all of the tubular structures with 000 silk. Close the sac and posterior lamina of the rectus sheath with interrupted 0 chromic or 00 Dexon suture. Prepare the anterior lamina of the rectus sheath for a distance of 1 to 2 cm all around the defect (Fig. 4.37).

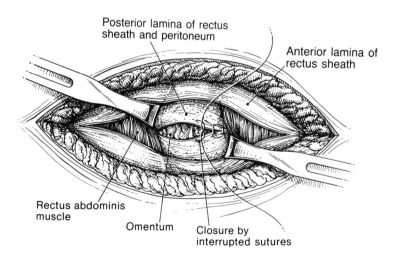

Posterior lamina of rectus sheath and peritoneum

Anterior lamina of rectus sheath

Rectus abdominis muscle

Omentum

Closure by interrupted sutures

Figure 4.37. (By permission of JE Skandalakis, SW Gray, AR Mansberger, et al, *Hernia: Surgical Anatomy and Technique*, New York: McGraw-Hill, 1989.)

Step 4. Gently separate the posterior lamina of the rectus sheath from the peritoneum. Close the defect transversely, with or without imbrication, with interrupted 0 Surgilon.

Step 5. Close the linea alba with interrupted sutures.

Step 6. Close the skin with interrupted sutures. Many surgeons close the defect longitudinally in the same way that they close a midline incision. Also, many surgeons incorporate the peritoneum and fascia in one layer.

■ OMPHALOCELE AND GASTROSCHISIS

In infants, repair of omphalocele (exomphalos) and gastroschisis belongs not to general surgeons but to pediatric surgeons.

■ SPIGELIAN (LATERAL VENTRAL) HERNIA

A Spigelian hernia is a spontaneous protrusion of preperitoneal fat, a peritoneal sac, or, less commonly, a sac containing a viscus, through the Spigelian zone (fascia) at any point along its length. The zone is bounded medially by the lateral margin of the anterior lamina of the rectus sheath and laterally by the muscular fibers of the internal oblique muscle.

The surgeon should be familiar with three entities in this area:

1. The semilunar line (of Spieghel) marks the lateral border of the rectus sheath and extends from the pubic tubercle to the tip of the costal cartilage of the 9th rib.

2. The semicircular line (arcuate line, fold, or line of Douglas) marks the caudal end of the posterior lamina of the aponeurotic rectus sheath, below the umbilicus and above the pubis. Unfortunately, the semilunar and semicircular lines are not easily seen in the operating room.

3. The Spigelian fascia (zone, aponeurosis) is composed of the aponeuroses of the external oblique, internal oblique, and transversus abdominis muscles. The region between these muscles and the lateral border of the rectus muscle defines the Spigelian fascia. For all practical purposes, the Spigelian fascia is formed by the approximation and fusion of the internal oblique and transversus abdominis aponeuroses. If the fusion of these aponeuroses is loose, a "zone" rather than a fascia is formed. The external oblique aponeurosis remains intact over the hernia. Fig. 4.38 shows the location of the hernias of the anterior abdominal wall: (A) is above the semicircular line, (B) is below the semicircular line.

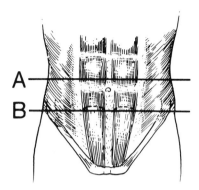

Figure 4.38. (By permission of JE Skandalakis, SW Gray, AR Mansberger, et al, *Hernia: Surgical Anatomy and Technique*, New York: McGraw-Hill, 1989.)

As illustrated in Fig. 4.39A, herniation usually begins with preperitoneal fat passing through defects in the transversus abdominis (A_1) and internal oblique (A_2) aponeuroses. In Fig. 4.39B, notice that the transversus abdominis and internal oblique are broken and that the aponeurosis of the external oblique muscle remains intact and, with the skin, forms the covering of the hernia.

Repair of Spigelian Hernia

Procedure:

Step 1. Make a transverse or vertical incision through the aponeurosis of the external oblique muscle over the palpable mass. If the mass is not palpable at examination, make a midline or vertical rectus incision. If the hernia is incarcerated, the ring should be incised medially toward the rectus abdominis muscle.

Step 2. Retract the aponeurosis of the external oblique muscle, revealing the internal oblique muscle and the hernial sac.

Step 3. Open the sac; inspect its contents, ligate, and push the sac into the abdomen.

Step 4. Free the ring of Spigelian fascia from preperitoneal fat and peritoneal adhesions (Fig. 4.40).

Step 5. Close the defect in the transversus abdominis and the internal oblique muscle with 0 or 00 Surgilon interrupted sutures.

Step 6. Close the defect in the aponeurosis of the external oblique muscle.

Step 7. Close the skin with interrupted sutures or clips.

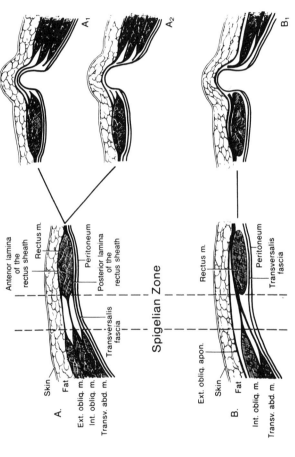

Figure 4.39. (A₁) Transversus abdominis and internal oblique broken; (A₂) Transversus abdominis and internal oblique broken. (B₁) Transversus abdominis and internal oblique broken. (By permission of JE Skandalakis, SW Gray, AR Mansberger, et al, *Hernia: Surgical Anatomy and Technique*, New York: McGraw-Hill, 1989.)

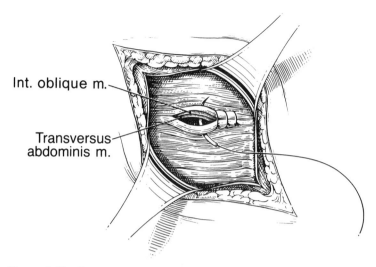

Int. oblique m.

Transversus abdominis m.

Figure 4.40. (By permission of JE Skandalakis, SW Gray, AR Mansberger, et al, *Hernia: Surgical Anatomy and Technique*, New York: McGraw-Hill, 1989.)

Inguinal (Groin) Hernias

Three types of hernia—direct inguinal, indirect inguinal, and external supravesical—may emerge through the abdominal wall by way of the external inguinal ring above the inguinal ligament. A fourth type, femoral hernia, emerges beneath the inguinal ligament by way of the femoral canal. These four hernias make up 90 percent of all hernias.

■ SURGICAL ANATOMY OF GROIN HERNIAS

Within the groin area are the inguinal and femoral canals. The inguinal canal is an oblique cleft about 4 cm long in the adult, lying about 4–5 cm above the inguinal ligament. The femoral canal below the inguinal ligament is 1.25–2 cm long and occupies the most medial compartment of the femoral sheath.

■ LAYERS OF THE LOWER ANTERIOR BODY WALL

In the inguinal region, the layers of the abdominal wall are:

1. Skin
2. Subcutaneous or superficial fasciae (Camper's and Scarpa's) containing fat

3. Innominate fascia (of Gallaudet). This is the superficial or external layer of fascia of the external oblique muscle. It is not always recognizable. Its absence is of no surgical importance.

4. External oblique aponeurosis, including the inguinal (Poupart's), lacunar (Gimbernat's), and reflected inguinal (Colles') ligaments

5. Spermatic cord in the male; round ligament of the uterus in the female

6. Transversus abdominis muscle and aponeurosis, internal oblique muscle, falx inguinalis (Henle), and the conjoined tendon (when present)

7. Transversalis fascia and aponeurosis associated with the pectineal ligament (Cooper's), iliopubic tract, falx inguinalis, and transversalis fascia sling

8. Preperitoneal connective tissue with fat

9. Peritoneum

10. Superficial and deep inguinal rings

■ FOSSAE OF THE ANTERIOR ABDOMINAL WALL (Fig. 4.41)

The inner (posterior) surface of the anterior body wall above the inguinal ligament and below the umbilicus is divided into three shallow fossae on

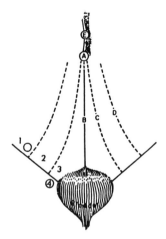

Figure 4.41. Diagram of the fossae of the anterior abdominal wall and their relation to the sites of groin hernias: (A) umbilicus; (B) median umbilical ligament (obliterated urachus); (C) medial umbilical ligament (obliterated umbilical arteries); (D) lateral umbilical ligament containing inferior (deep) epigastric arteries; and (E) falciform ligament. Sites of possible hernias: (1) lateral fossa (indirect inguinal hernia), (2) medial fossa (direct inguinal hernia), (3) supravesical fossa (supravesical hernia), and (4) femoral ring (femoral hernia). (By permission of JS Rowe, JE Skandalakis, and SW Gray, *Am Surg* 39(5):269–270; 1973.)

either side of a low ridge formed in the midline by the median umbilical ligament, the obliterated urachus. Each of these fossae is a potential site for a hernia. From lateral to medial, these fossae are:

- The *lateral fossa*, bounded medially by the inferior epigastric arteries. It contains the internal inguinal ring, the site of indirect inguinal hernia.

- The *medial fossa*, between the inferior epigastric artery and the medial umbilical ligament (remnant of the umbilical artery). It is the site of direct inguinal hernia.

- The *supravesical fossa*, between the medial and the median umbilical ligaments. It is the site of external supravesical hernia.

■ WALLS OF THE INGUINAL CANAL

- *Anterior:* The anterior wall is formed by the aponeurosis of the external oblique muscle with some participation of the internal oblique muscle laterally.

- *Posterior:* In about ¾ of subjects, the posterior wall is formed laterally by the aponeurosis of the transversus abdominis muscle and the transversalis fascia. In the remainder, the posterior wall is transversalis fascia only. Medially the posterior wall is reinforced by the internal oblique aponeurosis.

- *Superior:* The roof of the canal is formed by the arched fibers of the lower edge of the internal oblique muscle and by the transversus abdominis muscle and aponeurosis.

- *Inferior:* The wall of the canal is formed by the inguinal ligament (Poupart's) and the lacunar ligament (Gimbernat's).

The upper end of the inguinal canal is the internal or deep inguinal ring, which is a normal defect of the transversalis fascia. Its superior margin is formed by the transversus abdominis arch; its inferior margins are formed by aponeurotic fibers from the iliopubic tract, the inferior epigastric vessels, and the interfoveolar ligament (Hesselbach's). The inferior epigastric vessels penetrate the transversalis fascia.

The external or superficial inguinal ring is a triangular opening in the aponeurosis of the external oblique muscle. The superior and inferior crura, which form the margins of the ring, are held together and reinforced by intercrural fibers.

■ CONTENTS OF THE INGUINAL CANAL

Male

The spermatic cord in the male contains a matrix of connective tissue continuous with the preperitoneal connective tissue (see No. 8 in the list of layers of the anterior body wall, p. 164). The cord consists of:

- ductus deferens
- three arteries: the internal spermatic (testicular), deferential, and external spermatic (cremasteric)
- one venous plexus (pampiniform)
- the genital branch of the genitofemoral nerve
- the ilioinguinal nerve
- sympathetic fibers from the hypogastric plexus
- three layers of fascia: the external spermatic fascia, a continuation of the innominate fascia; the middle, cremasteric layer, continuous with the internal oblique muscle fibers and muscle fascia; and the internal spermatic fascia, an extension of the transversalis fascia.

Female

The inguinal canal includes the round ligament of the uterus, the genital branch of the genitofemoral nerve, the cremasteric vessels, the ilioinguinal nerve, and coverings as described for the male, although usually less distinct.

■ THE FEMORAL CANAL AND ITS SHEATH

The femoral sheath is formed anteriorly and medially by the transversalis fascia and some transversus aponeurotic fibers, posteriorly by the pectineus and psoas fasciae, and laterally by the iliacus fascia. The sheath forms three compartments, the most medial of which is the femoral canal, through which a femoral hernia may pass. The boundaries are:

- lateral: a connective tissue septum and the femoral vein
- posterior: the pectineal ligament (Cooper's)
- anterior: the iliopubic tract or the inguinal ligament or both
- medial: the aponeurotic insertion of the transversus abdominis muscle and transversalis fascia or, rarely, the lacunar ligament

In the 1990s, the operative treatment of groin hernia continues to be based on an accurate knowledge of anatomy. Understanding the endoabdominal (transversalis) fascia and its analogues (iliopubic tract/anterior femoral sheath) is the key to our knowledge of the etiology, development, diagnosis, and cure of these common problems.

The surgeon today must have the ability to modify the approach according to individual operative findings.

The various anatomical defects of inguinal hernia and the specific best operative care for each are as follows:

Excision of hernial sac and high ligation (in all except direct)

1. Small indirect	**a.** transversalis fascia repair of internal ring
2. Large indirect	**a.** iliopubic tract repair of posterior inguinal wall
	b. Cooper's ligament repair ad modum McVay
3. Small direct	**a.** iliopubic tract repair of posterior inguinal wall
4. Large direct	**a.** Cooper's ligament repair of posterior inguinal wall
	b. iliopubic tract repair with Marlex mesh buttress
5. External supravesical	as in direct
6. Pantaloon hernia	**a.** iliopubic tract repair of posterior inguinal wall plus transversalis fascia closure of internal ring
7. Femoral	**a.** preperitoneal approach and iliopubic tract repair
8. Sliding indirect	**a.** preperitoneal approach and iliopubic tract repair
	b. iliopubic tract repair (anterior approach)
	c. Cooper's ligament repair
9. Strangulated indirect or femoral	**a.** preperitoneal approach, bowel resection and anastomosis, iliopubic tract repair
10. Recurrent hernia	**a.** preperitoneal approach and iliopubic tract repair with Marlex mesh buttress

11. Massive hernia (loss of "right of domain")	**a.** 10-day pneumoperitoneum
	b. iliopubic tract repair of posterior inguinal wall with Marlex mesh buttress
	c. Cooper's ligament repair ad modum McVay

Today, surgeons also should be familiar with the Lichtenstein, Gilbert, and Stoppa procedures, which will be described.

■ INDIRECT INGUINAL HERNIA

An indirect inguinal hernia leaves the abdomen through the internal inguinal ring and passes down the inguinal canal a variable distance with the spermatic cord or round ligament.

Repair of Indirect Inguinal Hernia

Procedure:

Step 1. Incise the skin approximately 2–3 cm above and parallel to the inguinal ligament. (A transverse, gently curved incision following the lines of Langer is another option). The patient, male or female, will appreciate a symmetrical incision, with bilateral herniorrhaphy.

Incise the subcutaneous fascia (Camper's) and the fascia of Scarpa by sharp dissection. Open the aponeurosis of the external oblique muscle in the direction of its fibers. The external ring can be found with ease.

Remember:

✓ Ligate the large veins (superficial epigastric, superficial circumflex, and external pudendal) with plain catgut. Other small vessels may be treated by electrocoagulation.

✓ Protect the ilioinguinal nerve.

✓ If the hernia is recurrent, it will be necessary to excise the preexisting scar, both for cosmetic reasons and for good healing.

✓ Do not dissect too much medially and laterally to the incision of the aponeurosis of the external oblique muscle. Avoid dead spaces.

Step 2. Elevate the spermatic cord carefully and retract with a Penrose drain. Incise the posterior inguinal wall carefully. Such an incision will stimulate better healing (Fig. 4.42).

Step 3. Identify the sac located anterior to the spermatic cord, but do not separate from the cord. Dissect it at the internal ring and laterally to the deep epigastric vessels.

Step 4. Open the sac close to the internal inguinal ring.

Step 5. Perform a digital examination within the sac. Check for omental or viscus adhesions into the sac, possible femoral hernia, posterior wall weakness, and possible direct or external supra-vesical hernia (Fig. 4.43).

Step 6. Ligate and amputate the sac. Occasionally, if there is too much relaxation at the internal ring, the ligated sac will be fixed under the transversus abdominis muscle, which is the upper boundary of the internal ring. Leave the distal part of the sac in situ and open (Wantz procedure) to avoid anatomical complication.

We agree with Nyhus that a single technique is not appropriate for all patients. The following illustrates our technique:

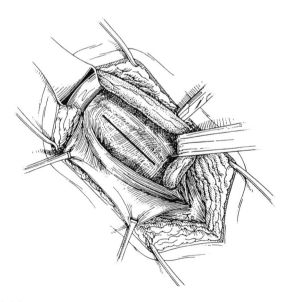

Figure 4.42. (By permission of JE Skandalakis, SW Gray, AR Mansberger, et al, *Hernia: Surgical Anatomy and Technique*, New York: McGraw-Hill, 1989.)

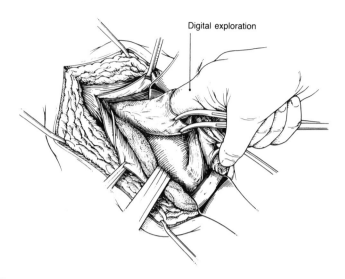

Digital exploration

Figure 4.43. (By permission of JE Skandalakis, SW Gray, AR Mansberger, et al, *Hernia: Surgical Anatomy and Technique*, New York: McGraw-Hill, 1989.)

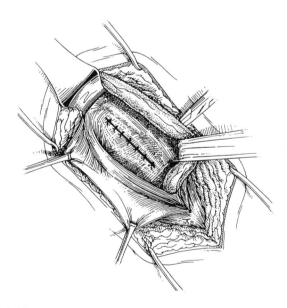

Figure 4.44. (By permission of JE Skandalakis, SW Gray, AR Mansberger, et al, *Hernia: Surgical Anatomy and Technique*, New York: McGraw-Hill, 1989.)

Step 7. **a.** Reapproximate the incision of the posterior inguinal wall with 3–0 silk (Fig. 4.44).

b. Suture the conjoined area to the ligament of Gimbernat with 0 Surgilon (Fig. 4.45).

c. Suture the conjoined area to the ligament of Cooper, including the iliopubic arch and, occasionally, the ligament of Poupart (shelving edge) if the ligament of Cooper is deep (Fig. 4.45).

d. After good palpation of the femoral arteries to avoid injury to the femoral vein, place this transitional suture as in **b** above, incorporating the femoral sheath.

e. Suture as above or suture the arch to the shelving edge of the inguinal ligament, including the iliopubic tract. The remainder of the sutures incorporate the arch, the iliopubic tract, and the inguinal ligament. Be careful with the deep inguinal ring. The suture in this area starts with the arch and incorporates the crura of the transversalis fascia (if present), the iliopubic tract, and/or the inguinal ligament,

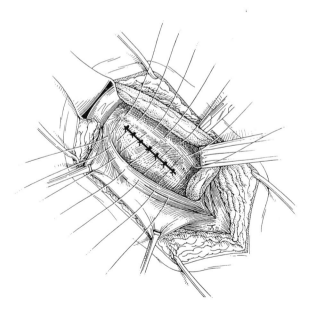

Figure 4.45. (By permission of JE Skandalakis, SW Gray, AR Mansberger, et al, *Hernia: Surgical Anatomy and Technique*, New York: McGraw-Hill, 1989.)

but not the transversus abdominis muscle, which must be protected. The distal phalanx of the 5th finger should be inserted with ease into the deep ring, thereby ensuring that the closure is not too snug.

Step 8. Tie all sutures. Close the aponeurosis of the external oblique muscle with interruped 00 Surgilon. Occasionally, we use deep bites to incorporate the arch, which was previously sutured to the inguinal ligament. The spermatic cord may be placed under or above the aponeurosis of the external oblique muscle. Close Scarpa's fascia with continuous or interruped 000 plain catgut. Close the skin with clips.

■ SLIDING INDIRECT INGUINAL HERNIA

A sliding indirect inguinal hernia contains the herniated viscus which makes up all or some of the posterior wall of the sac. The colon, ovaries, and uterine tube may be involved.

Repair of Sliding Indirect Inguinal Hernia

Communicating and noncommunicating sliding hernias are shown in Fig. 4.46. The internal ring is wider than usual due to the thick spermatic

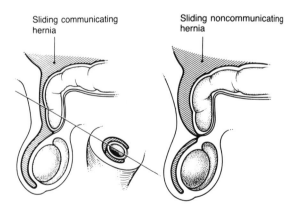

Figure 4.46. (By permission of JE Skandalakis, SW Gray, AR Mansberger, et al, *Hernia: Surgical Anatomy and Technique*, New York: McGraw-Hill, 1989.)

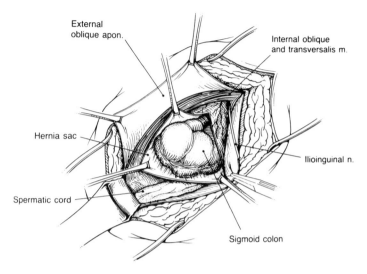

Figure 4.47. (By permission of JE Skandalakis, SW Gray, AR Mansberger, et al, *Hernia: Surgical Anatomy and Technique*, New York: McGraw-Hill, 1989.)

cord. Coincidental direct hernia or weakness of the posterior wall is a strong possibility.

The hernia sac is located anterior and medial to the cord, as in an indirect hernia. The descending viscus forms the posterior wall of the empty processus (Fig. 4.47).

Procedure:

Step 1. Mobilize the sac and open it high and anteriorly. Do not dissect the viscus from the posterior wall of the sac.

Step 2. If there is excess anterior wall of the sac, trim it carefully (Fig. 4.48).

Step 3. Close the remnants of the sac. Finish the repair as in indirect inguinal hernia.

■ DIRECT INGUINAL HERNIA

Direct inguinal hernia passes through the floor of the inguinal canal in Hesselbach's triangle, which is covered by the transversalis fascia and the aponeurosis of the transversus abdominis muscle, if present.

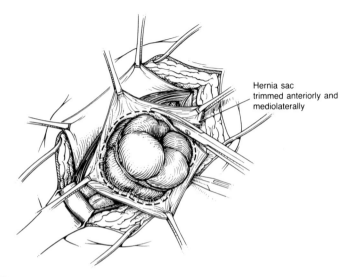

Hernia sac
trimmed anteriorly and
mediolaterally

Figure 4.48. (By permission of JE Skandalakis, SW Gray, AR Mansberger, et al, *Hernia: Surgical Anatomy and Technique*, New York: McGraw-Hill, 1989.)

Repair of Direct Inguinal Hernia

Hoguet's maneuver to convert a direct hernia sac to an indirect hernia is not described among the following procedures, since the direct hernia sac in some cases is not opened, but only closed by a purse string. However, we incise the posterior inguinal wall as we described previously. Cooper's ligament, the iliopubic tract, and also the conjoined area are used for the repair of practically all inguinofemoral hernias.

Procedure:

Step 1. Incision as in indirect.

Step 2. Bulging of the direct hernia with the cord pulled medially or laterally (Fig. 4.49).

Step 3. Using 000 silk, make a purse-string suture at the base of the unopened sac, or incise the posterior wall and sac carefully. Tie the suture.

Step 4. The suturing technique for direct inguinal hernia is the same as for indirect hernia. Follow the precautions outlined in Indirect Inguinal Hernia (pp. 168–173). Close Scarpa's fascia with continuous or interrupted 000 plain catgut.

Step 5. Close the skin with clips.

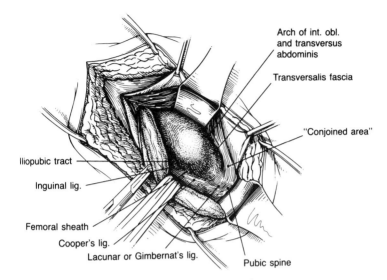

Figure 4.49. (By permission of JE Skandalakis, SW Gray, AR Mansberger, et al, *Hernia: Surgical Anatomy and Technique*, New York: McGraw-Hill, 1989.)

■ THE RELAXING INCISION (Fig. 4.50)

The surgeon should be familiar with the formation of the anterior lamina of the rectus sheath: Below the semicircular line (Douglas or arcuate) there is no posterior aponeurotic layer of the rectus sheath; the anterior layer is formed by the bilaminar aponeuroses of the internal oblique and transversus abdominis muscles and reinforced by the aponeurosis of the

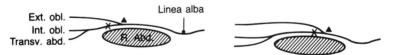

Figure 4.50. Diagrammatic drawing of the relaxing incision. X = point of relaxing incision at the anterior lamina of the rectus sheath. ▲ = "touch down" of the external oblique aponeurosis, always between the linea alba and semilunar line. (By permission of JE Skandalakis, SW Gray, AR Mansberger, et al. *Hernia: Surgical Anatomy and Technique*. New York: McGraw-Hill, 1989.)

external oblique muscle; the aponeurosis of the external oblique muscle may "touch down" at the lateral half or at the medial half of the anterior lamina. It almost never does so at the linea semilunaris (lateral border of the rectus abdominis) or at the linea alba.

The relaxing incision is made just lateral to the line of attachment ("touch down") of the external oblique aponeurosis to the anterior lamina of the sheath. This is at the point where the fused internal oblique and transversus abdominis aponeuroses form the rectus sheath.

The incision starts at the pubic crest and extends upward 5–8 cm. The length of the incision depends on the local anatomy and pathology.

A good anatomical relaxing incision will protect the external oblique aponeurosis and will not permit the rectus muscle to form a myocele.

Avoid the iliohypogastric nerve. Also avoid a linea alba incision or an incision at the linea semilunaris: this is done by careful elevation of the medial flap of the aponeurosis of the external oblique muscle (Fig. 4.50).

When the direct hernia repair is complete, the relaxing incision allows the transversus abdominis to slide inferiorly. As the incision opens, the rectus muscle is exposed, but the overlying intact superficial lamina (external oblique aponeurosis) of the rectus sheath prevents the development of a hernia.

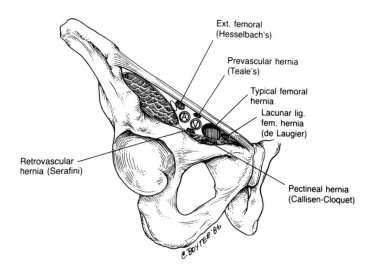

Figure 4.51. Femoral hernia. Typical and atypical pathways taken by the femoral hernial sac. Note the possible relations to the femoral artery (A) and femoral vein (V). (By permission of JE Skandalakis, SW Gray, AR Mansberger, et al, *Hernia: Surgical Anatomy and Technique*, New York: McGraw-Hill, 1989.)

■ EXTERNAL SUPRAVESICAL HERNIA

An external supravesical hernia leaves the peritoneal cavity through the supravesical fossa, which lies medial to the site of the direct inguinal fossae. Its subsequent course is that of a direct inguinal hernia.

The repair procedure is the same as for direct inguinal hernia. The surgeon should be careful to protect the iliohypogastric nerve, which is located medial to the superior edge of the surgical ellipse.

■ FEMORAL HERNIA

A femoral hernia is a protrusion of preperitoneal fat or intraperitoneal viscus through a weak transversalis fascia into the femoral ring and the femoral canal. Fig. 4.51 shows typical and atypical pathways taken by the femoral hernial sac, and Fig. 4.52 illustrates possible locations of aberrant obturator arteries.

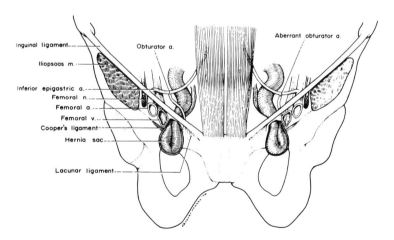

Figure 4.52. Femoral hernia. The left half of the drawing shows an aberrant obturator artery (40 percent) passing medial to the hernial sac, making it dangerous to incise the lacunar ligament. The right half of the drawing shows an aberrant obturator artery passing lateral to the hernial sac, making it safe to incise the lacunar ligament. (By permission of JE Skandalakis, SW Gray, and JT Akin, *Surg Clin NA* 54(6):1227–1246; 1974.)

Repair of Femoral Hernia Above the Inguinal Ligament

Procedure:

Step 1. Make an incision above the inguinal ligament as in direct hernia. Incise the internal oblique muscle, the transversus abdominis muscle, and the transversalis fascia without entering the peritoneum.

Blunt dissection in the preperitoneal space will direct the surgeon to the neck of the hernia sac, which should not be opened at this time.

Step 2. Isolate the sac under the inguinal ligament at the fossa ovalis, and with the index and middle finger of the other hand, gently push the unopened sac upward through the femoral canal into the inguinal canal (Fig. 4.53). The femoral hernia now becomes a direct hernia (Fig. 4.54).

If the hernia is not strangulated, this pressure is very useful. If the hernia is incarcerated or strangulated, the contents of the sac should be examined and not permitted to return to the abdominal cavity.

Step 3. Make a purse-string suture at the base of the unopened sac (Fig. 4.55). Tie the suture and continue the repair as for direct hernia (Fig. 4.55).

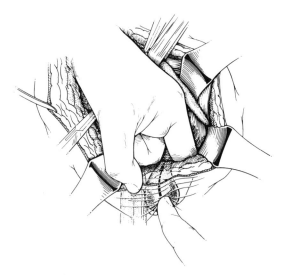

Figure 4.53. (By permission of JE Skandalakis, SW Gray, AR Mansberger, et al, *Hernia: Surgical Anatomy and Technique*, New York: McGraw-Hill, 1989.)

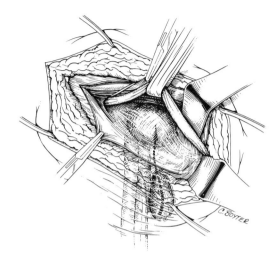

Figure 4.54. (By permission of JE Skandalakis, SW Gray, AR Mansberger, et al, *Hernia: Surgical Anatomy and Technique*, New York: McGraw-Hill, 1989.)

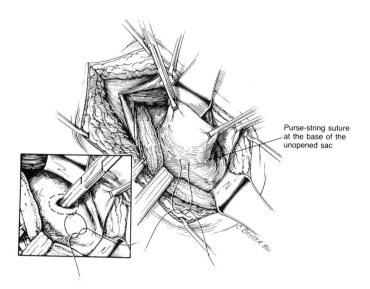

Purse-string suture at the base of the unopened sac

Figure 4.55. (By permission of JE Skandalakis, SW Gray, AR Mansberger, et al, *Hernia: Surgical Anatomy and Technique*, New York: McGraw-Hill, 1989.)

Note: An alternative method of repair accomplishes tightening of the femoral canal by suturing the iliopubic tract (above) to Cooper's ligament (below). Care must be taken to avoid constriction of the femoral vein.

If there is heavy fixation of the neck to the transversalis fascia, make a small incision at the transversalis fascia around the neck, free the sac, and using a purse-string suture, proceed to perform a direct herniorrhaphy. If the sac has remained in the upper part of Scarpa's triangle, use a Kelly clamp to bring the sac into the inguinal canal. If the hernia is strangulated, elevate the inguinal ligament by inserting a hemostat underneath it. Then make a little cut of the ligament to liberate the viscus. Another alternative method of reduction requires sectioning of the lacunar ligament. The surgeon must be certain that an aberrant obturator artery is not present before severing the ligament. Gently manipulate the sac into the posterior wall without losing the contents. An assistant should hold the mass firmly with the thumb and index finger. Open the sac and inspect the contents.

If the viscus is vital, trim and ligate the sac. Proceed with the repair as in direct inguinal hernia. If the viscus is not vital, resection and anastomosis with the usual repair should follow.

Femoral Hernia Repair Below the Inguinal Ligament

Procedure:

Step 1. Make a vertical or transverse incision just above the femoral swelling with extension of the subcutaneous tissues (Fig. 4.56).

Step 2. Isolate the swelling by careful sharp dissection and digital maneuver until the sac is exposed.

Step 3. Carefully open the sac. Fluid (which is always present) is sent to the lab for culture and sensitivity testing (Fig. 4.57).

Step 4. Inspect the contents of the sac. If viable, push the contents gently into the abdominal cavity. If constriction of the neck does not permit the return of the viscus into the peritoneal cavity, the hernia ring should be cut. It is our opinion that the best anatomical entity to sacrifice in this situation is the inguinal ligament, not the lacunar ligament.

Step 5. Ligate the sac with 00 Surgilon and excise it. Gently push the sac into the peritoneal cavity so that the canal is as clean as possible.

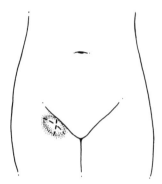

Figure 4.56. (By permission of JE Skandalakis, SW Gray, AR Mansberger, et al, *Hernia: Surgical Anatomy and Technique*, New York: McGraw-Hill, 1989.)

Step 6. Using 0 Surgilon, suture the inguinal ligament to the pectineal fascia or to Cooper's ligament. We prefer to use Cooper's ligament (Figs. 4.58 and 4.59).

Step 7. Close the subcutaneous fat and the skin. If the contents of the sac (bowel) are not viable, the assistant should keep the loop in situ, holding it firmly. Make a lower midline incision immediately; resection and anastomosis of the bowel must be done from above. Use of drains or closure of the wound depends upon whether there was any contamination of the fossa ovalis or the peritoneal cavity.

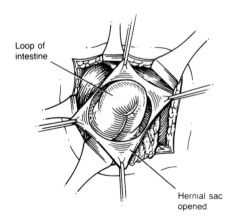

Loop of
intestine

Hernial sac
opened

Figure 4.57. (By permission of JE Skandalakis, SW Gray, AR Mansberger, et al, *Hernia: Surgical Anatomy and Technique*, New York: McGraw-Hill, 1989.)

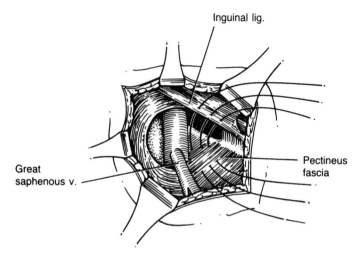

Figure 4.58. (By permission of JE Skandalakis, SW Gray, AR Mansberger, et al, *Hernia: Surgical Anatomy and Technique*, New York: McGraw-Hill, 1989.)

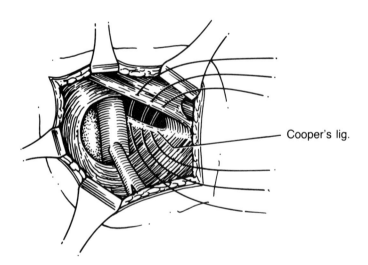

Figure 4.59. (By permission of JE Skandalakis, SW Gray, AR Mansberger, et al, *Hernia: Surgical Anatomy and Technique*, New York: McGraw-Hill, 1989.)

■ MALE AND FEMALE PEDIATRIC INGUINAL HERNIA, AND UNDESCENDED TESTIS

Both of these procedures should be done by a pediatric surgeon.

■ THE NYHUS PROCEDURE (PREPERITONEAL APPROACH AND ILIOPUBIC TRACT REPAIR)

Fig. 4.60 is a diagrammatic representation of important anatomical structures of the posterior inguinal wall as seen from the preperitoneal approach. Fig. 4.61 is the same view demonstrating sites of groin hernias.

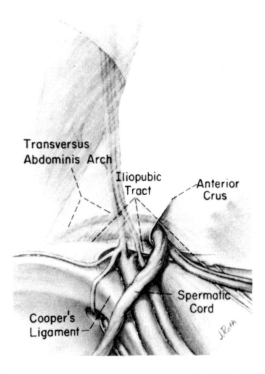

Figure 4.60. (By permission of LM Nyhus, The preperitoneal approach and iliopubic tract repair of inguinal hernia. In: Nyhus, LM, Condon, RL. *Hernia*. 3rd ed. Philadelphia: JB Lippincott, 1989.)

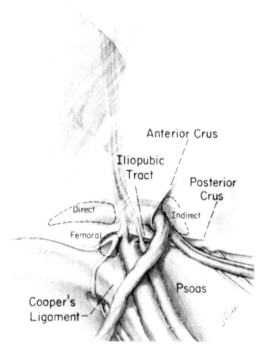

Figure 4.61. (By permission of LM Nyhus, The preperitoneal approach and iliopubic tract repair of inguinal hernia. In: Nyhus, LM, Condon, RL. *Hernia*. 3rd ed. Philadelphia: JB Lippincott, 1989.)

Fig. 4.62 shows the operative approach to the preperitoneal space. It is rarely necessary to ligate and sever the inferior epigastric artery and vein.

Nyhus Procedure, Iliopubic Tract Repair, Direct Inguinal Hernia

Procedure:

Step 1. Make a transverse skin incision two finger breadths above the symphysis pubis. (Some of the following description includes direct quotation from Dr. Nyhus).

Step 2. After the skin and subcutaneous tissues have been incised and the rectus sheath exposed, the level of the internal ring may be

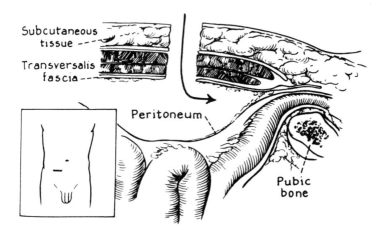

Figure 4.62. (By permission of LM Nyhus, The preperitoneal approach and iliopubic tract repair of inguinal hernia. In: Nyhus, LM, Condon, RL. *Hernia.* 3rd ed. Philadelphia: JB Lippincott, 1989.)

estimated by insertion of the left index finger into the external ring. This simple maneuver allows visualization of the location of the internal ring in the surgeon's mind's eye. The incision in the anterior rectus fascia should be placed so that it will pass just superior (cephalad) to the internal ring.

Step 3. Make a transverse fascial incision beginning over the midrectus of the affected side (Fig. 4.63).

Step 4. Enlarge the incision by separating and cutting the fascia and muscle fibers of the external oblique, internal oblique, and transversus abdominis muscles. The transversalis fascia is seen in the depth of the wound. When the transversalis fascia is cut, the preperitoneal space is entered and the proper plane of dissection is achieved.

Step 5. Isolate, but do not open, the sac and redundant peritoneum. Invert the sac, using a purse-string suture, if necessary. Suture the superior edge of the direct defect (transversalis fascia/transversus abdominis aponeurosis) above to the iliopubic tract below (Fig. 4.64).

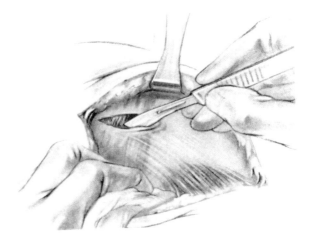

Figure 4.63. (By permission of LM Nyhus, The preperitoneal approach and iliopubic tract repair of inguinal hernia. In: Nyhus, LM, Condon, RL. *Hernia*. 3rd ed. Philadelphia: JB Lippincott, 1989.)

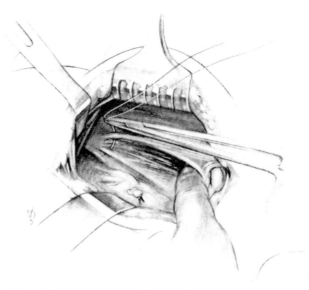

Figure 4.64. (By permission of LM Nyhus, The preperitoneal approach and iliopubic tract repair of inguinal hernia. In: Nyhus, LM, Condon, RL. *Hernia*. 3rd ed. Philadelphia: JB Lippincott, 1989.)

Nyhus Repair, Indirect Hernia

Procedure:

Step 1. The approach is the same as in direct hernia. Isolate, prepare, open, close, and excise the indirect sac.

Step 2. Close the defect medially by suturing the fused edge of the transversalis fascia and the transversus abdominis aponeurosis to the iliopubic tract. Also suture laterally, creating a new abdominal ring by suturing the anterior crus of the sling to the posterior crus (iliopubic tract). Use 00 silk.
The spermatic cord is resting in the area of the femoral vessels. Close the wound in layers with interrupted 0000 silk.

■ THE CONDON PROCEDURE (ANTERIOR ILIOPUBIC TRACT REPAIR)

Repair of Indirect Inguinal Hernia

Procedure:

Step 1. Reconstruct the posterior wall of the inguinal canal by suturing the transversus abdominis arch to the iliopubic tract from the pubic tubercle to the deep inguinal ring. Also suture lateral to the cord for reconstruction of the deep inguinal ring. Use 00 Dacron or nylon sutures.

Repair of Direct Inguinal Hernia

Procedure:

Step 1. Make an incision at the bulging posterior wall of the inguinal canal. Excise all redundant and weakened tissue.

Step 2. Place sutures between the transversus abdominis arch above and Cooper's ligament and the iliopubic tract below.

Step 3. Make a relaxing incision; use additional sutures if necessary (Fig. 4.65).

Step 4. Complete the relaxing incision. Tie the sutures that were placed previously.

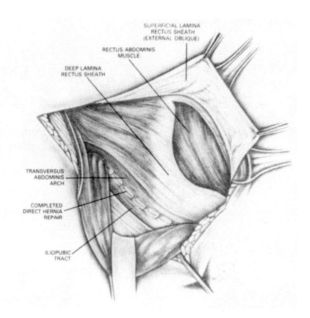

Figure 4.65. (By permission of RE Condon. Anterior iliopubic tract repair. In: Nyhus LM, Condon RL. *Hernia*, 3rd ed. Philadelphia: JB Lippincott, 1989.)

■ SHOULDICE TECHNIQUE

Procedure:

Steps 1-6. Follow steps 1-6 for indirect inguinal hernia repair (pp. 168-169).

Step 7. Incise the posterior wall of the inguinal canal from the internal ring, avoiding the deep epigastric vessels, and travel downward medially, ending at the pubic tubercle (Fig. 4.66).

Step 8. Elevate the narrower medial flap as much as possible, but do not elevate the lower lateral flap.

Step 9. Start the first suture line at the pubic bone. Use 000 continuous Prolene and approximate the deep part (white line) of the elevated medial flap to the free edge of the lateral flap. Tie the continuous suture at the internal ring, but do not cut (Fig. 4.67).

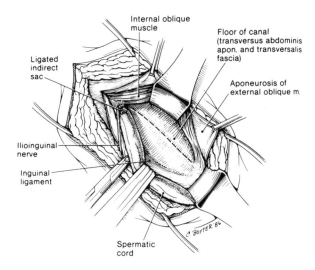

Figure 4.66. (By permission of JE Skandalakis, SW Gray, AR Mansberger, et al, *Hernia: Surgical Anatomy and Technique*, New York: McGraw-Hill, 1989.)

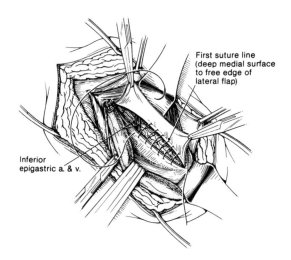

Figure 4.67. (By permission of JE Skandalakis, SW Gray, AR Mansberger, et al, *Hernia: Surgical Anatomy and Technique*, New York: McGraw-Hill, 1989.)

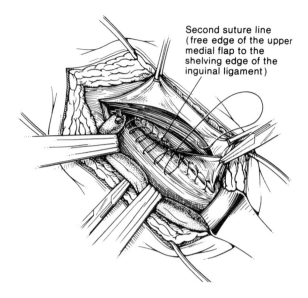

Second suture line
(free edge of the upper
medial flap to the
shelving edge of the
inguinal ligament)

Figure 4.68. (By permission of JE Skandalakis, SW Gray, AR Mansberger, et al, *Hernia: Surgical Anatomy and Technique*, New York: McGraw-Hill, 1989.)

Step 10. Using the same uncut suture, approximate the free edge of the medial flap in a continuous way to the shelving edge of the inguinal ligament, traveling downward from the internal ring to the pubic bone. Tie and cut the suture at the pubic bone (Fig. 4.68).

Step 11. Using 000 Prolene, start the third suture line at the internal ring, approximating the internal oblique and transversus arch and the conjoined area to the inguinal ligament. Tie the suture at the area of the pubic tubercle, but do not cut.

Step 12. Using the same suture, reapproximate the same anatomical entities as in step 11 from the pubic tubercle to the internal ring (Fig. 4.69).

Step 13. Close the external oblique aponeurosis above the spermatic cord. Occasionally, if there is too much tension, the aponeurosis is closed under the spermatic cord.

Step 14. Close the superficial fascia and skin as described previously.

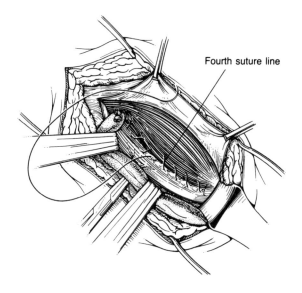

Fourth suture line

Figure 4.69. (By permission of JE Skandalakis, SW Gray, AR Mansberger, et al, *Hernia: Surgical Anatomy and Technique*, New York: McGraw-Hill, 1989.)

■ OTHER REPAIR PROCEDURES FOR INGUINAL HERNIA

The Use of Prosthesis

A sheet of Mersilene, Marlex mesh, or other synthetic prosthetic material is placed at the posterior wall of the inguinal canal and secured to the arch and conjoined area above and to the iliopubic tract and/or shelving edge of the inguinal ligament below with interrupted 0000 silk sutures.

Synthetic mesh also may be placed in intraperitoneal, preperitoneal, subaponeurotic, or subcutaneous locations as well.

■ RECURRENT INGUINAL AND FEMORAL HERNIA

A recurrent hernia is one that appears at the site of the initial operation with pathology identical to that for which repair was previously undertaken.

Procedure:

Step 1. Examine the inguinal area well.

Step 2. Try to understand the previous repair. Ask for the report of the repair or reread your own.

Step 3. Remove the skin scar.

Step 4. Carefully dissect to locate the spermatic cord in males. It is essential to locate, protect, and preserve the spermatic cord, thereby avoiding complications such as bleeding and possible atrophy or necrosis of the testis.

Step 5. The spermatic cord may be found

    a. under the skin and subcutaneous tissue

    b. under the aponeurosis of the external oblique muscle

    c. deep to the muscle layers in extremely rare cases

Step 6. Identify the inguinal ligament.

Step 7. Identify, if possible, the genital branch of the genitofemoral nerve, the ilioinguinal nerve, and the iliohypogastric nerve. To avoid neuroma, sacrifice the nerves if it is absolutely necessary.

Step 8. Palpate and locate the defect.

Step 9. Find the sac. In an indirect hernia, open the sac, perform a digital exploration, ligate the sac, and transfix it. In a direct or external supravesical hernia, if the sac is small, do not open it; instead, purse-string it. If the sac is large, incise it, and follow the steps of indirect or direct technique.

Step 10. Meticulously dissect the anatomical entities and strata involved by removing old sutures and scar tissue and by reaching good aponeurotic, not fascial, edges around the defect, if possible.

Step 11. Locate Cooper's ligament.

Step 12. Satisfy yourself that this is a recurrent hernia, not a new one.

Step 13. After you find the "good stuff," use whichever technique or modification will best restore the local distorted anatomy and personally satisfy you with the repair.

Step 14. The repair should be effected with no tension. If tension is anticipated, consider the use of a prosthesis, such as one or two layers of Marlex mesh; present philosophy advises prosthesis.

Here the surgeon should be familiar with the surgical ellipse. Unfortunately, in cases of recurrent hernia, some anatomical elements — such as the inguinal ligament, Cooper's ligament, or the iliopubic tract — are occasionally unidentifiable. Usually the superior medial (above) part of the ellipse is in better condition than the inferior lateral (lower) part. If the inguinal ligament, the iliopubic tract, or Cooper's ligament are unidentifiable, the prosthetic material can be anchored to the remnants of the conjoined area and the arch. The mesh should correspond to a line from the anterior superior iliac spine to the pubic tubercle, including, of course, the pectineal line. We believe, however, that in such a case the answer is the Stoppa procedure.

Step 15. If the patient is old or has had several procedures for recurrent hernia, do not hesitate to perform an orchiectomy. Removal, not severance, of the spermatic cord and testis will facilitate permanent closing of the internal ring.

■ LICHTENSTEIN'S TENSION-FREE HERNIORRHAPHY

In primary hernias, this procedure includes prosthetic implant without repair of the floor. For recurrent inguinal hernias and femoral hernias, it also includes a prosthetic plug.

To repair the primary hernia, suture the prosthesis with continuous 2–0 polypropylene suture, attaching it to the lacunar and inguinal ligaments and to the rectus sheath and the arch (Fig. 4.70).

For the repair of recurrent or femoral hernia, clean the defect, and dissect and invaginate the sac. Roll a strip of 10 × 2 cm polypropylene into a cylindrical plug and insert it into the defect until it fits snugly. Suture the plug to the edges of the defect with interrupted 2-0 polypropylene suture. If necessary to secure the plug, use more sutures (Fig. 4.71).

■ THE STOPPA PROCEDURE

This procedure uses the Giant Prosthetic Reinforcement of the Visceral Sac (GPRVS). The defect of the abdominal wall is not repaired, but it is reinforced with a large prosthesis placed in the properitoneal area (which is Bogros' space) that for all practical purposes, replaces or reinforces the endopelvic fascia.

The technique is essentially the same for unilateral and bilateral repair.

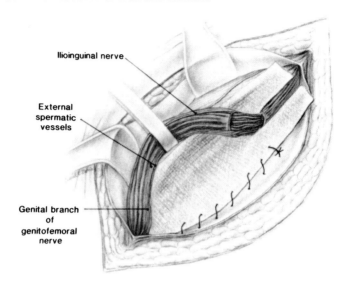

Figure 4.70. (By permission of PK Amid, AG Shulman, IL Lichtenstein, *Am J Surg* 165:369–371; 1993).

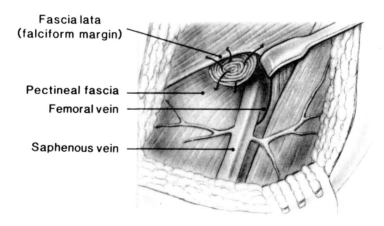

Figure 4.71. (Courtesy Dr. Irving L. Lichtenstein)

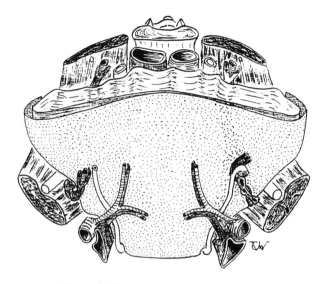

Figure 4.72. (Courtesy Dr. Rene F. Stoppa)

No sutures are used, but the intraabdominal pressure keeps the prosthesis in situ (Fig. 4.72).

■ THE GILBERT SUTURELESS MESH-PLUG REPAIR

Procedure:

Step 1. The indirect hernia sac is dissected and inverted into the abdominal ring.

Step 2. A folded conelike polypropylene mesh is inserted into the abdominal ring. Size the plug according to the diameter of the defect (Fig. 4.73).

Step 3. The floor of the inguinal canal is covered by another piece of flat polypropylene mesh. Superiorly, there is a slit in the mesh through which the spermatic cord exits laterally (Fig. 4.74).

Step 4. Dr. Gilbert does not use any sutures, but we prefer to secure the plug with two or three sutures and the flat mesh with several interrupted sutures medially and laterally.

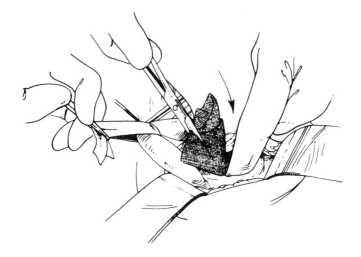

Figure 4.73. (Courtesy Dr. Arthur I. Gilbert and Hernia Institute of Florida)

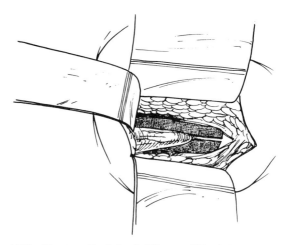

Figure 4.74. (Courtesy Dr. Arthur I. Gilbert and Hernia Institute of Florida)

■ HYDROCELE

A hydrocele is a collection of abnormal fluid within the sac of the tunica vaginalis. It may be associated with a hernia. There are several varieties.

If the hydrocele changes in size (as determined by patient observation), it is a communicating hydrocele and requires a high ligation of the sac in addition to partial excision of the hydrocele.

Repair of Adult Noncommunicating Hydrocele

Procedure:

Step 1. Make a transverse incision in the scrotum. The terminal vascular branches in the scrotum lie transversely; therefore, to minimize bleeding, a transverse incision is recommended for exploration.

Step 2. Carefully divide the three uppermost layers of the testis. Deliver the testis with its covering outside the scrotum.

Step 3. Withdraw the fluid from the sac and observe the spermatic cord (Fig. 4.75).

Step 4. Observe the covering of the spermatic cord.

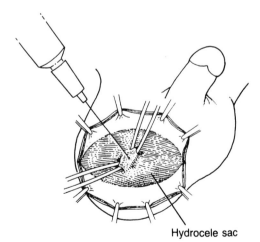

Hydrocele sac

Figure 4.75. (By permission of JE Skandalakis, SW Gray, AR Mansberger, et al, *Hernia: Surgical Anatomy and Technique*, New York: McGraw-Hill, 1989.)

Step 5. Open the tunica vaginalis and perform a subtotal or total removal of the sac.

Step 6. Approximate the dartos muscle and close the skin. Use only a few catgut sutures for the approximation, thereby avoiding skin inversion due to dartos retraction.

Repair of Pediatric Hydrocele—Inguinal Approach

This procedure should be done by a pediatric surgeon.

■ POSTERIOR (LUMBAR) BODY WALL

Surgical Anatomy of the Posterior (Lumbar) Body Wall

The lumbar area of the posterior body wall is bounded:

- superiorly: by the 12th rib
- interiorly: by the crest of the ilium
- posteriorly: by the erector spinae (sacrospinalis) muscles
- anteriorly: by the posterior border of the external oblique muscle

In this area, the body wall is composed of the following layers of muscle and fascia:

1. Thick, tough skin
2. Superficial fascia: two layers of fibrous tissue with fat between them
3. A superficial muscle layer composed of the latissimus dorsi muscle posterolaterally and the external oblique muscle anterolaterally
4. Thoracolumbar fascia containing three layers: posterior, middle, and anterior. The posterior and middle layers envelop the sacrospinalis muscle, and the middle anterior layer envelops the quadratus lumborum. Another characteristic of the middle layer of the thoracolumbar fascia is its lateral continuation to the transversus abdominis aponeurosis by fusion of all three layers. Therefore, the transversus abdominis aponeurosis should be accepted on faith as part of the thoracolumbar fascia.
5. A middle muscular layer of the sacrospinalis, internal oblique, and serratus posterior inferior muscles
6. The deep muscular layer, composed of the quadratus lumborum and psoas muscles
7. Transversalis fascia
8. Preperitoneal fat
9. Peritoneum

Within this area, two triangles may be described: the superior lumbar triangle (Grynfeltt's) and the inferior lumbar triangle (Petit's).

The base of the superior lumbar triangle is the 12th rib and the serratus posterior inferior muscle. The anterior (abdominal) boundary is the posterior border of the internal oblique muscle; the posterior (lumbar) boundary is the anterior border of the sacrospinalis muscle. The floor of the triangle is formed by the aponeurosis of the transversus abdominis muscle arising by fusion of the layers of the thoracolumbar fascia. The roof of the triangle is formed by the external oblique and latissimus dorsi muscles.

The base of the inferior lumbar triangle is the iliac crest. The anterior (abdominal) boundary is the posterior border of the external oblique muscle. The posterior (lumbar) boundary is the anterior border of the latissimus dorsi muscle. The floor of the triangle is formed by the internal oblique muscle with contributions from the transversus abdominis muscle and the posterior lamina of the thoracolumbar fascia. The triangle is covered by superficial fascia and skin.

The two triangles may be compared as follows:

Superior Triangle	Inferior Triangle
Inverted triangle (apex down)	Upright triangle (apex up)
Larger	Smaller
More constant	Less constant
Most common site of lumbar hernia	Less common site of lumbar hernia
12th thoracic nerve	No nerves
1st lumbar nerve	No nerves
Avascular	More vascular
Covered by latissimus dorsi muscle	Covered by superficial fascia and skin
Floor: union of the layers of the thoracolumbar fascia to form the aponeurosis of the transversus abdominis	Floor: thoracolumbar fascia, internal oblique muscle, and (partially) transversus abdominis muscle

Lumbar Hernia (Fig. 4.76)

Hernia through the Superior Lumbar Triangle

BOUNDARIES: If the hernia is small, the hernia ring is formed by the aponeurosis of the transversus abdominis only; if it is large, it may

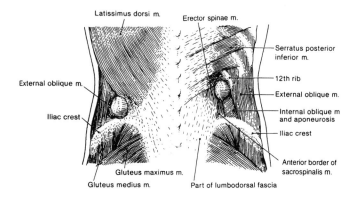

Figure 4.76. Left: An inferior hernia through Petit's triangle. The base of the triangle is formed by the iliac crest. Right: A superior hernia through Grynfeltt's triangle. The base of the inverted triangle is formed by the 12th rib. (By permission of JE Skandalakis, SW Gray, AR Mansberger, et al, *Hernia: Surgical Anatomy and Technique*, New York: McGraw-Hill, 1989.)

occupy the entire superior triangle. It may be necessary to enlarge the ring by a medial or lateral incision, or both, midway between the 12th rib and the crest of the ilium.

Hernia through the Inferior Lumbar Triangle

BOUNDARIES: If the hernia is small, the ring is formed by the thoracolumbar fascia and fibers of the internal oblique muscle. If it is larger, the ring may include the boundaries of the whole inferior triangle. Enlargement of the ring is by section of the fascia.

Repair of Lumbar Hernia (Dowd-Ponka Repair)

Procedure:

Step 1. Make an incision, oblique or vertical, over the hernia site. Remember that in the upper hernia, the sac lies beneath skin, superficial fascia, and latissimus dorsi muscle; in the lower hernia, there is no layer of muscle (Fig. 4.77).

Step 2. Using 000 silk, ligate the hernia sac, if present, and replace it in the abdomen. If a large lipoma is present, a purse-string suture or several interrupted sutures will keep the fat "down."

Step 3. Place a Marlex or Prolene patch over the defect, and suture to the external oblique and latissimus dorsi muscles and lumbar periosteum using 000 interrupted Surgilon (Fig. 4.78).

Incisions:

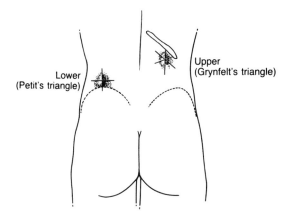

Figure 4.77. (By permission of JE Skandalakis, SW Gray, AR Mansberger, et al, *Hernia: Surgical Anatomy and Technique*, New York: McGraw-Hill, 1989.)

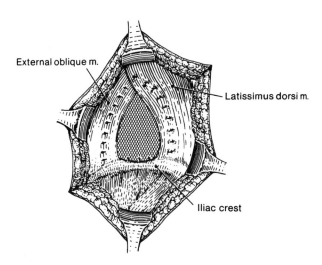

Figure 4.78. (By permission of JE Skandalakis, SW Gray, AR Mansberger, et al, *Hernia: Surgical Anatomy and Technique*, New York: McGraw-Hill, 1989.)

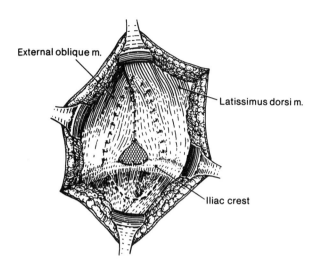

Figure 4.79. (By permission of JE Skandalakis, SW Gray, AR Mansberger, et al, *Hernia: Surgical Anatomy and Technique*, New York: McGraw-Hill, 1989.)

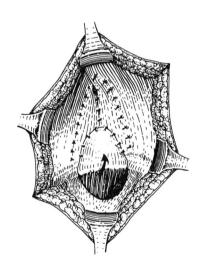

Figure 4.80. (By permission of JE Skandalakis, SW Gray, AR Mansberger, et al, *Hernia: Surgical Anatomy and Technique*, New York: McGraw-Hill, 1989.)

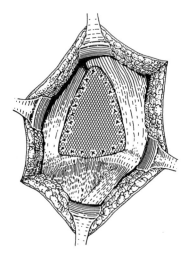

Figure 4.81. (By permission of JE Skandalakis, SW Gray, AR Mansberger, et al, *Hernia: Surgical Anatomy and Technique*, New York: McGraw-Hill, 1989.)

Step 4. Approximate the external oblique and latissimus dorsi muscles over the patch as far as possible without tension. Cut a flap of gluteal fascia, as shown by the dotted line in Fig. 4.79.

Step 5. Use the flap of gluteal fascia turned up to cover the defect remaining, and secure it to the present muscles with 000 Surgilon interrupted sutures. A large hernial ring may require a second layer of mesh sutured to the muscles (Figs. 4.80 and 4.81, Fig. 4.31).

Step 6. Close the subcutaneous fat and skin. Jackson-Pratt drains may be necessary.

5

Diaphragm

ANATOMY

The diaphragm is a musculomembranous entity separating the thorax from the abdomen. The muscular part originates anteriorly from the xiphoid process, laterally from the inner surface of the six lower cartilages, and posteriorly from the medial and lateral lumbosacral arches, the median arcuate ligament, and the bodies of the three upper lumbar vertebrae. The muscular part inserts on the central tendon.

■ THE CRURA

The crura arise from the anterior surface of the 1st to the 4th lumbar vertebrae on the right, and the first two or three lumbar vertebrae on the left. The crural fibers pass superiorly and anteriorly, forming the muscular arms that surround the openings for the aorta and the esophagus; they insert on the central tendon. At their origin on the vertebrae, the crura are tendinous, becoming increasingly muscular as they ascend into the diaphragm proper (Fig. 5.1). Posteriorly and medially, the crura also are tendinous; sutures to approximate the crura should always be placed through the tendinous portions.

The pattern of the crural arms at the esophageal hiatus is variable. In one-half or more, both right and left arms arise from the right crus (Fig. 5.2A). In one-third or more, the left arm arises from the right crus and the right arm arises from both crura (Fig. 5.2B). In the remaining, a variety of uncommon patterns is present. Hiatus hernia is not associated with any specific hiatal pattern.

205

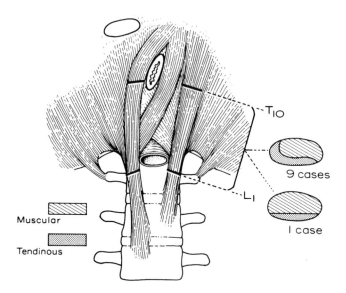

Figure 5.1. The crura consist of both tendinous and muscular tissue; only the tendinous portion holds sutures. In 9 out of 10 persons, the medial edge of the crura is tendinous. (By permission of SW Gray, JS Rowe, and JE Skandalakis, *Am Surg* 45(9):575–587, 1979.)

■ OPENINGS OF THE DIAPHRAGM

Hiatus of the Inferior Vena Cava

The hiatus of the inferior vena cava lies in the right part of the central tendon about 2.5 cm to the right of the midline and at the level of the 8th thoracic vertebra. The margins of the hiatus are fixed to the vena cava, which is accompanied by branches of the right phrenic nerve (Fig. 5.3).

Esophageal Hiatus

The elliptical esophageal hiatus is in the muscular portion of the diaphragm 2.5 cm or less to the left of the midline at the level of the 10th thoracic vertebra (Figs. 5.4 and 5.5). The anterior and lateral margins of

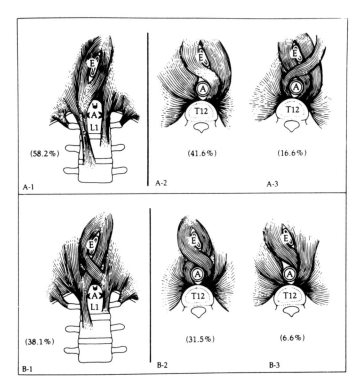

Figure 5.2. The most common pattern of the diaphragmatic crura. (A-1) and (B-1) seen from below. (A-2, A-3) and (B-2, B-3) seen from above. E = esophagus; A = aorta. (By permission of JE Skandalakis, SW Gray, JS Rowe, et al. In: Nyhus LM, Baker RJ. *Mastery of Surgery*, 2nd ed. Boston: Little, Brown, 1992, pp 377–396.)

the hiatus are formed by the muscular arms of the diaphragmatic crura, and the posterior margin is formed by the median arcuate ligament (Fig. 5.6). The anterior and posterior vagal trunks and the esophageal arteries and veins from the left gastric vessels pass through the hiatus with the esophagus.

Composition and Configuration of the Hiatal Ring

Regardless of its components, the normal hiatus should admit one or two of the surgeon's fingers if there is no folding of the peritoneum into the mediastinum.

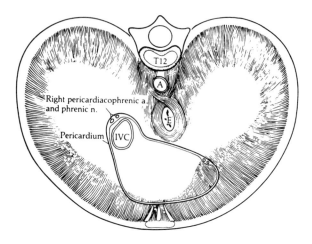

Figure 5.3. The diaphragm viewed from above. The area in contact with the pericardium is indicated. The pericardial fibrous tissue is continuous with that of the diaphragm. (By permission of JE Skandalakis, SW Gray, JS Rowe, et al. In: Nyhus, LM, Baker, RJ. *Mastery of Surgery*, 2nd ed. Boston: Little, Brown, 1992, pp 377–396.)

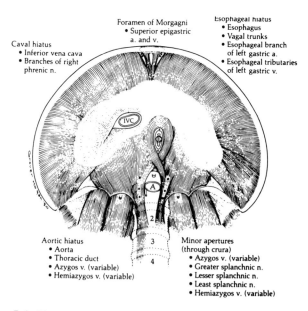

Figure 5.4. The apertures of the diaphragm seen from below and the structures traversing them. (By permission of JE Skandalakis, SW Gray, JS Rowe, et al. In: Nyhus, LM, Baker, RJ. *Mastery of Surgery*. 2nd ed. Boston: Little, Brown, 1992, pp 377–396.)

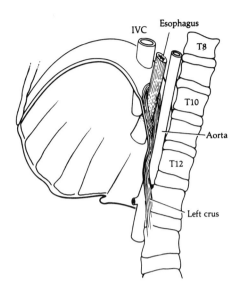

Figure 5.5. The diaphragmatic openings for the inferior vena cava (IVC), the esophagus, and the aorta as seen from the left. (By permission of JE Skandalakis, SW Gray, JS Rowe, et al. In: Nyhus, LM, Baker, RJ. *Mastery of Surgery*, 2nd ed. Boston: Little, Brown, 1992, pp 377–396.)

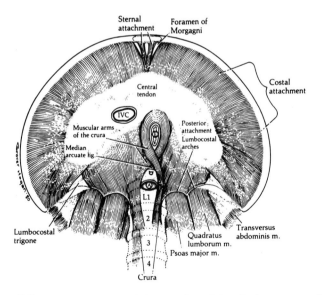

Figure 5.6. The attachments of the muscles of the diaphragm seen from below. (By permission of JE Skandalakis, SW Gray, JS Rowe, et al. In: Nyhus, LM, Baker, RJ. *Mastery of Surgery*, 2nd ed. Boston: Little, Brown, 1992, pp 377–396.)

The following means of narrowing the hiatus have been preferred:

1. Vertical posterior approximation of the crura (Fig. 5.7A). This is a commonly used method.

2. Vertical anterior approximation of the crura (Fig. 5.7B). Some surgeons recommend this type of repair. It has the following advantages: (a) it is easier than posterior approximation; (b) the crura are more tendinous anteriorly; and (c) the procedure accentuates the gastroesophageal angle.

3. Horizontal narrowing of the hiatus (Fig. 5.7C). In some patients, a transverse defect is apparent; hence a horizontal approximation is appropriate.

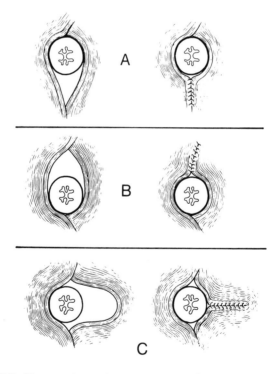

Figure 5.7. Three methods of narrowing the esophageal hiatus: (A) vertical with posterior approximation of the crura; (B) vertical with anterior approximation of the crura; (C) horizontal with shortening of one crus. (By permission of JE Skandalakis, SW Gray, and JR Rowe Jr. *Anatomical Complications in General Surgery*, New York: McGraw-Hill, 1983.)

The Aortic Opening

The oblique course of the aorta takes it behind the diaphragm rather than through it (Fig. 5.5). At the level of the 12th thoracic vertebra, the anterior border of the opening is the median arcuate ligament; laterally the diaphragmatic crura form its margins. The thoracic duct and sometimes the azygos vein accompany the aorta.

Other Openings in the Diaphragm

Anteriorly, the superior epigastric vessels pass through the parasternal spaces (foramina of Morgagni). In the dome of the diaphragm, the phrenic nerves pierce the upper surface to become distributed over the lower surface between the muscle and the peritoneum.

The azygos vein may pass behind the diaphragm with the aorta, to the right of the right crus, or it may pierce the right crus. Also passing through the crura are the greater, lesser, and least splanchnic nerves (Fig. 5.4).

The Median Arcuate Ligament

The esophageal hiatus is separated from the aortic hiatus by fusion of the arms of the left and right crura. If the tendinous portions of the crura are fused, the median arcuate ligament is present as a fibrous arch passing over the aorta, connecting the right and left crura. If the fusion is muscular only, the ligament is ill-defined or absent.

The median arcuate ligament passes in front of the aorta at the level of the 1st lumbar vertebra just above the origin of the celiac trunk (Fig. 5.6). In 16 percent, a low median arcuate ligament covers the celiac artery and may compress it.

In about 50 percent of the population, the ligament is sufficiently well developed to use in surgical repair of the esophageal hiatus. In the remainder, there is enough preaortic fascia lateral to the celiac trunk to perform a posterior fixation of the gastroesophageal junction. The celiac ganglion, just below the arcuate ligament, must be avoided.

■ DIAPHRAGMATIC–MEDIASTINAL RELATIONS

Over much of the anterosuperior surface of the diaphragm, the fibrous tissue of the central tendon is continuous with the fibrous pericardium (Fig. 5.3).

In addition to the pericardium, the mediastinum on the right contains the inferior vena cava, the right phrenic nerve, the right pulmonary ligament, the esophagus with the right vagal trunk, the azygos vein, the vertebral bodies, and the right sympathetic trunk (Fig. 5.8).

In the left mediastinum are the pericardium, the left phrenic nerve, the esophagus, the left vagal trunk, the descending aorta, the vertebral bodies, and the left sympathetic trunk. The triangle (of Truesdale) formed by the pericardium, aorta, and diaphragm contains the left pulmonary ligament and the distal esophagus. In sliding hiatus hernia, the stomach is in this triangle (Fig. 5.9).

The remainder of the superior surface of the diaphragm is covered with parietal pleura. The approximation of the right and left pleurae between the esophagus and the aorta forms the so-called mesoesophagus. The right pleura is in contact with the lower third of the esophagus almost down to the esophageal hiatus (Fig. 5.10). This creates the risk of accidental entrance into the pleural cavity during abdominal operations on the esophageal hiatus. In spite of this proximity of the right pleura, the surgeon, working on the right side of the operation table, is more likely to produce a pneumothorax or hemopneumothorax on the left.

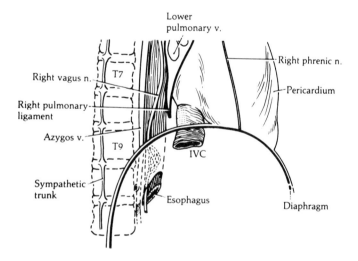

Figure 5.8. Structures in the inferior portion of the right mediastinum. (By permission of JE Skandalakis, SW Gray, JS Rowe, et al. In: Nyhus, LM, Baker, RJ. *Mastery of Surgery*, 2nd ed. Boston: Little, Brown, 1992, pp 377–396.)

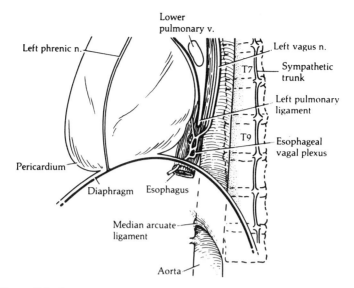

Figure 5.9. Structures in the inferior portion of the left mediastinum. (By permission of JE Skandalakis, SW Gray, JS Rowe, et al. In: Nyhus, LM, Baker, RJ. *Mastery of Surgery*. 2nd ed. Boston: Little, Brown, 1992, pp 377–396.)

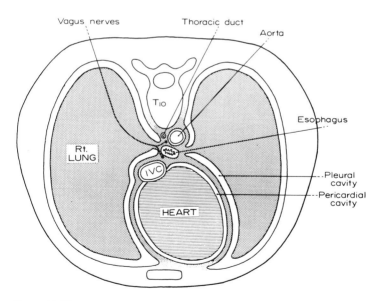

Figure 5.10. Cross section through the thorax at the level of T_{10} showing the relation of the pleura to the distal esophagus. (By permission of SW Gray, JS Rowe, and JE Skandalakis, *Am Surg* 45(9):575–587, 1979.)

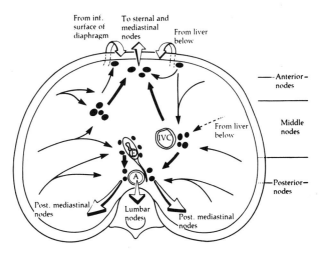

Figure 5.13. Lymphatic drainage of the diaphragm seen from above. The diaphragm receives lymph from the liver below and sends it to ascending sternal, anterior, and posterior mediastinal nodes. (By permission of JE Skandalakis, SW Gray, JS Rowe, et al. In: Nyhus, LM, Baker, RJ. *Mastery of Surgery*, 2nd ed. Boston: Little, Brown, 1992, pp 377–396.)

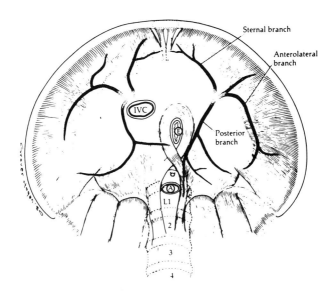

Figure 5.14. The major branches of the phrenic nerves from below. Each phrenic nerve divides just before entering the diaphragm from above. (By permission of JE Skandalakis, SW Gray, JS Rowe, et al. In: Nyhus, LM, Baker, RJ. *Mastery of Surgery*, 2nd ed. Boston: Little, Brown, 1992, pp 377–396.)

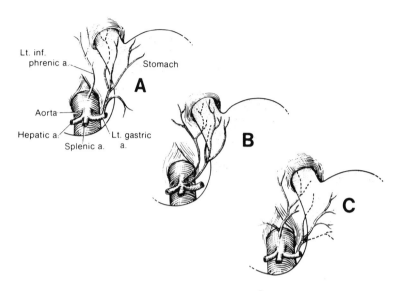

Figure 5.15. Variations in the blood supply to the distal esophagus and the esophageal hiatus. (A) The inferior phrenic artery supplies the margin of the hiatus. An esophageal branch of the left gastric artery supplies the esophagus and anastomoses with the thoracic esophageal arteries. This is the most frequent pattern. (B) The esophagus is supplied by esophageal branches of the left gastric and the inferior phrenic arteries without cranial anastomoses. (C) The esophagus is supplied entirely by a branch of the inferior phrenic artery, which anastomoses with the thoracic esophageal arteries. This pattern is rare. (By permission of JE Skandalakis, SW Gray, and JR Rowe Jr. *Anatomical Complications in General Surgery*, New York: McGraw-Hill, 1983.)

■ NERVE SUPPLY TO THE DIAPHRAGM

The right phrenic nerve enters the diaphragm through the central tendon just lateral to the opening for the inferior vena cava. Occasionally it passes through that opening with the vena cava. The left phrenic nerve pierces the superior surface of the muscular portion of the diaphragm just lateral to the left border of the heart (Fig. 5.14).

The peripheral portions of the pleura and peritoneum have an independent sensory innervation that arises from the 7th to the 12th intercostal nerves.

■ STRUCTURES AT OR NEAR THE ESOPHAGEAL HIATUS (Fig. 5.15)

A number of structures lie close to the esophageal hiatus of the diaphragm and hence may be injured in surgical procedures on the hiatus. They are:

- left inferior phrenic artery and left gastric artery
- left inferior phrenic vein
- left gastric (coronary) vein
- aberrant left hepatic artery, if present
- other vessels (celiac trunk, aorta, inferior vena cava)
- vagal trunks (Fig. 5.16)
- celiac ganglia
- thoracic duct
- subphrenic spaces
- lower esophagus

Extensive mobilization or skeletonization of the lower esophagus may result in perforation during a surgical procedure, or afterward, from subsequent local ischemia.

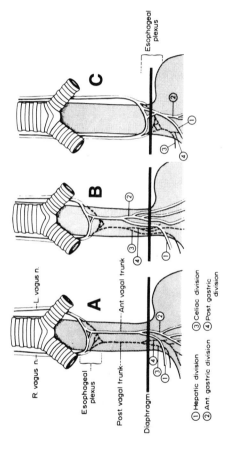

Figure 5.16. Where four or more vagal structures emerge through the hiatus, they may be (A) divisions that have separated just above the diaphragm, (B) divisions and their branches that arise above the diaphragm, or (C) elements of the esophageal plexus that extend below the diaphragm. The vagal trunks are entirely within the abdomen. (By permission of JE Skandalakis, JS Rowe, SW Gray, et al., *Surg* 75(2):233–237, 1974.)

TECHNIQUE

■ DIAPHRAGMATIC HERNIA

Hiatus hernia is a protrusion of a portion of the stomach into the thoracic mediastinum through the esophageal hiatus of the diaphragm. It includes a hernial sac (Table 5.1).

Five types of hernia are recognized today: sliding hiatus, paraesophageal hiatus, combined sliding and paraesophageal, congenital short esophagus, and traumatic diaphragmatic.

In sliding hiatus hernia, the esophagus moves freely through the hiatus, with the gastroesophageal junction in the thorax or in the normal position at different times. Sliding hernias make up 90 percent of all hiatus hernias (Fig. 5.17B). A sac is present.

An uncommon type of sliding hernia is one that becomes secondarily fixed in the thorax by adhesions. The esophagus in such patients appears to be too short to reach the diaphragm because of contraction of the longitudinal muscle coat.

In paraesophageal hiatus hernia, the gastroesophageal junction remains in its normal location. The gastric fundus cardia and greater curvature bulge through the hiatus beside the esophagus; a sac is present. Volvulus of the herniated stomach is a major complication (Fig. 5.17C).

A combined sliding and paraesophageal hernia occurs when the gastroesophageal junction is displaced upwards, as in a sliding hernia, and the fundus and greater curvature are herniated, as in a paraesophageal hernia (Fig. 5.17D).

Much debate centers around the classification of the congenital short esophagus. Three conditions must be considered. (1) In the *grossly normal esophagus*, the lower portion of the esophagus is lined by gastric mucosa (Barrett esophagus). This may be described also as heterotopic gastric mucosa. (2) In the *irreducible partially supradiaphragmatic true stomach*, the stomach has herniated into the thorax through an enlarged diaphragmatic esophageal hiatus and become fixed. This is true fixed hiatus hernia. (3) *Partially supradiaphragmatic true stomach* exists from birth and is not reducible. This is true "congenital short esophagus" (Fig. 5.17E) and is very rare.

When performing surgery for esophageal hernia, **remember** to:

✓ Avoid injury to the vagus nerves.

✓ Avoid injury to the mediastinal pleura.

✓ Avoid injury to the left hepatic vein.

✓ Avoid perforation of the esophagus.

Table 5.1 Hernia through the Esophageal Hiatus

Hernia	Anatomy	Sac and contents	Remarks
Sliding hiatus hernia Fixed hiatus hernia	Congenital potential hernia. G-E junction and cardia are displaced upwards to enter the mediastinum above the diaphragm. The phrenoesophageal membrane is attenuated. The herniated stomach may move freely or become fixed in the thorax.	Sac lies anterior and to the left of herniated stomach. Contents: cardia, stomach.	A large hiatus (admitting three fingers) may be a predisposing factor. Actual herniation usually occurs in middle life but has been seen in newborn.
"Pure" paraesophageal hernia	Congenital potential hernia. The G-E junction and cardia are in normal position. The fundus has herniated through the hiatus into the thorax beside the esophagus.	Sac lies anterior to esophagus and posterior to pericardium. Contents: cardia and fundus of stomach.	An enlarged hiatus may be a predisposing factor. Actual herniation occurs in adult life.
Combined sliding and paraesophageal hernia	Congenital potential hernia. The G-E junction, cardia and much of the greater curvature of stomach have herniated into the thorax.	Sac lies anterior to esophagus and posterior to pericardium in right posteroinferior mediastinum. Sac may contain fundus and body of stomach, omentum, transverse colon, spleen.	A hiatus already enlarged by a hiatus hernia. Progresses to complete thoracic stomach with volvulus.
Congenital short esophagus	Congenital hernia. The G-E junction and cardia are displaced upwards and fixed in the thorax.	No sac present.	This lesion is rare. It appears to result from failure of the embryonic esophagus to elongate enough to bring the G-E junction into the abdomen.

(By permission of SW Gray, LJ Skandalakis, and JE Skandalakis. Classification of hernias through the esophageal hiatus. In: Jamieson, GG (ed.) *Surgery of the Esophagus.* Edinburgh: Churchill Livingstone, 1988, pp. 143–148.)

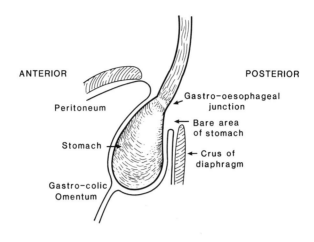

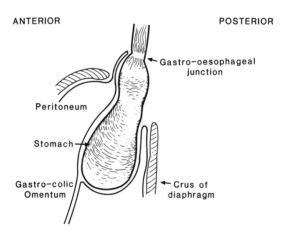

Figure 5.17. Esophageal hiatus in sagittal section with (a) normal anatomy and (b–e) the various abnormalities described in the text: (b) sliding hiatus hernia, (c) paraesophageal hiatus hernia, (d) combined sliding and paraesophageal hiatus hernia, (e) congenital short esophagus. (By permission SW Gray, LJ Skandalakis and JE Skandalakis. In: Jamieson, GG (ed). *Surgery of the Esophagus*. Edinburgh: Churchill Livingstone, 1988, pp 143–148.)

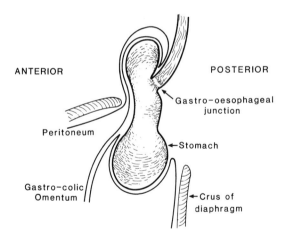

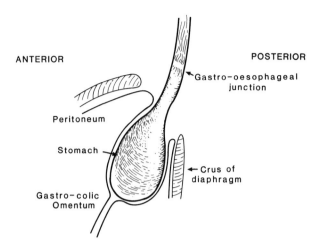

ANTERIOR

POSTERIOR

Gastro-oesophageal
junction

Peritoneum

Stomach

Crus of
diaphragm

Gastro-colic
Omentum

Figure 5.17 Continued.

✓ Avoid perforation of the esophagus.

✓ Watch for an aberrant blood supply to the left triangular ligament.

✓ Watch for accessory bile ducts.

✓ Consider inserting a bougie.

✓ Consider the necessity of gastropexy or gastrostomy.

✓ Consider the necessity of an antireflux procedure.

Note: Congenital diaphragmatic hernias such as Morgagni's and Bochdalek's should be repaired by a pediatric surgeon.

Repair of Sliding Hiatus Hernia

Procedure:

Step 1. A transverse, oblique, or vertical midline incision may be used. Incise the triangular ligament and retract the left lobe of the liver. Incise the peritoneal coverings of the esophagus; then pass a Penrose drain beneath the esophagus for traction.

Step 2. Dissect the greater curvature of the stomach, beginning at the cardia and continuing toward the gastrosplenic ligament and the vasa brevia. One or two vasa brevia may be divided, but damage to the spleen must be avoided (Fig. 5.18).

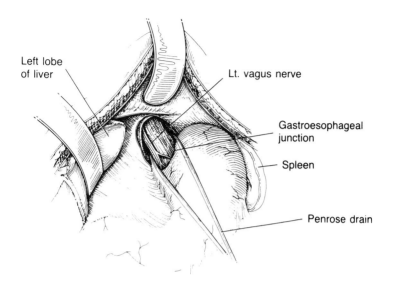

Figure 5.18. (By permission of JE Skandalakis, SW Gray, AR Mansberger, et al, *Hernia: Surgical Anatomy and Technique*, New York: McGraw-Hill, 1989.)

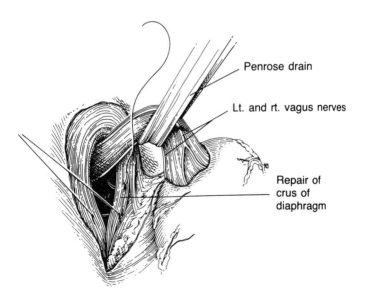

Figure 5.19. (By permission of JE Skandalakis, SW Gray, AR Mansberger, et al, *Hernia: Surgical Anatomy and Technique*, New York: McGraw-Hill, 1989.)

Step 3. Dissect the diaphragm and the tissue beneath the esophagus. At this stage, a widened hiatus can be repaired with 0 Surgilon sutures, carefully avoiding the underlying aorta, celiac axis, and pleura. Do not constrict the esophagus (Fig. 5.19).

Step 4. Nissen Fundoplication. The anesthesiologist passes a No. 50 French dilator into the esophagus to prevent constriction by an excessively tight fundic wrap.

Remember:

✓ Avoid the gas-bloat syndrome by protecting the vagus nerve and maintaining an adequate lumen in the distal esophagus.

✓ If the vagus nerve is transected, do a pyloroplasty.

✓ If the pylorus is stenotic, pyloroplasty is again recommended.

✓ If chronic peptic ulcer disease (duodenal ulcer) is present, vagotomy and pyloroplasty should be performed.

✓ It is nearly impossible to make a Nissen fundoplication too loose, and very easy to make it too tight, so err to the former.

Step 5. Wrap the fundus of the stomach 360 degrees around the lower esophagus, and insert 00 silk sutures from the stomach to the esophagus to the stomach (Fig. 5.20).

Step 6. Place at least four sutures to complete the wrap and place collar sutures between the wrap and the esophagus (at the upper portion) and between the wrap and the stomach (at the lower portion) (Fig. 5.21).

Step 7. Perform a Stamm gastrostomy and close the abdominal wall.

Note: When the wrap is completed and prior to placing the lower collar suture, the surgeon should be able to place one finger between the wrap and the anterior esophageal area (see Fig. 5.27).

Repair of Paraesophageal Hernia

Precedure:

Step 1. Open the abdomen as for sliding hiatus hernia. Incise the left triangular ligament of the liver.

Step 2. Reduce the stomach and esophagus into the abdomen (Fig. 5.22).

Step 3. Open the hernia sac and expose the esophagus. Protect the anterior vagal trunk, and excise the sac (Fig. 5.23).

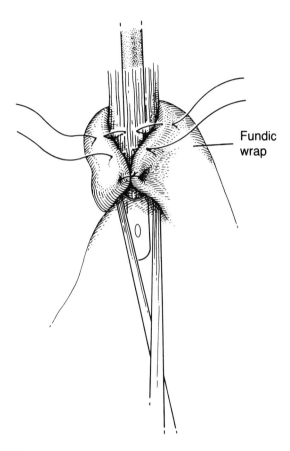

Figure 5.20. (By permission of JE Skandalakis, SW Gray, AR Mansberger, et al, *Hernia: Surgical Anatomy and Technique*, New York: McGraw-Hill, 1989.)

Step 4. Perform anterior approximation of the crura with interrupted 0 Surgilon sutures (Fig. 5.24). Alternatively, perform posterior approximation of the crura. Occasionally the lesser curvature of the stomach is sutured to the left crus posteriorly with interrupted 00 silk sutures. The diaphragm should admit one finger between it and the esophagus (Figs. 5.25–5.27).

Step 5. The fundus of the stomach may be sutured to the undersurface of the diaphragm with 000 silk to add stability to the anatomical repair (Fig. 5.26).

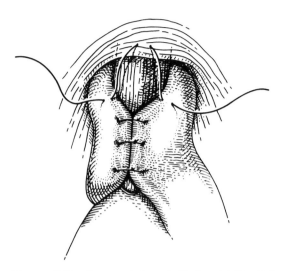

Figure 5.21. (By permission of JE Skandalakis, SW Gray, AR Mansberger, et al, *Hernia: Surgical Anatomy and Technique*, New York: McGraw-Hill, 1989.)

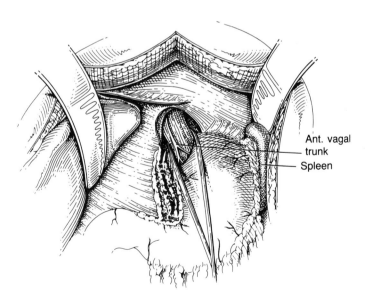

Ant. vagal
trunk
Spleen

Figure 5.22. (By permission of JE Skandalakis, SW Gray, AR Mansberger, et al, *Hernia: Surgical Anatomy and Technique*, New York: Mc-Graw-Hill, 1989.)

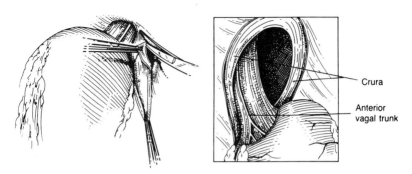

Figure 5.23. (By permission of JE Skandalakis, SW Gray, AR Mansberger, et al, *Hernia: Surgical Anatomy and Technique*, New York: McGraw-Hill, 1989.)

Step 6. A fundic wrap (see Nissen Fundoplication, step 4 of Repair of Sliding Hiatus Hernia, p. 226) may be added to the repair in those unusual instances where a mixed paraesophageal hernia with reflux is present (Fig. 5.27).

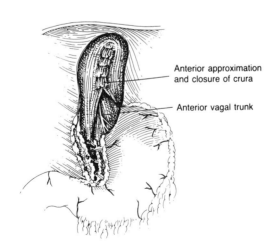

Figure 5.24. (By permission of JE Skandalakis, SW Gray, AR Mansberger, et al, *Hernia: Surgical Anatomy and Technique*, New York: McGraw-Hill, 1989.)

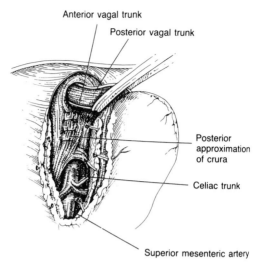

Figure 5.25. (By permission of JE Skandalakis, SW Gray, AR Mansberger, et al, *Hernia: Surgical Anatomy and Technique*, New York: McGraw-Hill, 1989.)

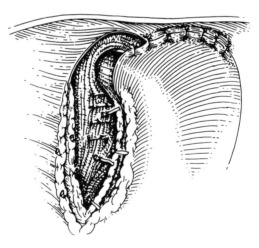

Figure 5.26. (By permission of JE Skandalakis, SW Gray, AR Mansberger, et al, *Hernia: Surgical Anatomy and Technique*, New York: McGraw-Hill, 1989.)

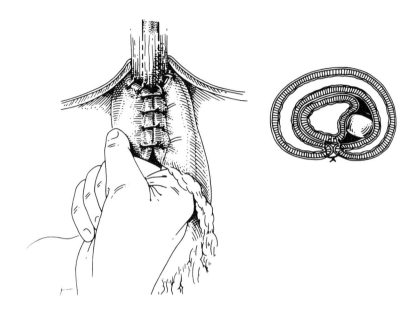

ə 5.27. (By permission of JE Skandalakis, SW Gray, AR Mansberger, et
ˈnia: *Surgical Anatomy and Technique*, New York: McGraw-Hill, 1989.)

Repair of Traumatic Diaphragmatic Hernia

Procedure:

Step 1. Explore the abdomen through an upper midline incision.

Step 2. Identify the defect and determine its extent. Inspect the intestines and other organs in the abdominal cavity for injury.

Step 3. Approximate the edges of the diaphragm with interrupted 0 Surgilon or Mersilene sutures.

Step 4. Insert a chest tube.

6

Esophagus

ANATOMY

■ GENERAL DESCRIPTION OF THE ESOPHAGUS

Length of the Esophagus

The esophagus is about 25 cm in length. The most useful reference point is the upper incisors, which are about 15 cm above the pharyngoesophageal junction; if the external nares are included, 2–3 cm must be added. In defining the esophagus, it is adequate to divide it into cervical, thoracic, and abdominal segments.

Constrictions of the Esophagus

Major Constrictions

There are three major constrictions:

1. The cricopharyngeal or pharyngoesophageal constriction (diameters 1.7 × 2.3 cm).

2. The bronchoaortic constriction. Anatomically there are two separate constrictions: the aortic at the level of T_4 with diameters of 1.9 × 2.3 cm, and the bronchial at the level of T_5 with diameters of 1.7 × 2.3 cm.

3. The diaphragmatic constriction at the level of T_9 or T_{10} with a diameter of 2.3 cm.

These constrictions define two regions of dilatation: superior (between the cricopharyngeal and bronchoaortic constrictions) and inferior (between the bronchoaortic and diaphragmatic constrictions).

Minor Constrictions (seen occasionally)

1. A retrosternal constriction may lie between the pharyngoesophageal and the aortic constrictions.

2. A cardiac constriction may lie behind the pericardium and is produced if right atrial enlargement is present, as in mitral stenosis.

3. A supradiaphragmatic constriction may be produced by a tortuous, arteriosclerotic aorta.

Curves of the Esophagus

The esophagus has three gentle curves: in the neck, behind the left primary bronchus; below the bifurcation of the trachea; and behind the pericardium. In terms of vertebral levels, the esophagus is to the left of the midline at T_1, to the right at T_6, and to the left again at T_{10}.

Remember the three Cs: three constrictions and three curves. Most esophageal pathology (e.g., lodgment of foreign bodies, burns from caustic chemicals, and cancer) is located at or close to these constrictions. The bronchoaortic constriction is the most frequently involved.

■ TOPOGRAPHY AND RELATIONS OF THE ESOPHAGUS

The tubercle of the cricoid cartilage is the single constant landmark of the upper esophageal opening.

The Pharyngoesophageal Junction

The muscular pharyngeal wall is formed by three overlapping muscles: the superior, middle, and inferior pharyngeal constrictors.

The inferior constrictor muscle blends inferiorly with the sphincter-like transverse cricopharyngeal muscle, which blends with the circular, muscular esophageal wall (Fig. 6.1). Posteriorly, there are two areas of weakness above and below the cricopharyngeal muscle (Fig. 6.1). These areas may become the site of acquired pulsion diverticula (Zenker's, above; Laimer's, below). They also are the sites of possible perforation by an esophagoscope.

There are two anatomical entities at this point which contribute to narrowing of the esophageal lumen: internally, the hypopharyngeal fold, and externally, the cricopharyngeal muscle. Instrumental perforation, lodging of foreign bodies, spasm, and neoplasms tend to occur at this location.

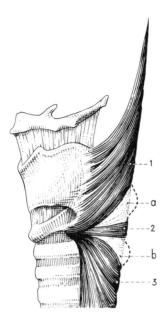

Figure 6.1. The lateral aspect of the pharyngoesophageal junction showing: (a) the upper weak area; (b) the lower weak area; (1) the oblique fibers of the inferior constrictor muscle; (2) the cricopharyngeal muscle; (3) the muscularis of the esophagus. (From J Terracol and RH Sweet. *Diseases of the Esophagus.* Philadelphia: WB Saunders, 1958.)

The cricopharyngeal muscle and the lower border of the cricoid cartilage demonstrate the end of the pharynx and the start of the esophagus. The so-called inferior constrictor of the pharynx, the cricopharyngeal muscle, originates from the thyroid and cricoid cartilages. It is composed of two parts, the upper oblique and the lower transverse; the lower transverse is probably the cricopharyngeal sphincter.

Between the two parts of the cricopharyngeal muscle is the weak area (triangle) of Killian. There is another weak area between the lower transverse and the muscular coat of the esophagus (Fig. 6.1).

Logically, a diverticulum above the transverse portion of the cricopharyngeal muscle should be recognized as pharyngeal, and one originating below as esophageal, but in the literature this distinction is not always made (Figs. 6.2A and B). For example, a diverticulum originating above the junction, which should be called Zenker's, may instead be referred to as pharyngoesophageal or esophageal, causing confusion.

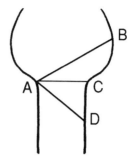

Figure 6.2A. Highly diagrammatic presentation of the musculature of the pharyngoesophageal junction, demonstrating also weakness and the formation of diverticulae. AB = oblique muscle; AC = transverse muscle; AD = muscular coat; ABC = Killian's triangle (1908) = pharyngeal diverticulum; ABD = Zenker's (1878) = pharyngoesophageal diverticulum; ACD = esophageal weakness = esophageal diverticulum. A congenital diverticulum has a wide neck and all layers. An acquired diverticulum has a narrow neck and no muscular coat.

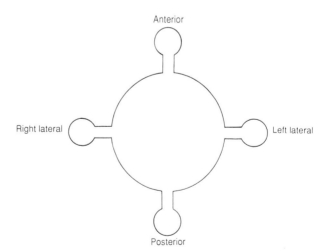

Figure 6.2B. Highly diagrammatic presentation of diverticulae. Note: The anterior diverticulum is a rare congenital condition.

Cervical Esophagus

The cervical esophagus is approximately 5–6 cm long and extends from C_6 to T_1, or from the cricoid cartilage and cricopharyngeal muscle to the thoracic inlet at the level of the sternoclavicular joints. The carotid tubercle (of Chassaignac), which is the palpable anterior tuberosity of the transverse process of C_6, is a good anatomical landmark. It projects somewhat to the left of the trachea, and incisions are commonly made on this side to approach the esophagus.

Anteriorly, the cervical esophagus is covered by the larynx and trachea.

Anterolaterally, there are four anatomical entities related to the esophageal wall on each side (see Fig. 2.15). From the periphery inward they are: the carotid sheath, the inferior thyroid artery, the lobe of the thyroid gland, and the recurrent laryngeal nerve. Also related to the distal cervical esophagus on the left side is the thoracic duct.

Posteriorly, the cervical esophagus is related to: the alar fascia, the prevertebral fascia, the longissimus cervicis muscle, and the vertebrae.

Between the alar fascia and the prevertebral fasica is the retrovisceral space, the so-called danger space which extends down the mediastinum and ends approximately at the level of T_4.

Pretracheal Space

The space in front of the trachea is not related directly to the esophagus. It is related clinically, however, since perforations of the anterior esophageal wall may open into the pretracheal space and therefore the mediastinum, producing a serious or even fatal mediastinitis.

Thoracic Esophagus

This portion of the esophagus extends from the level of T_1 to T_{10} or T_{11}.

A knowledge of the anatomy of the mediastinum is essential to successful esophageal surgery. We remind the reader, however, that the thoracic esophagus is located in the superior and posterior mediastinum. The key structure of the superior mediastinum is the aortic arch. The posterior mediastinum displays venous structures on the right, arterial structures on the left.

The anterior relations of the thoracic esophagus from above downward are the following structures: trachea and aortic arch, right pulmonary artery, left main bronchus, esophageal plexus below the tracheal bifurcation, pericardium and left atrium, anterior vagal trunk, and esophageal plexus and esophageal hiatus.

The posterior relations of the thoracic esophagus are: vertebral column, longus colli muscle, right posterior intercostal arteries, left thoracic duct obliquely from T_7 to T_4, right pleural sac, azygos vein, hemiazygos vein, accessory hemiazygos vein, anterior wall of the aorta, esophageal plexus of the vagus nerve below the tracheal bifurcation and sometimes the posterior vagal trunk.

The lateral relations on the right are: mediastinal pleura, azygos vein, right main bronchus, root of right lung, right vagus nerve, and esophageal plexus (Fig. 6.3).

The lateral relations on the left are: aortic arch, left subclavian artery, left recurrent laryngeal nerve, left vagus nerve, thoracic duct from T_4 to C_7, pleura, and descending thoracic aorta (Fig. 6.4).

The following structures are between the esophagus and the left mediastinal pleura: left common carotid artery, left subclavian artery, aortic arch, and descending aorta. The entire length of the thoracic esophagus is directly related to the right mediastinal pleura except where the arch of the azygos vein crosses above the right main bronchus.

Surgical Considerations

✔ From a surgical standpoint, lesions of the upper half of the thoracic esophagus should be explored through a right thoracotomy to avoid technical problems with the aortic arch. Lesions of the lower

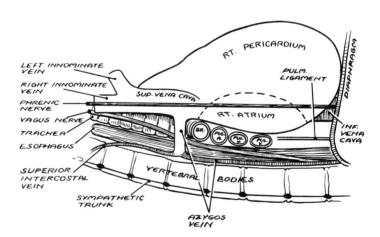

Figure 6.3. Highly diagrammatic view of the right mediastinum showing the disposition of its contents. (By permission of JE Skandalakis, SW Gray, and LJ Skandalakis. In: Jamieson, GG. *Surgery of the Esophagus*. Edinburgh: Churchill Livingstone, 1988, pp 19–35.)

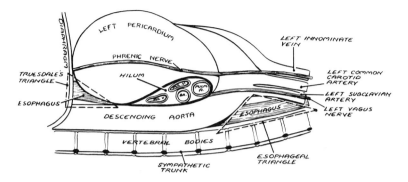

Figure 6.4. Highly diagrammatic view of the left mediastinum showing the disposition of its contents. (By permission of JE Skandalakis, SW Gray, and LJ Skandalakis. In: Jamieson, GG. *Surgery of the Esophagus.* Edinburgh: Churchill Livingstone, 1988, pp 19–35.)

half of the thoracic esophagus can be explored through a left or a right thoracotomy.

✓ With the right-sided approach, the azygos vein should be ligated and divided where it crosses the right wall of the esophagus to empty into the posterior wall of the superior vena cava. The azygos vein may be ligated with impunity. However, ligation of the superior vena cava between the atrium and the azygos vein cannot be tolerated if the azygos vein has been ligated.

✓ The esophageal triangle in the left side of the mediastinum is formed by the descending arch of the aorta, the subclavian artery, and the vertebral column. The floor of the triangle is formed by the left mediastinal pleura beneath which the esophagus is located (Fig. 6.4).

✓ The lower end of the thoracic esophagus, covered by pleura, may be found in the triangle of Truesdale, which is formed by the diaphragm below, the pericardium above and anteriorly, and the descending aorta posteriorly (Fig. 6.4). The posterior approximation of the right and left pleurae betwen the esophagus and the aorta forms the so-called mesoesophagus. The right pleura is in contact with the lower ⅓ of the esophagus, almost to the diaphragmatic hiatus. This proximity of the right pleura to the hiatus introduces the risk of pneumothorax during abdominal operations on the hiatus. The anterior approximation of the two pleurae is at the sternal angle (see Fig. 5.10).

Anatomical Weak Points

Two anatomically weak areas of the esophageal wall, one above and one below the cricoid muscle, have been mentioned. They may become the sites of pulsion diverticula. Another weak area, the left lateral posterior wall of the esophagus near the diaphragm, is occasionally the site of spontaneous idiopathic rupture of the healthy esophagus.

Abdominal Esophagus and Gastroesophageal Junction (Fig. 6.5)

External Junction

The gastroesophageal junction lies in the abdomen just below the diaphragm.

The abdominal esophagus is said to be from 0.5 to 2.5 cm in length, and occasionally as long as 7 cm. The surgeon has access to an appreciable length of esophagus below the diaphragm.

The abdominal esophagus lies at the level of the 11th or 12th thoracic vertebra, and is partially covered by peritoneum in front and on its left lateral wall. Relations with surrounding structures are as follows:

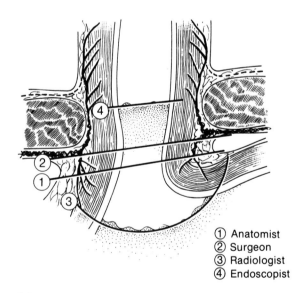

① Anatomist
② Surgeon
③ Radiologist
④ Endoscopist

Figure 6.5. Views of the "gastroesophageal junction" by four specialties. Each is correct. (By permission of JE Skandalakis, SW Gray, and JR Rowe, *Anatomical Complications in General Surgery*, New York: McGraw-Hill, 1983.)

ANTERIOR: The posterior surface of the left lobe of the liver, the left vagal trunk, and the esophageal plexus

POSTERIOR: One or both crura of the diaphragm, the left inferior phrenic artery, and the aorta

TO THE RIGHT: The caudate lobe of the liver

TO THE LEFT: The fundus of the stomach

Internal Junction

The histological junction between esophagus and stomach is marked by an irregular boundary between stratified squamous epithelium and simple columnar epithelium. Above the boundary, islands of columnar gastric epithelium may be present at all levels of the esophagus. The lower esophagus may occasionally be lined by gastric mucosa. A biopsy specimen to identify histological changes in the mucosa should be taken more than 2 cm above the epithelial junction to avoid most of these patches.

Part of the problem of defining the gastroesophageal junction is the fact that this mucosal boundary does not coincide with the external junction described above. In the living patient, the situation is even less simple. The submucosal connective tissue is so loose that the mucosa moves freely over the underlying muscularis. Even at rest, the junctional level may change. Fig. 6.5 shows the internal gastroesophageal junction from the point of view of four specialties.

"Cardiac Sphincter"

There is a sphincter at the cardiac orifice of the stomach that normally permits swallowing but not reflux. A slight thickening of the circular musculature of the distal esophagus has been described.

Several other structures have been held responsible for closing the cardia: the angle (of His) at which the esophagus enters the stomach, the pinchcock action of the diaphragm, a plug of loose esophageal mucosa (mucosal rosette), the phrenoesophageal membrane, and the sling of oblique fibers of the gastric musculature.

Esophageal Hiatus and the Crura (see Chapter 5, Diaphragm)

Surgical Considerations

Placement of 0 silk deep sutures in the crura, including the attached pleura, is absolutely necessary for narrowing the hiatus. The surgeon must be certain the sutures are in the tendinous portions of the crura and not in the muscular part only.

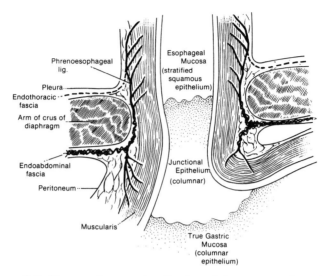

Figure 6.6. Diagram of a coronal section through the gastroesophageal junction and the esophageal hiatus of the diaphragm. (By permission of JE Skandalakis, SW Gray, and JR Rowe, *Anatomical Complications in General Surgery*, New York: McGraw-Hill, 1983.)

Phrenoesophageal Ligament (Fig. 6.6)

Where the esophagus passes from the thorax into the abdomen through the diaphragmatic hiatus, a strong, flexible, airtight seal is necessary. The seal must be strong enough to resist abdominal pressure that tends to push the stomach into the thorax and flexible enough to give with the pressure changes incidental to breathing and the movement incidental to swallowing. A seal known as the phrenoesophageal ligament or membrane consists, in principle, of the following elements: pleura, subpleural (endothoracic) fascia, phrenoesophageal fascia (of Laimer), transversalis (endoabdominal subdiaphragmatic) fascia, and peritoneum.

The first and last of these elements provide the requirement for airtightness, the middle three provide flexibility and strength. The ligament exists in infants, it is attenuated in adults, and it does not exist in adult patients with hiatal hernia.

The development of the phrenoesophageal ligament can be summarized as follows:

1. In newborn infants, the phrenoesophageal ligament is present.

2. In adults, the ligament is attenuated and subperitoneal fat accumulates at the hiatus.

3. In adults with hiatal hernias, the ligament for all practical purposes does not exist.

SURGICAL CONSIDERATIONS: Dividing the phrenoesophageal ligament will mobilize the cardia, but the surgeon undertaking a Hill procedure must be prepared to find the ligament ill-defined or absent.

Peritoneal Reflections

HEPATOGASTRIC (GASTROHEPATIC) LIGAMENT: The abdominal esophagus is contained between the two layers of the hepatogastric ligament. The ligament contains the following structures: left gastric artery and vein; hepatic division of left vagus trunk; lymph nodes; occasionally, both vagal trunks; occasionally, branches of the right gastric artery and vein; the left hepatic artery when it arises from the left gastric artery (in 23 percent of cases).

GASTROSPLENIC (GASTROLIENAL) LIGAMENT: The hepatogastric ligament encloses the abdominal esophagus on the right; its leaves rejoin on the left of the esophagus to form the gastrosplenic ligament. The lesser sac lies behind these ligaments. (For more information, see Chapter 15, Spleen.)

GASTROPHRENIC LIGAMENT (SEE CHAPTER 7, STOMACH)

The Structure of the Esophageal Wall (Fig. 6.7)

Mucosa

The esophagus is lined with a thick layer of nonkeratinizing, stratified squamous epithelium continuous with the lining of the oropharynx.

Submucosa

A layer of loose connective tissue lies external to the mucosa. *The thick submucosa is the strongest part of the esophageal wall.* It is this layer with the lamina propria that the surgeon must count on for a sound esophageal anastomosis.

Muscularis Externa

The chief muscles of the esophagus are an internal circular layer and an external longitudinal layer. Both layers in the upper quarter of the esophagus are large striated (voluntary) muscle fibers. In the second quarter, striated and smooth (involuntary) fibers are mingled; the lower half contains only smooth fibers (Fig. 6.8).

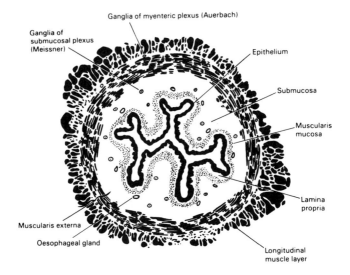

Figure 6.7. Cross section of the esophagus showing the layers of the wall. The longitudinal and circular layers of the muscularis externa contain striated muscle fibers decreasing distally. (By permission of JE Skandalakis, SW Gray, and LJ Skandalakis. In: Jamieson, GG. *Surgery of the Esophagus*. Edinburgh: Churchill Livingstone, 1988, pp 19–35.)

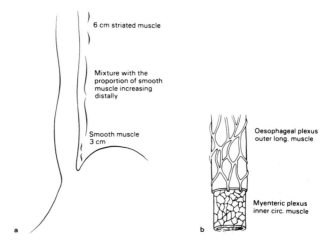

Figure 6.8. (a) Relative distribution of smooth and striated muscle in the esophagus. (b) The extrinsic and intrinsic nerves of the esophagus. (By permission of JE Skandalakis, SW Gray, and LJ Skandalakis. In: Jamieson, GG. *Surgery of the Esophagus*. Edinburgh: Churchill Livingstone, 1988, pp 19–35.)

Adventitia

The connective tissue of the mediastinum around the esophagus is not a true layer of that organ and it does not provide the surgeon with a firm anchorage for sutures. It is the lack of a serosa that contributes to the complication of anastomotic disruption following esophageal resection and anastomosis.

Nerve Supply to the Esophagus

Intrinsic Nerve Supply

Within the esophageal wall three are two plexuses of nerves: Meissner's plexus in the submucosa and Auerbach's plexus in the connective tissue between the circular and longitudinal muscularis externa.

Extrinsic Nerve Supply

The esophagus receives nerves from three sources: cerebrospinal, sympathetic, and parasympathetic (vagal).

Blood Supply of the Esophagus

The blood supply, segmental or not, is adequate for intramural anastamoses. Poor technique, not poor blood supply, is responsible for leakage (Tables 6.1 and 6.2).

Lymphatics of the Esophagus

The esophageal lymphatics form plexuses in the mucosa (lamina propria), submucosa, muscularis, and adventitia.

Lymph nodes are generously distributed along the esophagus, and groups of nodes have been named by their relations to adjacent organs (Fig. 6.9). "Skip areas" of up to 8 cm between lymph nodes involved in cancer may be encountered.

A few generalities about "unpredictable" drainage may be stated. Nodes of the cervical esophagus drain to internal jugular, supraclavicular, and upper paratracheal nodes. Nodes of the posterior thoracic region drain to posterior mediastinal, intercostal, and paraesophageal nodes. Nodes of the anterior thoracic region drain to tracheal, hilar, subcarinal, paracardial, and celiac nodes. Cancer involves paratracheal nodes on the right more often than those on the left. Posterior hilar nodes are more often involved than are other nodes at the carina.

Table 6.1 Arterial Supply of the Esophagus

Esophageal segment	Primary	Secondary or occasional
Cervical	Br. of inferior thyroid aa.	Br. of pharyngeal aa.
	Anterior: trachea and esophagus	Br. of subclavian a.
	Posterior: Esophagus and longi-tudinal trachea and transverse anastomoses	Br. of bronchial a. Superior thyroid a.
Upper thoracic	Br. of subclavian a. or lower branches of inferior thyroid a.	Ant. esophagotracheal a. from aortic arch
Mid thoracic	L. bronchial a. ascending br. to esophagus and trachea; de-scending br. to esophagus.	R. internal thoracic R. costocervical trunk R. subclavian a.
	R. bronchial a. branches as L. but smaller.	
	Ascending and descending branches may arise directly from aortic arch	
Lower thoracic	Superior and inferior esophageal aa. from aorta	Branches from R. inter-costal aa.
Abdominal	Branches of L. gastric a. L. inferior phrenic a.	Variable: R. inferior phre-nic a. Branches from splenic a. Branches from superior suprarenal a. Accessory L. hepatic a. Celiac trunk

(By permission of JE Skandalakis, SW Gray, LJ Skandalakis. Surgical anatomy of the esophagus. In: Jamieson, GG. *Surgery of the Esophagus*. Edinburgh: Churchill Living-stone, 1988, pp 19–35.)

Among patients with carcinoma of the cervical and upper thoracic esophagus, celiac nodes are involved in 10 percent. In cases of carcinoma of the middle ⅓, the celiac nodes are involved in 44 percent. In view of the anatomical distribution of lymphatics, less than subtotal esophagec-tomy is not a sound procedure. For better results, esophageal resection from 6 to 10 cm above and below the tumor is mandatory.

Table 6.2 Venous Drainage of the Esophagus

Esophageal Segment	Venous drainage	Termination
Cervical and superior innominate vein		Inferior thyroid vein
Thoracic (upper ⅓)		Bronchial vein
Superior vena cava	Highest intercostal vein	
Thoracic (middle ⅓)	Azygos and hemiazygos veins	Superior vena cava
Inferior thoracic and abdominal (lower ⅓)	Branch of left gastric vein	Hepatic portal vein
	Branches of splenic vein	
	Left inferior phrenic vein	

(By permission of JE Skandalakis, SW Gray, LJ Skandalakis. Surgical anatomy of the esophagus. In: Jamieson, GG. *Surgery of the Esophagus*. Edinburgh: Churchill Livingstone, 1988, pp. 19–35.)

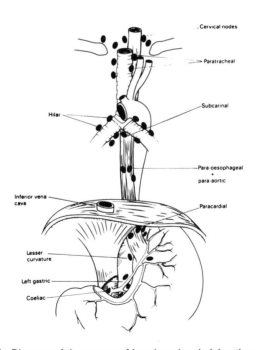

Figure 6.9. Diagram of the groups of lymph nodes draining the esophagus. There is no standard terminology. (By permission of JE Skandalakis, SW Gray, LJ Skandalakis. Surgical anatomy of the esophagus. In: Jamieson, GG. *Surgery of the Esophagus*. Edinburgh: Churchill Livingstone, 1988, pp. 19–35.)

Lymphatic Drainage of the Gastroesophageal Junction

It has been stated that cancer at the cardia spreads by lymphatics and usually appears first below the diaphragm among the gastrohepatic, gastrophrenic, gastrosplenic, and gastrocolic lymph nodes. Early metastasis to the liver may follow invasion of the gastric veins. Extension to the peripancreatic nodes is unusual. Isolated involvement of the diaphragm can occur. One study found that splenic hilar nodes were involved in 11 percent of spleens of patients with cancer of the gastroesophageal junction.

Metastatic spread above the diaphragm is less common, though not rare. Tumors of the esophagus just above the diaphragm may metastasize to the gastrohepatic nodes and liver.

Thus, the lymphatic channels at the cardia follow the arteries; the left gastric with its esophageal branches, and the splenic with its left gastroepiploic and vasa brevia. Unorthodox dissemination, however, must not be overlooked.

TECHNIQUE

■ PHARYNGOESOPHAGEAL DIVERTICULUM

Procedure:

Step 1. Incise as in thyroidectomy, but with extension to the right or the left according to the location and presentation of the diverticulum and less to the opposite side. Divide the subcutaneous fascia (fat and platysma) and use special retractors for traction (Fig. 6.10).

Step 2. Retract the sternocleidomastoid muscle laterally and isolate the carotid sheath. The ansa hypoglossi, which is located in front of or within the sheath, should be saved if possible, and sacrificed only if absolutely necessary. We like to divide the omohyoid muscle and ligate the middle thyroid vein. As in thyroidectomy, the thyroid lobe is retracted medially, and the recurrent nerve is found and protected. Ligate and divide the inferior thyroid vein if necessary (Fig. 6.11).

Step 3. At this point, the upper part of the diverticulum may be seen located medial to the sternocleidomastoid, lateral to the thyroid lobe and to the recurrent nerve but between the inferior pharyngeal constrictor above and the esophagus below (Fig. 6.12).

Step 4. By blunt dissection, separate the diverticulum from all surrounding structures. Elevate it, carefully clean its neck, clamp it with two clamps, and remove it (Figs. 6.12 and 6.13).

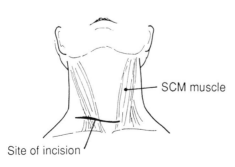

SCM muscle

Site of incision

Figure 6.10

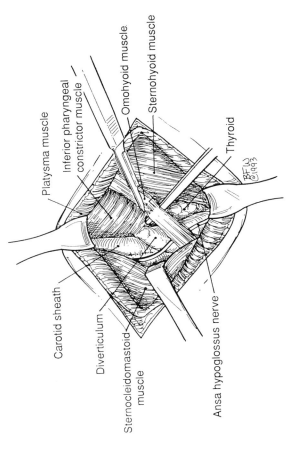

Platysma muscle

Inferior pharyngeal
constrictor muscle

Omohyoid muscle

Sternohyoid muscle

Thyroid

Carotid sheath

Diverticulum

Sternocleidomastoid
muscle

Ansa hypoglossus nerve

BFW
©1993

Figure 6.11

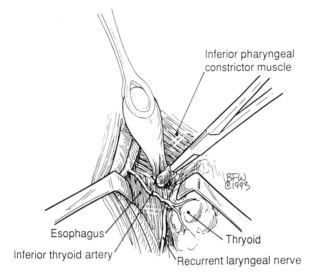

Figure 6.12

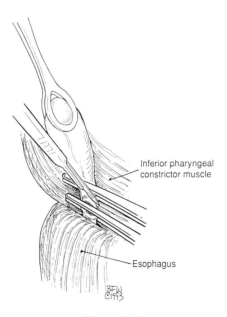

Figure 6.13

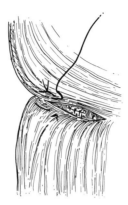

Figure 6.14

Step 5. Close the diverticulum base with 4–0 synthetic absorbable interrupted suture material. Close the cricopharyngeal muscle
with mattress interrupted 3–0 synthetic nonabsorbable sutures
(Fig. 6.14).

Step 6. Close the wound as in thyroidectomy. Drainage is up to the
surgeon.

Another method of amputation of the diverticulum is the use of TA-30
or TA-55 staples longitudinally or transversely. Be sure to proceed as
follows:

1. Establish good myotomy.

2. Isolate the neck of the diverticulum, if present.

3. Insert 40F Maloney dilator into the esophagus, if it has not been
inserted previously.

■ ACHALASIA OR CARDIOSPASM

Modified Heller's Procedure

Procedure:

Step 1. Make a transverse incision of the phrenoesophageal ligament.
The abdominal esophagus is further prepared by blunt and
sharp dissection, exposing the periesophageal space. Isolate
both vagi. Slowly use the index finger to penetrate the avascu-

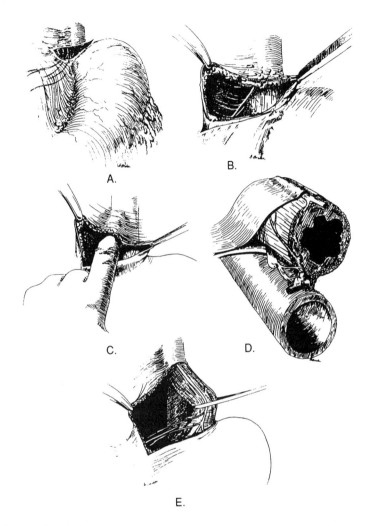

A.

B.

C.

D.

E.

Figure 6.15A-E. (By permission of PE Donahue, LM Nyhus, *Surg Gynecol Obstet* 152:218–220, 1981.)

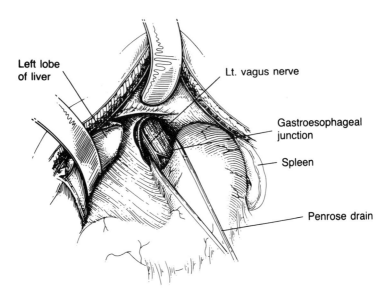

Figure 6.16. (By permission of JE Skandalakis, SW Gray, AR Mansberger, et al, *Hernia: Surgical Anatomy and Technique*, New York: McGraw-Hill, 1989.)

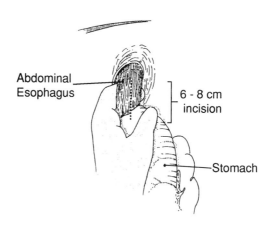

Figure 6.17

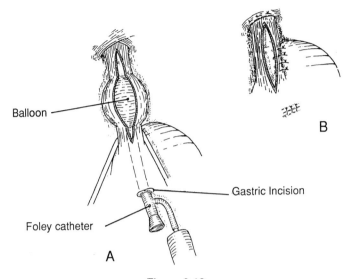

Balloon

Gastric Incision

Foley catheter

B

A

Figure 6.18

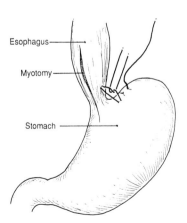

Esophagus

Myotomy

Stomach

Figure 6.19

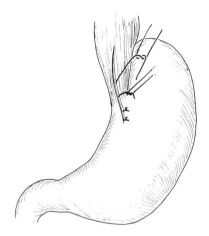

Figure 6.20

lar ligaments of the gastroesophageal junction (Figs. 16.15A–E).

Step 2. Pass a Penrose drain through for traction. Now the posterior mediastinum, as well as the stenotic segment of the abdominal esophagus with dilated proximal segments, is in view (Fig. 6.16).

Step 3. Insert a Foley catheter through a small gastric incision. The balloon should be located above the stenotic segment; this will help divide all fibrous and muscular elements (Fig. 6.17 [The dotted line indicates the incision for the esophagomyotomy]).

Step 4. Use the Penrose drain or the index finger for downward traction of the gastroesophageal junction. The incision of the esophageal musculature should be over the dilated esophageal segment. Using a curved Mixter, extend the incision proximally and distally to a length of 6–8 cm. It is recommended that the incision extend 1–2 cm to the stomach (Figs. 6.18A and B).

Step 5. For a partial fundoplasty (valvuloplasty), suture the gastric fundus at the posterior esophageal wall, as well as to the left and right margin of the myotomy (Figs. 6.19 and 6.20). Alternatively, a Nissen fundoplication may be done.

Step 6. Close the anterior gastric and abdominal walls.

7

Stomach

ANATOMY

■ THE TWO GASTRIC UNITS

From the viewpoint of a surgeon, the stomach is composed of two gastric systems or units. The first may be called the proximal gastric unit, which contains the proximal stomach, the distal esophagus, and the esophageal hiatus of the diaphragm (Fig. 7.1). The second is the distal gastric unit, which includes the gastric antrum and pylorus, together with the first part of the duodenum.

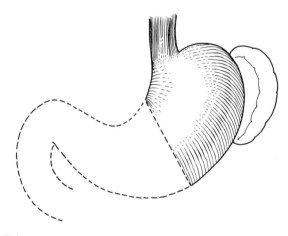

Figure 7.1. The proximal gastric surgical unit. The two ends of the stomach have different lesions, and operations require different methods. (By permission of JE Skandalakis, SW Gray, and JR Rowe, *Anatomical Complications in General Surgery*, New York: McGraw-Hill, 1983.)

The Proximal Gastric Surgical Unit

The length of the abdominal esophagus is given as from 0.5 to 2.5 cm. Its relations with surrounding structures are:

ANTERIOR: The posterior surface of the left lobe of the liver

POSTERIOR: The right crus of the diaphragm and aorta

RIGHT: The caudate (Spigelian) lobe of the liver

LEFT: The fundus of the stomach

The cardiac orifice is the gastroesophageal junction. The fundus, for all practical purposes, is the upper part of the body, which in the supine position augments upward. The body is the part of the stomach between the antrum and the fundus.

The Distal Gastric Surgical Unit

The gastric antrum, the pylorus, and the first portion of the duodenum form a unit from an embryonic, physiological, and certainly surgical viewpoint (Fig. 7.2).

Gastric Antrum

In the opened stomach, the antrum is easily distinguished from the body of the stomach by its mucosa, which is flatter, without rugae, and histo-

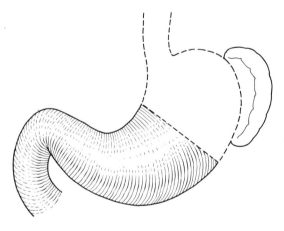

Figure 7.2. The distal gastric surgical unit. Most gastric surgery takes place in this area. (By permission of JE Skandalakis, SW Gray, and JR Rowe, *Anatomical Complications in General Surgery*, New York: McGraw-Hill, 1983.)

logically distinct, being without chief cells and parietal (acid-producing) cells. The margin is irregular but definite. Externally the antrum is difficult to demarcate. The boundary on the lesser curvature usually lies at the incisura angularis; usually it is easily found in textbook drawings, but it is inconstant and often absent in the operating room.

The surgeon who does not plan a gastrotomy to locate the antral margin may use as a landmark the "crow's foot" of the anterior descending vagal trunk; the antrum may be considered to begin 3–4 cm cranial to this, about 8–10 cm proximal to the pylorus. On the greater curvature, there is no good landmark. On the average, the boundary extends from a point on the lesser curvature ⅔ of the way from the pylorus to the esophagus to a point on the greater curvature ⅛ of the distance from the pylorus to the esophagus.

Pylorus

The pylorus is a region of the stomach variously called the pyloric canal, pyloric ring, or pyloric valve. Proximally, it merges into the gastric antrum without a definite external boundary; distally, it ends abruptly at the thin-walled duodenum.

At the pyloroduodenal junction, the continuity of the circular musculature is interrupted by a ring-shaped septum that arises from the connective tissue of the submucosa. Proximal to this ring, the circular muscle layer is thickened to form the pyloric sphincter; distal to the ring, the circular muscle coat at the duodenum is thinner.

First Part of the Duodenum

The distal gastric surgical unit includes only the first 2.5 cm of the duodenum. (For more information, see Chapter 8, Duodenum.)

Relations of the Distal Gastric Surgical Unit

Posteriorly the unit is related to the:

- floor of the lesser sac
- transverse mesocolon
- head and neck of the pancreas
- aorta and celiac trunk and its branches
- celiac ganglion and plexus
- hepatic triad
- gastroduodenal artery

Anteriorly the unit is related to:

- anterior abdominal wall
- medial segment of the left lobe and the anterior segment of the right lobe of liver
- transverse mesocolon if the stomach is empty
- neck of the gallbladder

■ GASTRIC WALL

The gastric wall consists of: (1) the serosa, (2) a muscular layer, (3) the submucosal layer, and (4) the mucosal layer.

The mucosa of the distal esophagus consists of stratified squamous epithelium, and the abdominal esophagus consists of both squamous epithelial and mucous cells. Simple columnar cells compose the mucosal layer of the cardia. The mucosal layer of the fundus and body consists of two types of cells: parietal (oxyntic), which secrete acid, and chief, which secrete pepsin.

■ LIGAMENTS

Gastrohepatic Ligament (Lesser Omentum)

The gastrohepatic ligament is the proximal part of the lesser omentum; it extends from the porta hepatis to the lesser curvature of the stomach and upward as the ventral mesentery of the abdominal esophagus. The ligament contains:

REGULARLY: Left gastric artery and vein, hepatic division of the anterior vagal trunk, anterior and posterior gastric divisions of the vagal nerve (nerves of Latarjet), and lymph nodes

OCCASIONALLY: Branches of the right gastric artery and vein, and an aberrant left hepatic artery (23 percent of individuals)

Hepatoduodenal Ligament

The hepatoduodenal ligament is the distal part of the lesser omentum extending from the liver to the first 2.5 cm of the duodenum. The free edge envelops the hepatic triad of the hepatic artery, portal vein, and extrahepatic bile ducts, as well as the hepatic plexus and lymph nodes.

Gastrocolic Ligament

The gastrocolic ligament is a portion of the greater omentum passing from the greater curvature of the stomach and the first part of the duodenum to the transverse colon.

Gastrosplenic Ligament (See Chapter 15, Spleen)

Gastrophrenic Ligament

The gastrophrenic ligament is a continuation of the gastrohepatic ligament to the left of the esophagus as the dorsal mesentery. It has an avascular area through which the surgeon's finger may safely pass and through which a Penrose drain may be inserted around the cardia to pull down the esophagus. This is a useful maneuver in vagotomy. The upper part of the ligament is avascular, and the lower part contains short gastric arteries and veins, and lymph nodes.

■ THE BLOOD SUPPLY OF THE STOMACH (Fig. 7.3)

These are the arteries of the stomach:

- inferior phrenic artery
- left gastric artery
- right gastric artery
- gastroduodenal artery
- right gastroepiploic artery
- left gastroepiploic artery
- posterior gastric artery
- short gastric arteries

The veins, for all practical purposes, follow the arteries.

The stomach can survive after ligation of all but one of its primary arteries, and general surgeons also know that extragastric ligation will not control bleeding from a gastric ulcer.

■ LYMPHATIC DRAINAGE OF THE STOMACH

The lymphatic drainage of the stomach consists of four zones as follows (Fig. 7.4):

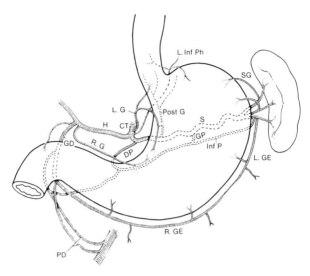

Figure 7.3. The arterial supply to the stomach: L.Inf Ph = left inferior phrenic artery; SG = short gastric artery; L.GE = left gastroepiploic artery; R.GE = right gastroepiploic artery; S = splenic artery; GP = great pancreatic artery; Inf P = inferior pancreatic artery; PD = pancreaticoduodenal artery; DP = dorsal pancreatic artery; GD = gastroduodenal artery; R.G = right gastric artery; H = hepatic artery; CT = celiac trunk; L.G = left gastric artery; Post G = posterior gastric artery. (By permission of JE Skandalakis, SW Gray, and JR Rowe, *Anatomical Complications in General Surgery*, New York: McGraw-Hill, 1983.)

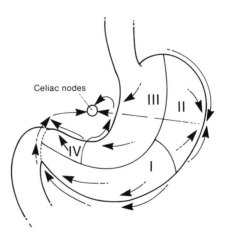

Figure 7.4. Diagram of the lymphatic drainage of the stomach. Most of the drainage finds its way to the celiac nodes: the "vortex of the metastatic whorl." (By permission of JE Skandalakis, SW Gray, and JR Rowe, *Anatomical Complications in General Surgery*, New York: McGraw-Hill, 1983.)

- Zone I (inferior gastric): draining into the subpyloric and omental nodes
- Zone II (splenic): draining into the pancreaticosplenic nodes
- Zone III (superior gastric): draining into the superior gastric nodes
- Zone IV (hepatic): draining into the suprapyloric nodes

■ VAGUS NERVE

The left and right vagus nerves descend parallel to the esophagus and form an esophageal vagal plexus between the level of the tracheal bifurcation and the level of the diaphragm. From this plexus, two vagal trunks, anterior and posterior, form and pass through the esophageal hiatus of the diaphragm. Each trunk subsequently separates into two divisions (Fig. 7.5).

From the anterior trunk, the hepatic division passes to the right in the lesser omentum, branching before it enters the liver. One branch turns downward to reach the pylorus and sometimes the first part of the duodenum. The second division, the anterior gastric, descends along the lesser curvature of the stomach, giving branches to the anterior gastric wall.

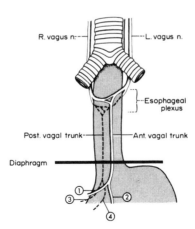

Figure 7.5. The terminology of vagal structures of the thorax and abdomen. In this example, two vagal trunks pass through the hiatus to enter the abdomen. 1 = hepatic division; 2 = anterior gastric division; 3 = celiac division; 4 = posterior gastric division. (By permission of JE Skandalakis, JS Rowe, and SW Gray, *Surg* 75(2):233–237, 1974.)

From the posterior trunk arises the celiac division, which passes to the celiac plexus, and the posterior gastric division, which supplies branches to the posterior gastric wall.

Identification of Vagal Structures at the Hiatus

The basic configuration and variations are well known, but the thoracic pattern is not visible to the abdominal surgeon, who must proceed on the basis of the structures that can be seen.

1. **Two vagal structures only (88 percent)** (Fig. 7.5). These will be the anterior and posterior vagal trunks, which have not yet split to form the four typical divisions. Both trunks are usually to the right of the midline of the esophagus. The posterior trunk lies closer to the aorta than to the esophagus (Fig. 7.6).

2. **Four vagal structures (7 percent)** (see Fig. 5.18A). These will be the

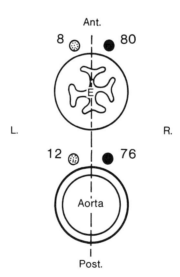

Figure 7.6. The relation of the anterior and posterior vagal trunks to the aorta and the esophagus, showing the number of specimens with vagal trunks lying to the right or left of the midline. In most but not all of the 88 specimens, the trunks are to the right of the midline. Note that the anterior trunks are closer to the esophagus than the posterior trunks. (By permission of JE Skandalakis, JS Rowe, and SW Gray, *Surg* 75(2):233–237, 1974.)

four divisions of the vagal trunks. Division has occurred above the diaphragm.

3. More than four vagal structures (5 percent). These may be (a) divisions and branches of divisions (Fig. 5.18B) (the anterior and posterior trunks lie entirely within the thorax), and (b) elements of the esophageal vagal plexus (Fig. 5.18C) (the anterior and posterior trunks lie entirely within the abdomen).

Distribution of the Vagus Nerves to the Stomach

Anterior Gastric Division

The separation of the anterior gastric and hepatic divisions occasionally occurs above the diaphragm, but they usually lie on the abdominal esophagus or the cardia.

In almost all cases, a major branch of the anterior gastric division forms the principal anterior nerve of the lesser curvature (anterior nerve of Latarjet). It usually lies from 0.5 to 1.0 cm from the lesser curvature.

From 2 to 12 branches pass from the principal nerve to the stomach wall. In our subjects, the average was 6.

Constant landmarks on the stomach are difficult to obtain. The position of the incisura angularis often has to be estimated.

Although we have often seen the nerve of Latarjet branch in the "crow's foot" formation, this pattern is far from constant, being equivocal in some cases and absent in many (Fig. 7.7).

Hepatic Division

The hepatic division of the anterior vagal trunk usually separates from the anterior gastric division at the level of the abdominal esophagus (Fig. 7.8). It lies between the leaflets of the avascular portion of the gastrohepatic ligament. It is frequently found in multiple and usually closely parallel branches.

Posterior Gastric Division

In most subjects, the posterior gastric division forms the principal posterior nerve of the lesser curvature (posterior nerve of Latarjet). As a rule, the posterior nerve appears to terminate slightly higher on the lesser curvature and possesses fewer gastric branches than does the anterior nerve. In no case did a posterior nerve reach the duodenum.

Celiac Division

The celiac division is the largest of the four vagal divisions. It lies in the gastropancreatic peritoneal fold. In all cases, it was single and led directly

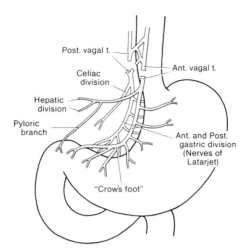

Figure 7.7. Truncal vagotomy results in vagal denervation of all abdominal organs. A concomitant drainage procedure is required for gastric stasis. (By permission of JE Skandalakis, SW Gray, and JR Rowe, *Anatomical Complications in General Surgery*, New York: McGraw-Hill, 1983.)

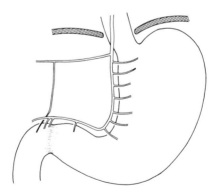

Figure 7.8. "Typical" distribution of anterior gastric and hepatic divisions of the vagus. (Modified by permission of JE Skandalakis, SW Gray, RE Soria, et al., *Am Surg* 46(3):130–139, 1980.)

to the celiac plexus. This division may follow the left gastric artery or the right crus of the diaphragm or take an intermediate position in the triangle bounded by the artery, the crus, and the right margin of the stomach.

■ SYMPATHETIC NERVES

Parietal cell vagotomy destroys the sympathetic nerves to the lesser curvature. The sympathectomy is partial, since fibers from the celiac ganglion to the greater curvature remain intact. The specific effects of this partial sympathectomy are not known.

TECHNIQUE

■ GASTROSTOMY

Stamm Gastrostomy

The surgeon chooses the type of incision, and a good preoperative evaluation helps greatly in the decision. The authors favor a small upper-midline incision, which may be extended, if necessary.

Procedure:

Step 1. With Babcock clamps, elevate the anterior wall of the stomach approximately 6–10 cm from the gastroduodenal junction. Then place and tie two purse-string sutures of 3-0 silk or Vicryl 120 degrees from each other (Fig. 7.9).

Step 2. Make a very small stab incision (usually 0.5 cm in length) in the center of the designated area of the purse-string sutures and insert an 18–22 Foley balloon catheter (Fig. 7.9).

Step 3. Insert the catheter and inflate the balloon. Tie the inner purse string very tightly, then tie the outer purse string; do not cut it or remove the needles (Fig. 7.10).

Step 4. Pull the catheter until it reaches the gastric mucosa at the gastric stab wound. Use gentle movements to ensure that the balloon is well attached to the gastric mucosa. Stitch the purse-string sutures to the anterior abdominal wall. To make certain

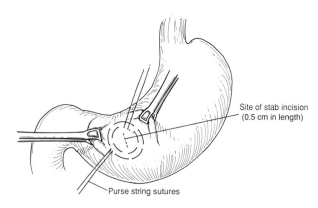

Site of stab incision (0.5 cm in length)

Purse string sutures

Figure 7.9

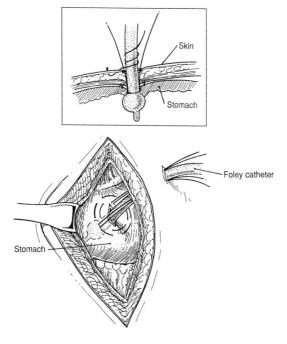

Figure 7.10

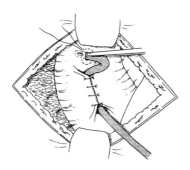

Figure 7.11

that dead space does not exist, use a third 3–0 silk suture to fix the gastric wall to the anterior abdominal wall. Close the skin and use a 2–0 silk suture to secure the gastrostomy tube to the skin of the abdominal wall.

Note: There are other types of gastrostomies, including Witzel and Janeway. They are seldom used today.

Witzel Gastrostomy

Procedure:

Step 1. Insert an 18–22 Foley balloon catheter into the stomach, but use only one purse-string suture to secure the catheter (Fig. 7.11).

Step 2. Close the anterior gastric wall with interrupted 3–0 silk sutures twice over the distal part of the Foley, creating a tunnel (Fig. 7.12).

■ JEJUNOSTOMY

The procedure is similar to gastrostomy, using a loop close and distal to the ligament of Treitz.

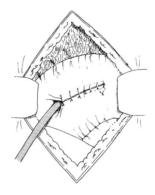

Figure 7.12

■ GASTROJEJUNOSTOMY

Retrocolic

Procedure:

Step 1. Make an upper-midline incision or incision of the surgeon's choice.

Step 2. The location of the stoma should be close to the pylorus at the most dependent area of the greater curvature. Place a Babcock clamp in an oblique fashion at the lesser curvature and at the greater curvature (Fig. 7.13).

Step 3. Lift the transverse colon to evaluate its mesocolon. To protect the middle colic artery, note its location. Identify an avascular area, which should be incised; in most cases, it will be to the left of the middle colic artery. The posterior wall of the stomach projects through the opening in such a way that the lesser curvature is located at the lowest corner of the mesenteric opening. Using interrupted 4-0 silk, suture the mesentery to the gastric wall at this point (Fig. 7.14).

Step 4. Again using interrupted 4-0 silk sutures, attach a jejunal loop, approximately 4-5 inches distal to the ligament of Treitz, to

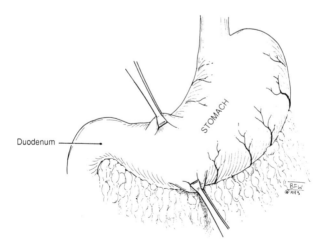

Figure 7.13

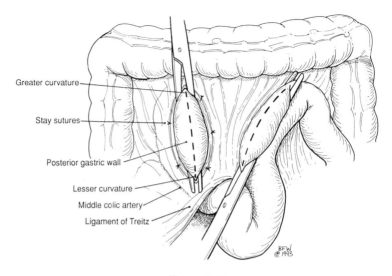

Greater curvature

Stay sutures

Posterior gastric wall

Lesser curvature

Middle colic artery

Ligament of Treitz

Figure 7.14

the gastric wall, proximal to the lesser curvature. Anastomose the loop to the posterior gastric wall in two layers using a running 3-0 chromic suture for the mucosa layer and a 3-0 silk interrupted suture for the seromuscular layer (Figs. 7.15–7.17).

Note: Alternatively, a stapled anastomosis is acceptable.

Step 5. Close the abdominal wall.

Antecolic (Fig. 7.18)

Follow steps as in the retrocolic gastrojejunostomy. The jejunal loop is anterior to the colon; therefore, attach it to the posterior wall of the stomach at the most dependent part of the greater curvature through an opening of the gastrocolic ligament.

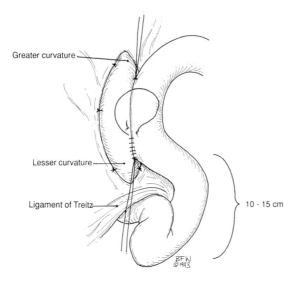

Figure 7.15

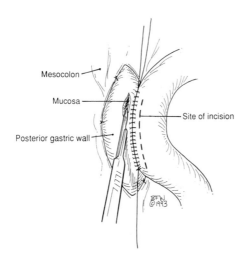

Figure 7.16

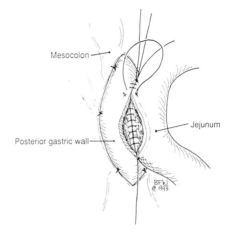

Figure 7.17

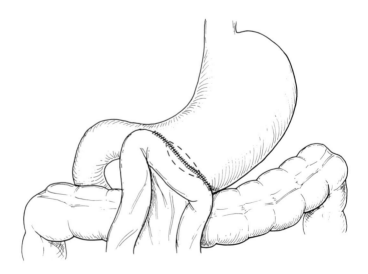

Figure 7.18

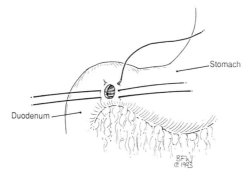

Figure 7.19

■ PERFORATED PEPTIC ULCER

Duodenal Graham Patch (Figs. 7.19 and 7.20)

Procedure:

Step 1. Perform detailed and complete cleansing by irrigating the peritoneal cavities. Be sure to pay special attention to the suprahepatic and subhepatic areas. The right and left pericolic gutters should be cleaned and the pelvis should be irrigated vigorously.

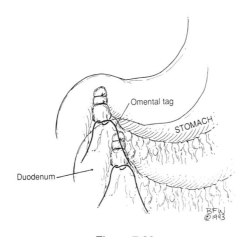

Figure 7.20

Step 2. Using no more than two or three sutures, plug the perforated ulcer with omentum. Then using a 3–0 silk or synthetic absorbable, take a full-thickness bite of duodenum on each side of the perforation. Tie the sutures above the omental piece.

Step 3. Irrigate, then close in layers using repeated irrigation. Drainage is up to the surgeon. Intravenous antibiotics, which were started prior to surgery, should be continued for at least 48 hours.

Notes:

✓ Occasionally, the perforated ulcer is associated with partial obstruction, bleeding, or both. Sometimes, especially 6 hours after the onset of perforation, local edema exists and interferes with the approximation or closure of the perforation with sutures. In very rare cases, the answer is a T-tube inserted into the perforation hole, with a definitive procedure taking place later on. Correction of the obstruction is not necessary, since the obstruction will disappear as soon as the inflammation subsides.

✓ If bleeding is present, it is probably arising from a posterior wall ulcer penetrating the gastroduodenal artery. Therefore, the patient has two problems: an anterior perforated ulcer and a posterior bleeding ulcer. Suture the artery superficially. **Remember:** The duct of Santorini is under the artery and in 10 percent of cases it is the only duct of the exocrine pancreas. If the suture incorporates the duct, pancreatitis can result. Again, occasionally in early perforation, a truncal or superselective vagotomy with pyloroplasty could be indicated or, perhaps, a truncal vagotomy with Billroth II procedure.

✓ Be sure to administer intravenous antibiotics prior to incision and for 24–48 hours postoperatively.

Perforated Gastric Ulcer

Since most gastric neoplasms are malignant, the surgeon should always remember that a perforated gastric ulcer could be of benign or malignant origin.

Procedure:

Step 1. Clamp the perforated ulcer with a Babcock clamp. After the peritoneal cavity has been thoroughly cleansed, remove the ulcer and send it to the lab for frozen section. During this time, irrigation of the peritoneal cavity continues, and the surgeon devises the patient's treatment strategy.

Step 2. If the ulcer is benign, close the gastric wall in two layers: the first with through-and-through absorbable suture, and the second with Lembert seromuscular suture of 3-0 or 4-0 silk. If the ulcer is malignant, the surgeon should consider performing a subtotal gastrectomy, especially if the perforation took place within 6 hours of surgery.

■ HIGH ANTERIOR OR POSTERIOR SUBCARDIAL GASTRIC ULCER

It is the authors' policy to excise the ulcer in toto and send it to the lab for frozen section.

An ulcer of the *anterior gastric wall* may be excised by making a circumferential incision around it. The procedure is aided by deep seromuscular sutures proximal and distal to the ulcer. If the ulcer is benign, close in two layers; if malignant, perform a proximal, subtotal Billroth II gastrectomy (surgical philosophy is never to use a Billroth I with gastric malignancy).

When working with an ulcer of the *posterior gastric wall*, which is very high and close to the gastroesophageal junction, establish good proximal mobilization of the stomach and abdominal esophagus. Turn the stomach in such a way that the greater curvature lies posterior and the lesser lies anterior. From this point, the procedure is the same as for an anterior gastric wall ulcer excision. Again, additional procedures depend upon the benignity or malignancy of the ulcer.

■ PYLORIC STENOSIS (Fig. 7.21)

Although this procedure is generally performed by a pediatric surgeon, we will present the technique because it is done occasionally by general surgeons.

Procedure:

Step 1. Make a right upper quadrant muscle-splitting incision.

Step 2. Deliver the pylorus and the pyloric tumor from the peritoneal cavity.

Step 3. Hold the tumor firmly with the thumb and index finger in such a way that the proximal duodenum is pushed up to the distal pylorus, protecting the duodenal mucosa.

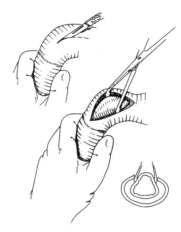

Figure 7.21

Step 4. Carefully incise the serosa and pyloric muscle. Using the Benson spreader with extreme care, further separate the muscle. With the pyloric mucosa exposed, check for mucosal perforation and, if present, close with 4–0 silk.

Step 5. Close the abdominal wall.

■ PYLOROPLASTY

Heineke-Mikulicz Pyloroplasty

Procedure:

Step 1. Put two sutures, one laterally and the other medially, at the middle of the hypothetical longitudinal pyloroduodenal incision (Fig. 7.22).

Step 2. Longitudinally incise the pylorus, including the stenosed duodenal segment. Close the wound transversely by traction of the two previously placed sutures in two layers using 3–0 absorbable sutures and 3–0 silk.

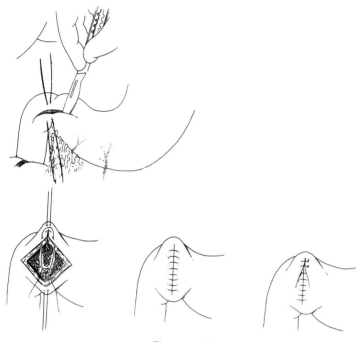

Figure 7.22

Finney Pyloroplasty (Fig. 7.23)

Procedure:

Step 1. Mobilize the first and second portions of the duodenum.

Step 2. With interrupted Lembert suture of 3–0 silk, appose the pyloric area of the stomach and the first portion of the duodenum.

Step 3. Make a U-shaped, inverted incision including the distal pyloric antrum and the proximal second portion of the duodenum. Locate the ulcer and excise it.

Step 4. Close the gastroduodenal opening in layers. Truncal vagotomy may be done if surgery is performed immediately after the perforation of the ulcer.

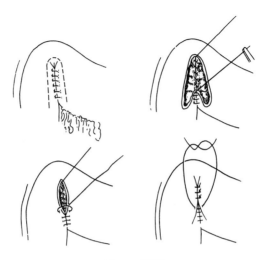

Figure 7.23

■ GASTRECTOMIES

Determination of Some Anatomical Boundaries

Some arbitrary guidelines on which to base gastric resections have been proposed (Fig. 7.24). All may be helpful; none are completely satisfactory.

Guides for 50 Percent Gastric Resection

1. A line starting on the lesser curvature at the 3rd vein down from the gastroesophageal junction to the greater curvature at the point where the left gastroepiploic vessels come closest to the gastric wall.

2. A line starting on the lesser curvature at the first descending branch of the left gastric artery to the greater curvature at the midpoint of the left gastroepiploic artery.

3. See Guide for Antrectomy below and Fig. 7.24.

Guide for 75 Percent Gastric Resection

A line starting on the lesser curvature at the first branch of the left gastric artery to a point on the greater curvature approximately 2.5 cm below the spleen or to a point in the avascular area between the short gastric artery and the left gastroepiploic artery (Fig. 7.24).

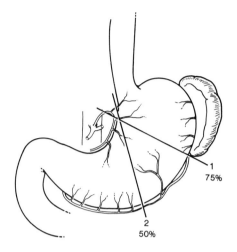

Figure 7.24. Some arbitrary landmarks for partial gastric resection: (line 1) 75 percent resection; (line 2) 50 percent resection. (By permission of JE Skandalakis, SW Gray, and JR Rowe, *Anatomical Complications in General Surgery*, New York: McGraw-Hill, 1983.)

Guide for Antrectomy

The classical external landmarks for the antrum have been the incisura angularis proximally and the pyloric sphincter distally. The proximal landmark is vague and inconsistent. An alternative solution follows:

✓ A line starting on the lesser curvature at the origin of the ascending esophageal branch of the left gastric artery (2–3 cm from the esophagus) to the greater curvature at the anastomosis between the right and left gastroepiploic arteries. This anastomosis is, unfortunately, neither obvious nor constant. The line is usually drawn at the midpoint of the greater curvature. This will remove the antrum together with a small cuff of distal fundus. This is about equal to a 50 percent resection and has the advantage of leaving none of the antral gastrin-producing cell area (Fig. 7.24).

The Location of the Antral Boundary

Deciding how much stomach to resect would be easy if one knew the location of the boundary between the acid-producing gastric glands and the gastrin-producing pyloric glands.

Gastrotomy with Direct Observation

Some feel that there is an internally visible demarcation between the relatively smooth surface of the antral mucosa and the rugose surface of the body mucosa. Others have found this apparent difference to be misleading. Present evidence is that the antral junction may be an irregular line of demarcation or, more often, a zone of transition about 2 mm wide at the lesser curvature and about 3 mm wide at the greater curvature.

Determining the boundary in dogs by using Congo red indicator and electrostimulation of the vagal trunks is a useful method but requires gastrotomy.

Estimation Based on Averages

The boundary starts on the lesser curvature ⅖ of the distance from the pylorus to the cardia. It ends on the greater curvature ⅛ of the distance from the pylorus to the cardia.

Some other factors must be considered (Fig. 7.25). The position of the junction may shift with the pathologic state of the stomach. Also, the area of gastrin-producing antral mucosa appears to expand in the presence of a gastric ulcer, while remaining unchanged in the presence of a duodenal ulcer.

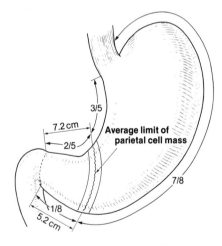

Figure 7.25. The antrum–body junction in the "average stomach" is found at ⅖ of the distance from the pylorus to the cardia along the lesser curvature and ⅛ of the same distance along the greater curvature. (By permission of JE Skandalakis, SW Gray, and JR Rowe, *Anatomical Complications in General Surgery*, New York: McGraw-Hill, 1983.)

Estimation Based on Landmarks

Three landmarks may be used to help determine the junction of antrum and fundus: the pylorus, the "crow's foot" of the gastric divisions of the vagus nerve, and the incisura angularis.

1. The boundary of the antrum starts on the lesser curvature 6–10 cm proximal to the pyloric valve.

2. The boundary of the antrum starts on the lesser curvature 3–4 cm proximal to the "crow's foot."

3. The boundary of the antrum starts at the incisura angularis (which may or may not be present).

4. There are no landmarks on the greater curvature.

As one can see, the preceding guidelines are arbitrary and unsatisfactory.

Mobilization of the Stomach

Mobilization of the stomach may be obtained by (1) incising the gastrosplenic ligament and leaving the spleen in place, (2) mobilizing the spleen and preserving the short gastric arteries, or (3) removing the spleen.

Further mobilization of the stomach may be achieved by incision of the phrenoesophageal ligament to permit the distal esophagus to be brought into the abdomen. Inconstant avascular adhesions between the posterior surface of the stomach and the pancreas may require division.

Mobilization of the Duodenum

The first step is the method of Kocher. The peritoneum lateral to the duodenum is sectioned from the epiploic foramen downward, and the duodenum and head of the pancreas are raised from the underlying vena cava. A laparotomy pad may be placed behind the duodenum and pancreas. Further mobilization may be obtained by separating the first part of the duodenum from the pancreas.

In performing an esophagoduodenectomy after total gastrectomy, as much as 3.5 cm can be gained by sectioning the cystic duct and artery (with removal of the gallbladder), partially releasing the common bile duct, and allowing the duodenum to be rotated.

Complications of Ligation of the Left Gastric Arteries

Ischemia of the Gastric Remnant

Following a radical subtotal gastrectomy, the blood supply to the remaining gastric pouch comes from:

- ascending branches of the left gastric artery
- anterior short gastric arteries
- left inferior phrenic artery
- descending branches from thoracic esophageal branches
- posterior gastric artery

Ischemia Resulting in Gastric Necrosis with Subsequent Anastomotic Leakage and Peritonitis

T-closure of Stomach or Duodenum

T-closures of the stomach or duodenum are not recommended because the blood supply to the resulting corners may be inadequate. A long gastrotomy incision for the management of massive upper gastrointestinal bleeding should not extend past the pylorus, so that if a subsequent gastric resection seems desirable, a T-closure of the duodenal stump may be avoided. Similarly, if the surgeon believes a pyloroplasty may be required, a long exploratory incision might force him to make a T-closure of the pylorus. Fig. 7.26 shows the recommended exploratory incisions for evaluating gastroduodenal hemorrhage.

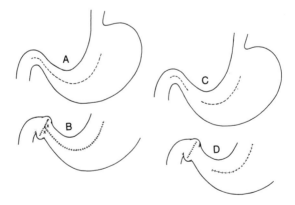

Figure 7.26. Gastrostomy incisions: (A) long incision extending into pylorus; (B) closure of long incision resulting in corners (x) that may become ischemic; (C) two separate incisions; (D) closure avoids the corners of the preceding incision. (By permission of JE Skandalakis, SW Gray, and JR Rowe, *Anatomical Complications in General Surgery*, New York: McGraw-Hill, 1983.)

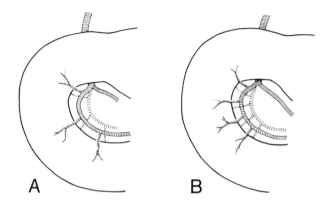

Figure 7.27. Variations of arteries to the duodenum: (A) widely spaced arterial branches; (B) closely spaced arterial branches. These branches should be treated as end arteries, and as many as possible should be preserved. (By permission of JE Skandalakis, SW Gray, and JR Rowe, *Anatomical Complications in General Surgery*, New York: McGraw-Hill, 1983.)

It has been demonstrated that the entire stomach can be perfused through the right gastroepiploic artery alone.

Ischemia of the Duodenal Cuff

The duodenal branches of the pancreaticoduodenal arcades should be treated as end arteries and preserved if possible. This may be especially important in those patients having few, widely spaced (2–3 cm) duodenal branches (Fig. 7.27).

To be within the zone of safety, the minimum length required for anastomosis is 1–2 cm.

Control of Hemorrhage from the Gastroduodenal Artery

The rich submucosal vasculature of the stomach and duodenum becomes a disadvantage in the control of massive hemorrhage from ulcerative erosion of the gastroduodenal artery.

Careful suture ligation of the bleeding site from the inside is the only procedure recommended.

The retroduodenal portion of the gastroduodenal artery is about 2.5 cm from the pylorus and separated by about 0.8 cm (range 0.4–1.2 cm) of pancreatic tissue.

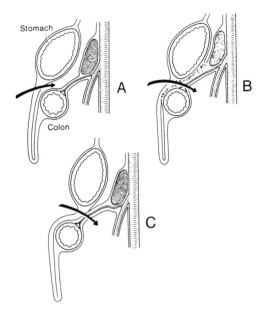

Figure 7.28. Entrance to the lesser sac. (A) Normal anatomy. The arrow indicates entrance through the greater omentum. The middle colic artery in the transverse mesocolon is in no danger. (B) Pathologic fixation of the omentum and posterior wall of the stomach with the transverse mesocolon. (C) Normal anatomy, but entrance so far inferior may injure the middle colic artery. (By permission of JE Skandalakis, SW Gray, and JR Rowe, *Anatomical Complications in General Surgery*, New York: McGraw-Hill, 1983.)

The Middle Colic Artery

A gastrectomy requires the surgeon to enter the lesser peritoneal cavity. Typically, entrance is obtained through the anterior leaf of the greater omentum (Fig. 7.28A). With reasonable care, the surgeon usually avoids perforating the transverse mesocolon, in which lies the middle colic artery.

In the presence of pathology, such as gastric ulcer or pancreatitis, the posterior leaf of the greater omentum and the posterior wall of the stomach may have become fixed to the transverse mesocolon and pancreas, thus eliminating the cavity of the lesser sac and giving the surgeon no warning that the mesocolon has been penetrated (Fig. 7.28B).

Even in the absence of abnormal fixation, should surgeons attempt to enter the lesser sac too far inferiorly, they will pass through the fused anterior leaf and transverse mesocolon (Fig. 7.28C). Under either circumstance, the middle colic vessels may be inadvertently ligated and divided along with the gastroepiploic branches.

The Posterior Gastric Artery

A posterior gastric artery as much as 2 mm in diameter may arise from the proximal or middle third of the splenic artery. It supplies the posterior wall of the upper body, the fundus, and the cardia. Unrecognized, it may be a source of troublesome hemorrhage.

Because there are numerous types of gastrectomies and modifications (antecolic, retrocolic, large stoma [Polya's], small stoma [Hofmeister], Roux-en-Y, etc.), presentation of all of them is not possible within the scope of this book (Figs. 7.29 and 7.30). We have included subtotal distal gastrectomy (Billroth I and Billroth II), the difficult duodenal stump, total gastrectomy for cancer, vagotomy, and highly selective (or proximal gastric) vagotomy.

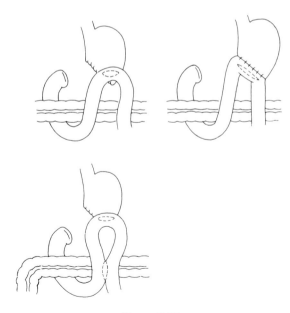

Figure 7.29

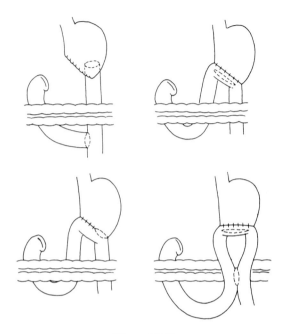

Figure 7.30

Subtotal Distal Gastrectomy

Billroth I (Figs. 7.31–7.33)

Procedure:

Step 1. Mobilize the distal stomach by careful ligation of the arteries and veins of the lesser and greater curvature, distal to the point of the gastric transection. The surgeon now decides whether to perform an 80 percent or 50 percent gastrectomy or antrectomy and ligates the vessels accordingly.

    a. Ligation of the gastrocolic ligament.
Start in the vicinity of the origin of the left gastroepiploic vessels by carefully dividing the ligament between clamps. Ligate with 2-0 silk, proceeding from left to right to reach the gastroduodenal junction.

    b. Remember that the middle colic artery is within the leaflets of the transverse mesocolon. Carefully separate the transverse mesocolon from the posterior gastric wall to

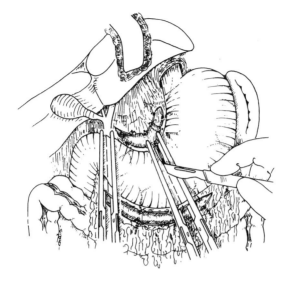

Figure 7.31

avoid injuring this vessel, which occasionally is not anastomosed with the marginal artery and, therefore, may cause problems for the transverse colon.

c. Use small, curved mosquito clamps to skeletonize the gastroduodenal area by ligating the vessel with 3-0 or 4-0 silk.

Step 2. Ligate the vessels of the lesser curvature and the right gastric artery. (To avoid duodenal ischemia, ligate only the number of vessels necessary to perform the anastomosis.) Continue dissecting and ligating toward the left gastric artery, which should be doubly ligated.

Step 3. Place two seromuscular sutures just below the duodenal transection line and a Kocher clamp just distal to the pylorus, but not in the duodenum. Divide the duodenum just distal to the Kocher clamp; this will insure that no gastric mucosa is left at this level. We prefer not to use any clamps at the duodenum.

Step 4. At the designated line of gastric division, place clamps: noncrushing proximally and crushing (Kocher) distally, directed toward the lesser curvature. Then divide the stomach and remove the specimen. Place a suture, as an indicator, at a point

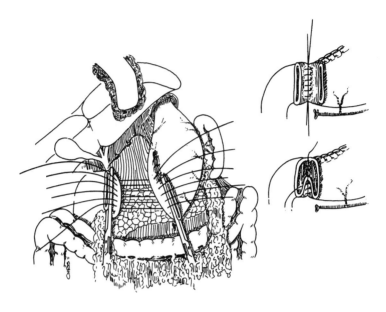

Figure 7.32

of the noncrushing clamp designating the two areas of the gastric remnant, one toward the lesser curvature (which will be closed), and one toward the greater curvature (which will be anastomosed to the duodenum). The first area should be closed with two layers, using 3-0 chromic continuous oversewn, and after removal of the clamp, with 3-0 interrupted silk. Alternatively, a TA-90 stapler may be used for closing the lesser curvature. We like to cover the staple line with 3-0 silk Lembert sutures.

Step 5. Because of some peculiar mobility of the gastric mucosa, we apply Babcock clamps, bringing the mucosal and submucosal layers together so the gastric mucosa will not retract. Obtain hemostasis. Using interrupted 3-0 silk, approximate the gastric and duodenal wall posteriorly. Remove clamps and anastomose the gastric opening (including the gastric wall in toto) to the duodenum. Use a running 3-0 chromic for the mucosae and interrupted 3-0 silk seromuscular for the outside.

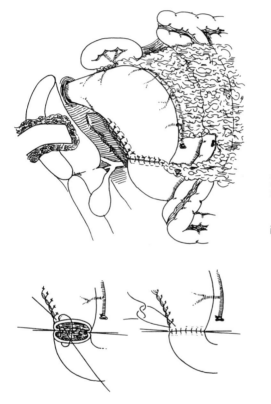

Figure 7.33

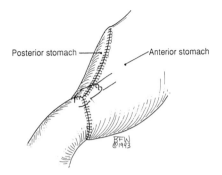

Posterior stomach —   ⟋Anterior stomach

Figure 7.34

Remember the Angle of Sorrow:

✓ This is where three suture lines come together at the lesser curvature area where the stomach and duodenum are anastomosed. This should be reinforced with 3-0 silk, taking seromuscular bites of both sides of the lesser curvature and the duodenum (Fig. 7.34).

Billroth II

Procedure:

Step 1. Mobilize the stomach for 80 percent or 50 percent gastrectomy, or antrectomy as described before for Billroth I. Also, mobilize the first portion of the duodenum to allow enough room for a two-layer closure or for use of the TA-55 stapler across the duodenum. We always support the staple line with interrupted 3-0 silk Lembert sutures. Also, we like to cover the suture line with any piece of fat that may be present in the vicinity.

Step 2. There are many modifications of the Billroth II gastrectomy. The surgeon may decide to use the opening of the gastric remnant in toto or to use part of it as we described in Billroth I. We present only the retrocolic method in Figs. 7.35–7.46, but the antecolic method is acceptable on rare occasions.

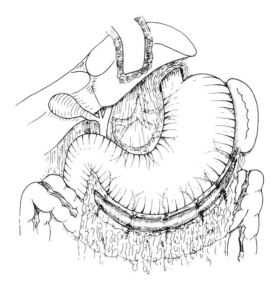

Figure 7.35. Mobilization of the stomach and first part of the duodenum.

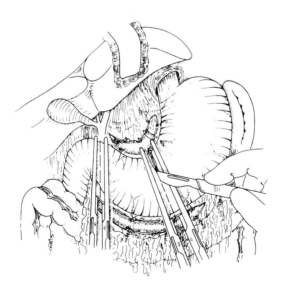

Figure 7.36. Transect and remove the distal stomach and a small part of the first portion of the duodenum.

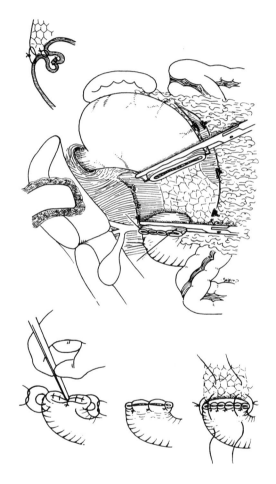

Figure 7.37. The specimen is removed and the duodenum opening is closed in two layers.

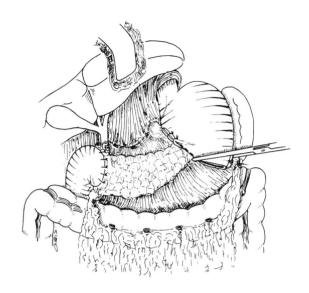

Figure 7.38. Partial closure of the gastric opening at the lesser curvature side.

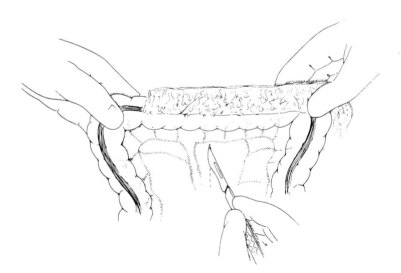

Figure 7.39. Elevate the transverse colon, and through an avascular area of the mesocolon, insert a proximal jejunal loop if a retrocolic anastomosis is desired.

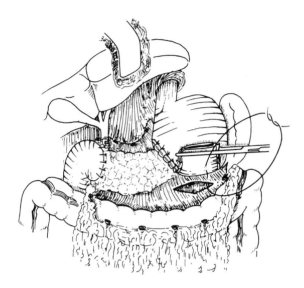

Figure 7.40. Suturing of the mesocolon to the posterior gastric wall close to the opening.

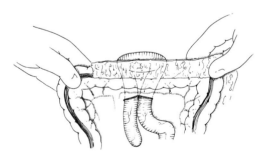

Figure 7.41. The proximal loop is inserted through the opening of the mesocolon.

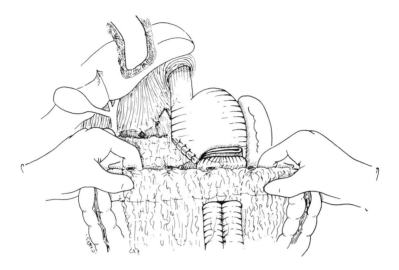

Figure 7.42. The four-layer anastomosis (see also Figs. 7.43 and 7.44).

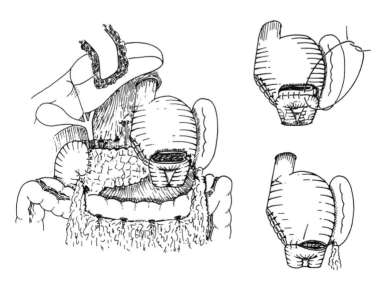

Figure 7.43. The four-layer anastomosis (continued in Fig. 7.44).

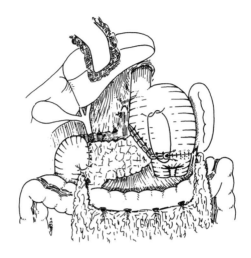

Figure 7.44. Completion of the four-layer anastomosis.

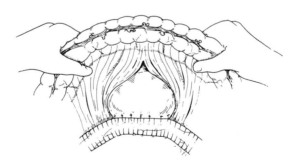

Figure 7.45. Figs. 7.45 and 7.46: An alternative method of anastomosis, bringing the stomach down the mesocolic opening and securing the gastric wall with interrupted sutures to the transverse mesocolon.

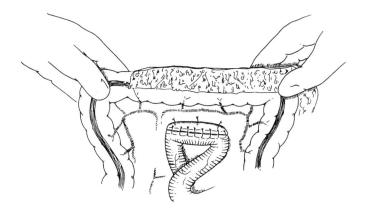

Figure 7.46

The Difficult Duodenal Stump

Procedure:

Step 1. Close the duodenal stump as perfectly as possible. We prefer to make a small abdominal wall incision close to the duodenal stump and insert an 18–22 French Foley catheter with balloon. Make a small cut distal to the suture line of the stump in the duodenal wall and insert the tip of the catheter, directed downward to the second portion of the duodenum. Use a 3–0 purse-string silk suture at the site of the duodenostomy tube and cover the area with an omental piece. Then use one or two more 3–0 silk sutures to bring the duodenostomy tube area to the abdominal wall to eliminate dead space between it and the duodenal stump. Secure the tube to the skin with a 2–0 silk suture.

Another method is to place the catheter into the duodenal stump and close the stump around the catheter in two layers, and to wrap the stump and tube with omentum. Remember to avoid dead space.

Total Gastrectomy for Cancer

Note:

The specimen should include the following: (Fig. 7.47)

- gastroesophageal junction
- lesser omentum (hepatogastric and partial hepatoduodenal ligaments)
- distal pancreas, as required
- greater omentum, including gastrocolic ligament, but protecting the transverse mesocolon, which contains the middle colic artery
- spleen
- left lobe of the liver, if required by the presence of local extension
- other neighboring anatomical entities involved by metastasis or by direct extension
- all the lymphovascular tissue around the stomach

Procedure:

Step 1. Approach the gastroesophageal area and, with the index finger, penetrate the local avascular ligaments. Insert a Penrose drain for traction of the abdominal esophagus (Fig. 7.48).

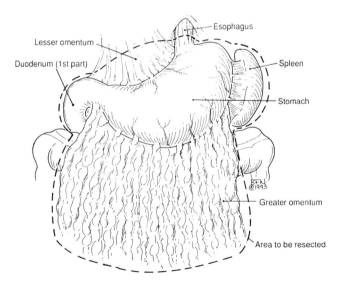

Figure 7.47

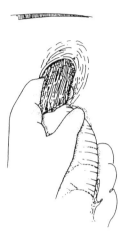

Figure 7.48

Step 2. Elevate the greater omentum and carefully separate it from the transverse colon (Figs. 7.49 and 7.50). Treat the duodenum and the lower pole of the spleen with care. If the surgeon decides to perform a splenectomy, the splenic veins and ligaments should be ligated and cut. Continue the upward dissection of the greater omentum, with ligation of the upper short gastric vessels.

Step 3. Remove the lesser omentum. Ligate doubly the right and left gastric arteries. We prefer sharp and blunt dissection, pushing all the tissues from the porta hepatis toward the greater curvature (Fig. 7.51).

Step 4. With complete gastric mobilization from the gastroesophageal junction to the proximal portion of the second part of the duodenum, divide the duodenum and the abdominal esophagus (Fig. 7.52). Place 3-0 silk stay sutures on each side of the esophagus (Fig. 7.53). Remove the specimen.

Step 5. Perform duodenal closure as described previously. Gastrointestinal continuity is accomplished by a Roux-en-Y esophagojejunal anastomosis as follows: Divide the jejunum between the GIA stapler. Sacrifice one or two (preferably, one) arterial arcades. Pass the distal end of the divided bowel through a small hole of the transverse colon. Anastomose end-to-side or end-to-end with the esophagus using 4-0 interrupted silk (Fig.

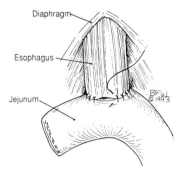

Figure 7.53

7.54). Be careful that the esophageal mucosa retracts upward, and be sure to include all the esophageal layers in your bites. Before the anterior layer is closed, pass the nasogastric tube into the jejunal loop. We protect the anastomosis with two or three interrupted silk sutures, anchoring the jejunal wall just

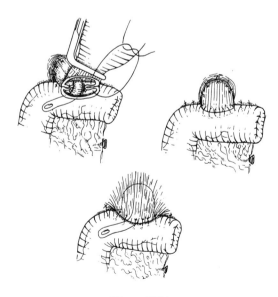

Figure 7.54

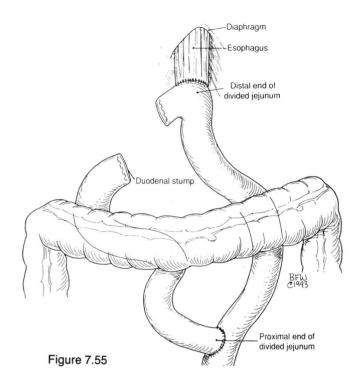

Figure 7.55

below the suture line to the esophageal hiatus. We prefer the end-to-side anastomosis.

Step 6. Anastomose the opening of the proximal jejunum to the jejunal loop in two layers. Fix the opening of the transverse mesocolon to the jejunum with a few 4-0 silk interrupted sutures (Fig. 7.55).

Step 7. Close the abdomen.

■ THE VAGOTOMIES

There are four types of vagotomy: truncal, selective, parietal cell, and extended proximal.

Truncal Vagotomy

A truncal vagotomy is performed by sectioning the anterior and posterior trunks within the abdomen (Fig. 7.7). This procedure destroys the vagal innervation to the stomach and all other abdominal viscera. Identification is subordinate in this procedure; complete transection is the goal.

Complete skeletonization of the abdominal esophagus is mandatory, and pyloric drainage is usually necessary.

Selective Vagotomy

In selective vagotomy, only the anterior and posterior descending nerves of the gastric divisions (nerves of Latarjet) are divided. The hepatic branch of the anterior division, including the pyloric branch, and the celiac branch of the posterior division are preserved (Fig. 7.56). Thus, the stomach is denervated, while the vagal fibers to the pylorus, the biliary tract, and the intestines remain intact.

Parietal Cell Vagotomy

A parietal cell vagotomy may also be called "highly selective vagotomy," "superselective vagotomy," "proximal gastric vagotomy," or "acidosecretive vagotomy." The goal is denervation of the proximal ⅔ of the stomach only, preserving the antral and pyloric innervation as well as the hepatic and celiac divisions. Denervation is accomplished by sectioning of the proximal gastric branches of the descending anterior and posterior

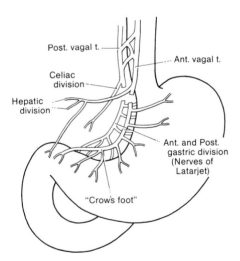

Figure 7.56. Selective vagotomy preserves the celiac and hepatic divisions but will not denervate the pylorus, biliary tract, and remaining intestinal tract. (By permission of JE Skandalakis, SW Gray, and JR Rowe, *Anatomical Complications in General Surgery*, New York: McGraw-Hill, 1983.)

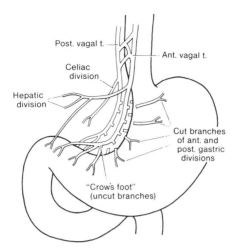

Figure 7.57. Parietal cell (superselective) vagotomy preserves antropyloric as well as celiac and hepatic innervation. There is some risk of perforation as a result of ischemia of the lesser curvature. (By permission of JE Skandalakis, SW Gray, and JR Rowe, *Anatomical Complications in General Surgery*, New York: McGraw-Hill, 1983.)

nerves of Latarjet while preserving the distal branches to the antrum and pylorus (Fig. 7.57).

The distal extent of a highly selective vagotomy is to the left of the "crow's foot," about 7 cm from the pylorus. This may or may not coincide with the location of the boundary between the antrum and the body of the stomach. Various authors state that the distal limit of dissection should be between 5 and 10 cm from the pylorus.

Extended Proximal Vagotomy

Extended proximal vagotomy for complete gastric denervation as shown in Fig. 7.58 consists of vagal denervation of the gastric fundus and greater curvature of the stomach.

Incomplete Vagotomy

Vagotomy may be said to be complete if no areas of parietal cell activity can be found with a pH probe; if activity is found, the vagotomy is

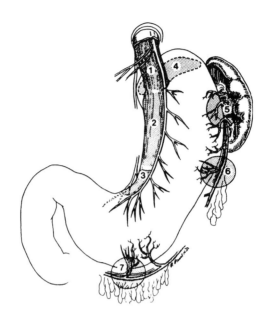

Figure 7.58. The seven areas of vagotomy. Preganglionic efferent vagus nerves reach the parietal cell mass in seven areas. Area 1 is the periesophageal region; area 2 is the lesser curve of the stomach; area 3 is the crow's foot area; area 4 is represented by the broken line, as the gastropancreatic fold is not visible anteriorly; area 5 is the region of short gastric vessels; area 6 is the left gastroepiploic pedicle; and area 7 is the right gastroepiploic pedicle. Areas 3, 4, 6, and 7 are divided routinely during extended highly selective vagotomy. Area 5 is preserved because the nerves at this site cannot be divided without sacrificing essential blood supply to the proximal part of the stomach. (By permission of PE Donahue, HM Richter, KJM Liu, et al., *Surg Gynecol Obstet* 1: 176, 1993.)

incomplete. Clinically, vagotomy may be considered complete if there is no recurrence of an ulcer.

Gastric branches arising from vagal trunks proximal to the separation of the major division may be present and, if so, must be sectioned. The first and highest of such posterior branches is the "criminal nerve of Grassi."

■ SURGICAL PROCEDURES

Truncal Vagotomy

Procedure:

Step 1. Mobilize the abdominal esophagus by peritoneal incision of the gastroesophageal junction. Palpate the abdominal esophagus. Locate the anterior vagus nerve and mobilize it with a nerve hook. Remove a segment of the nerve, clip the proximal and distal ends, and send the specimen to the lab for frozen section (Fig. 7.59).

Step 2. Palpate the posterior area. The nerve may be located close to the aorta between the right and left diaphragmatic crura and slightly right of the midline. Again, remove a segment of the nerve, clip the proximal and distal ends, and send to the lab for frozen section (Fig. 7.60).

Step 3. Because the vagus nerve exhibits many vagaries, it is important to skeletonize the esophagus.

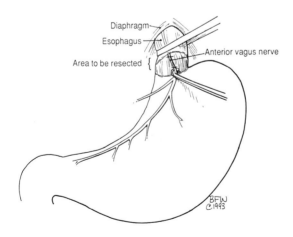

Figure 7.59

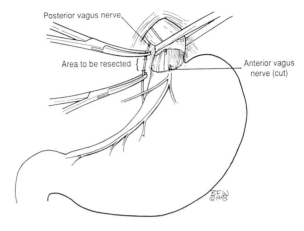

Figure 7.60

Parietal Cell Vagotomy

Procedure:

Step 1. Mobilize the abdominal esophagus at the periesophageal space. Localize the right and left vagus nerves, which should be protected. Localize the nerves of Latarjet. Protect the hepatic division and celiac divisions.

Step 2. Mobilize the distal half of the greater curvature. Starting approximately 6 cm from the pylorus, begin an upward dissection of the neurovascular elements between the inner curve and the nerve of Latarjet, by dividing and ligating them with 4–0 silk. Continue dissection toward the cardiac angle.

Remember:

✓ Protect the trunks
✓ Protect the nerves of Latarjet
✓ Protect the pyloric branch
✓ Protect the crow's foot

Step 3. Re-peritonealization.
Re-peritonealize the lesser curve by approximating the anterior and posterior walls with interrupted 3–0 silk.

8

Duodenum

ANATOMY

■ GENERAL DESCRIPTION OF THE DUODENUM

The first portion of the duodenum passes slightly upward from the pylorus to the neck of the gallbladder. The proximal end is movable and enclosed by the same peritoneal layers that invest the stomach. The distal half of the first portion becomes retroperitoneal. Posteriorly, this portion is related to the common bile duct, the portal vein, the gastroduodenal artery, and the inferior vena cava.

The second (descending) portion lies posterior to the transverse mesocolon and anterior to the right kidney and the inferior vena cava. The left border is attached to the head of the pancreas.

The common bile and pancreatic ducts open into the left side of this portion of the duodenum.

Typically the third portion of the duodenum (about 7.5 cm long) is horizontal and the fourth portion (2.5–5.0 cm long) is ascending.

The third and fourth portions of the duodenum lie inferior to the transverse mesocolon. Their cranial surfaces are in contact with the uncinate process of the pancreas (Fig. 8.1). The parietal peritoneum covering the fourth portion of the duodenum contains folds beneath which are blind recesses or paraduodenal fossae.

The third, or horizontal, portion of the duodenum passes to the left and slightly upward, crossing anterior to the inferior vena cava and posterior to the superior mesenteric artery and vein.

The fourth, or ascending, portion passes upward and slightly to the left, crossing the spine anterior to the aorta. It may cover the origin of the inferior mesenteric artery from the aorta. The duodenum ends at the duodenojejunal flexure where it is fixed by the suspensory ligament (of Treitz). The flexure usually lies immediately to the left of the aorta.

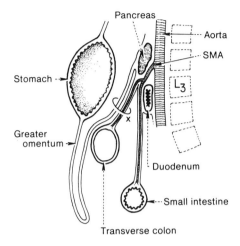

Figure 8.1. Diagrammatic sagittal section showing the position of the duodenum in relation to the aorta and the superior mesenteric artery. The transverse mesocolon is marked by an X. (Modified by permission of SW Gray, JT Akin, JH Milsap, et al., *Contemp Surg* 10:33–56, 1977.)

■ SURGICAL ANATOMY OF THE DUODENUM

At the gastroduodenal junction, the continuity of the circular musculature is interrupted by a ring-shaped septum of connective tissue derived from the submucosa. Proximal to this ring, the circular muscle layer is thickened to form the pyloric sphincter of the stomach; distal to the ring there is an abrupt decrease in the thickness of the circular muscle to form the relatively thin-walled duodenum. This decrease results in a pyloric "os pylorus" surrounded by a duodenal fornix. This arrangement must be kept in mind when performing pyloromyotomy.

Internally, the appearance of the submucosal glands of Brunner marks the gastroduodenal junction. This may not agree with the muscular junction. In humans, the submucosal glands may extend a few centimeters into the pylorus, and occasionally, antral gastric mucosa may prolapse through the pylorus, producing a radiological finding but not a true clinical syndrome. The duodenojejunal junction is marked externally by the attachment of the suspensory ligament of Treitz.

The suspensory muscle or ligament is a fibromuscular band that arises from the right crus of the diaphragm and inserts on the upper surface of the duodenojejunal flexure. It passes posterior to the pancreas and the splenic vein and anterior to the left renal vein.

The suspensory ligament usually inserts on the duodenal flexure and the third and fourth portions of the duodenum (Fig. 8.2B). It may insert on the flexure only (Fig. 8.2A), or on the third and fourth portions only (Fig. 8.2C). There may also be multiple attachments (Fig. 8.2D).

■ DUODENAL VASCULAR SYSTEM

Arteries

The blood supply of the duodenum is confusing due to origin, distribution and individual variations (Figs. 8.3–8.5). This is especially true of the blood supply of the first portion of the duodenum.

The first part of the duodenum is supplied by the supraduodenal artery and the posterior superior pancreaticoduodenal branch of the gastroduodenal artery (retroduodenal artery of Edwards, Michel, and Wilkie), which is a branch of the common hepatic artery.

The remaining three parts of the duodenum are supplied by an anterior and a posterior arcade. From the arcades spring pancreatic and duodenal branches. Those supplying the duodenum are called arteriae rectae; they may be embedded in the substance of the pancreas.

Four arteries contribute to the pancreaticoduodenal vascular arcades. The anterior superior pancreaticoduodenal arteries (commonly two in number) arise from the gastroduodenal artery on the ventral surface of the pancreas. The second, the posterior superior pancreaticoduodenal (retroduodenal) artery, usually passes in front of the common bile duct and descends on the posterior surface of the pancreas, then crosses behind the bile duct and joins the posterior branch of the inferior pancreaticoduodenal artery. The anterior inferior and posterior inferior pancreaticoduodenal arteries, the 3rd and 4th arteries, arise from the superior mesenteric artery or its first jejunal branch, either separately or from a common stem.

The surgeon should be sure to ligate only one of the two arcades, superior or inferior only.

Veins

The veins of the lower first part of the duodenum and the pylorus usually open into the right gastroepiploic veins (Figs. 8.6 and 8.7).

The venous arcades draining the duodenum follow the arterial arcades and tend to lie superficial to them.

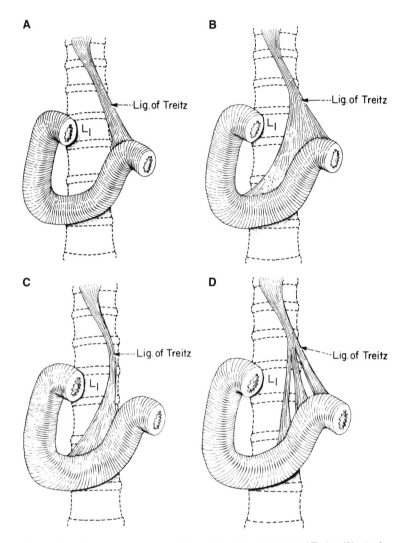

Figure 8.2. Four configurations of the suspensory ligament of Treitz: (A) attachment to the duodenojejunal flexure; (B) attachments to the flexure and the third
and fourth portions of the duodenum; (C) attachments to the third and fourth
portions only; (D) multiple separated attachments of the suspensory ligament.
(By permission of JE Skandalakis, JT Akin, JH Milsap, et al., *Contemp Surg*, 10:
33–56, 1977.)

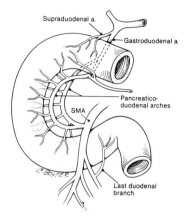

Figure 8.3. Major arterial supply to the duodenum. (By permission of SW Gray, GL Colborn, LB Pemberton, LJ Skandalakis, JE Skandalakis, *Am Surg* 15(4):257–261; 15(5):291–298; 15(7):469–473; 15(8):492–494, 1989.)

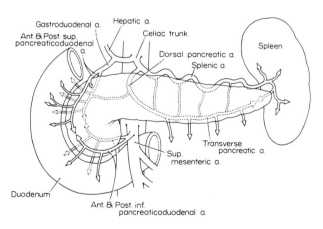

Figure 8.4. Anterior view of arterial supply of the duodenum and pancreas. (By permission of JE Skandalakis, SW Gray, JS Rowe, et al., *Contemp Surg* 15(5):17–40 and 15(6):21–50, 1979.)

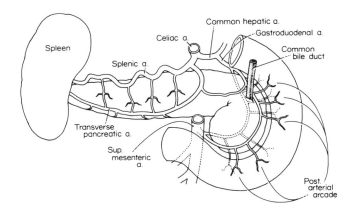

Figure 8.5. Posterior view of arterial supply of the duodenum and pancreas. (By permission of JE Skandalakis, SW Gray, JS Rowe, et al., *Contemp Surg* 15(5):17–40 and 15(6):21–50, 1979.)

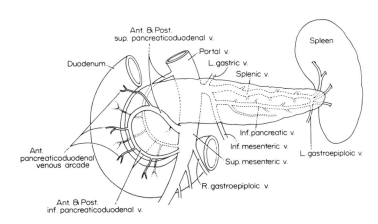

Figure 8.6. The venous drainage of the duodenum and pancreas: anterior view. (By permission of JE Skandalakis, SW Gray, JS Rowe, et al., *Contemp Surg* 15(5):17–40 and 15(6):21–50, 1979.)

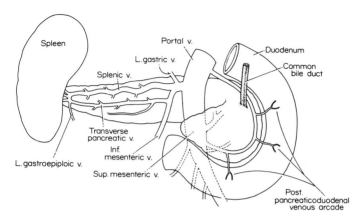

Figure 8.7. The venous drainage of the duodenum and pancreas, and formation of the hepatic portal vein: posterior view. (By permission of JE Skandalakis, SW Gray, JS Rowe, et al., *Contemp Surg* 15(5):17–40 and 15(6):21–50, 1979.)

Lymphatic Drainage

The duodenum is richly supplied with lymphatics (Fig. 8.8). Collecting trunks pass over the anterior and posterior duodenal wall toward the

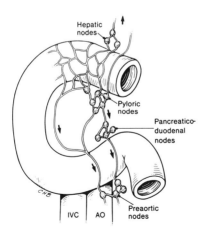

Figure 8.8. Diagrammatic presentation of duodenal lymphatica. (By permission of SW Gray, LB Pemberton, LJ Skandalakis, et al., *Am Surg* 55, 1989.)

lesser curvature to enter the anterior and posterior pancreaticoduodenal lymph nodes.

Although lymphatics of the pancreas have received some attention, those of the duodenum have received very little.

■ NERVE SUPPLY OF THE DUODENUM

Within the duodenal wall, there are two plexuses. Meissner's plexus is in the submucosa, and Auerbach's plexus is between the circular and the longitudinal layers of the muscularis externa. In six of the 100 specimens we examined, nerves from the hepatic division of the anterior vagal trunk gave rise to one or more branches that innervated the first part of the duodenum. In most specimens, such branches could only be traced to or above the gastric incisura. The vagus nerve has numerous vagaries.

TECHNIQUE

Surgery of the duodenum includes duodenotomy, duodenostomy, duodenal resection, partial anastomosis with stomach or jejunum, etc. Most of these surgical techniques are described in other chapters in connection with other organs such as the stomach (Chapter 7) and the pancreas (Chapter 9). The authors present here only the duodenal exposure and the superior mesenteric artery syndrome (vascular compression of the duodenum).

■ SURGICAL APPLICATIONS

First Part of the Duodenum

Good results from surgical procedures in the first part of the duodenum can be anticipated if the surgeon has good anatomical knowledge and practices good technique and conservative skeletonization. The blood supply to this area is questionable.

Second Part of the Duodenum

Because of the fixation of the duodenum and pancreas, the common blood supply for both organs (superior and inferior pancreaticoduodenal arcades), and the opening of the common bile duct and pancreatic ducts, the duodenum is one of the most difficult areas to approach when operating. A pancreaticoduodenectomy should be performed when malignant disease is found; but with benign disease, a more conservative approach, such as segmental resection, is the preferred treatment.

Third Part of the Duodenum

The proximal third of the duodenum is difficult to deal with because of its relationship to the head of the pancreas and the uncinate process. It is important to be aware of the superior mesenteric vessels, the transverse mesocolon with its marginal artery and the middle colic artery, and the inferior mesenteric artery, which in most cases is covered by the third portion of the duodenum. The surgeon should proceed slowly dealing with the uncinate process, which is closely related to the superior mesenteric vessels. The inferior pancreaticoduodenal arcades yield many small vessels, and small twigs from the superior mesenteric artery are present.

Fourth Part of the Duodenum

The fourth portion of the duodenum is related to two important anatomical entities: the ligament of Treitz and the inferior mesenteric vein, located to the left of the paraduodenal fossae. This portion is a useful place to begin exploring the distal duodenum (third and fourth portions), and the surgeon should remember that mobilization of the right colon and transection of the ligament of Treitz are necessary for good exposure of the distal duodenum. The divisions of the intestinal branches of the superior mesenteric artery provide the blood supply, which is similar to that of the rest of the small bowel. The arteries have no collateral circulation and the wall has the least efficient blood supply in the antimesenteric border. (The duodenum does not have a mesentery; the middle of the anterior wall, which is covered by peritoneum, should be considered "antimesenteric.")

■ EXPOSURE AND MOBILIZATION OF THE DUODENUM (Figs. 8.9–8.11)

It may be necessary to expose the duodenum to search for traumatic injury, for pancreatic procedures, for exploration of the distal common bile duct, for section of the suspensory ligament to relieve duodenal compression, or to reduce a redundant proximal loop of a gastrojejunostomy above the transverse mesocolon. Exposure can be accomplished by the following maneuvers:

1. Mobilization of the second and proximal third portions of the duodenum is obtained by incising the parietal peritoneum along the descending duodenum (second portion) and retracting it medially; this is the Kocher maneuver. The posterior wall of the duodenum can be examined and the retroduodenal and pancreatic portions of the common bile duct can be explored.

2. An incision through the transverse mesocolon or the gastrocolic omentum, or reflection of the right half of the colon, exposes the third portion of the duodenum, proximal to the superior mesenteric vessels; this is the Cattell maneuver (Fig. 8.11).

3. Incision through the gastrocolic omentum and further reflection of the right colon provides exposure of the duodenum distal to the

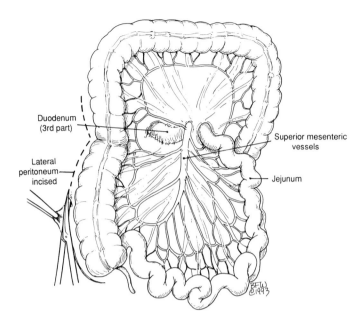

Figure 8.9. Mobilization of the right colon by incision of the lateral peritoneum and exposure of the 3rd part of the duodenum by incision of the transverse mesocolon. Note that the superior mesenteric vein is not shown.

superior mesenteric vessels. By dividing the parietal fold just inferior to the paraduodenal fossa, the distal duodenum can be visualized. The duodenum can be further mobilized by transection of the suspensory muscle.

Surgical notes to remember:

✓ It is impossible to perform duodenectomy alone because the head of the pancreas is fixed to the duodenal loop; the only practical procedure is pancreaticoduodenectomy.

✓ It is important not to ligate both the superior and the inferior pancreaticoduodenal arteries. The result may be necrosis of the head of the pancreas and of a great part of the duodenum.

✓ The accessory pancreatic duct (of Santorini) passes under the gastrointestinal artery. To avoid injury to or ligation of the duct, ligate the artery away from the anterior medial duodenal wall where the papilla is located. "Water under the bridge" applies to the gastroduodenal artery and the accessory pancreatic duct as well as to the

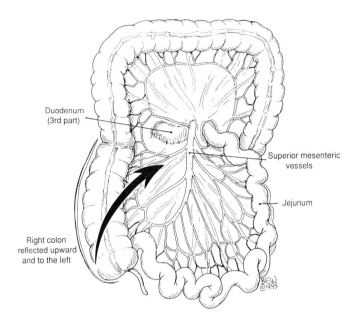

Figure 8.10. Arrow indicating medial retraction of the right colon. Note that the superior mesenteric vein is not shown.

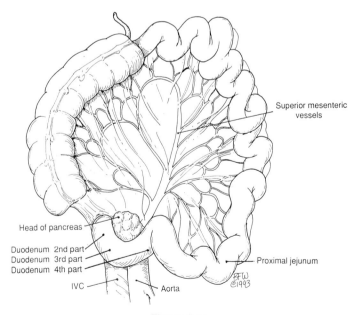

Figure 8.11

relation of the uterine artery and ureter. In 10 percent of cases, the duct of Santorini is the only duct draining the pancreas; therefore, it would be catastrophic if the duct were ligated accidentally along with the gastroduodenal artery.

✓ No more than 2 cm of the first part of the duodenum should be skeletonized. If more is done, it may necessitate a duodenostomy to avoid blowup of the stump secondary to poor blood supply.

✓ The suspensory ligament may be transected and ligated with impunity.

✓ When dealing with a large, penetrating posterior duodenal or pyloric ulcer, the surgeon should remember that: the proximal duodenum shortens because of the inflammatory process (duodenal shortening); the anatomical topography of the distal common bile duct as well as the opening of the duct of Santorini and the ampulla of Vater is distorted; leaving the ulcer in situ is a wise decision; and useful procedures include careful palpation or visualization of the location of the ampulla of Vater or common bile duct exploration with a catheter insertion into the common bile duct and the duodenum.

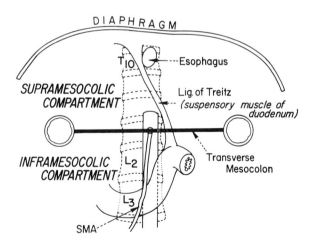

Supra and Inframesocolic Compartments

Notice the origin of lig. of Treitz and the normal location of duodenum.

Figure 8.12. (By permission of JE Skandalakis, JT Akin, JH Milsap, et al., *Contemp Surg* 10:33–56, 1977.)

✓ The common bile duct, in most cases, is located to the right of the gastroduodenal artery at the posterior wall of the first portion of the duodenum. In many cases, the artery crosses the supraduodenal portion of the common bile duct anteriorly or posteriorly, a phenomenon also observed with the posterosuperior pancreaticoduodenal artery, which crosses the common bile duct ventrally and dorsally.

■ SURGICAL ANATOMY AND REPAIR OF THE VASCULAR COMPRESSION OF THE DUODENUM (Figs. 8.2 and 8.12–8.16)

Procedure:

Step 1. Isolate, ligate, and divide the ligament of Treitz. This allows the duodenum to drop far enough for the surgeon to insert two fingers between the duodenum and the origin of the superior mesenteric artery.

Step 2. If the duodenum does not fall sufficiently, then a duodenojejunostomy is the next step.

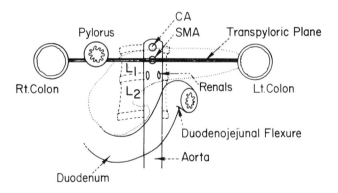

Transpyloric Plane

With a little imagination the pancreas and transverse mesocolon are at the same line.

Figure 8.13. (By permission of JE Skandalakis, JT Akin, JH Milsap, et al., *Contemp Surg* 10:33–56, 1977.)

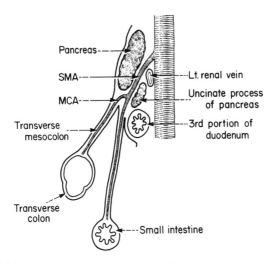

Figure 8.14. Diagrammatic sagittal section showing the duodenum between the superior mesenteric vessel and the aorta. (By permission of JE Skandalakis, JT Akin, JH Milsap, et al., *Contemp Surg* 10:33–56, 1977.)

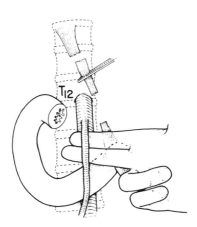

Figure 8.15. Section of the ligament of Treitz will usually allow the duodenum to drop far enough to admit two fingers between the superior mesenteric artery and the aorta. (By permission of JT Akin, JH Milsap, SW Gray, et al., *Contemp Surg* 10:33–56, 1977.)

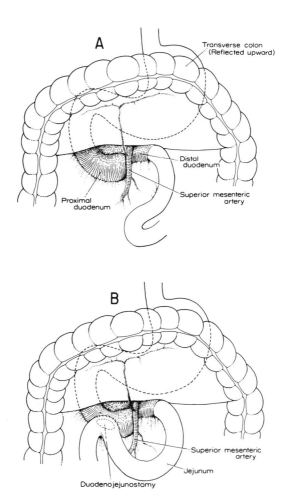

Figure 8.16. (A) Note the dilated proximal duodenum. (B) Duodenojejunostomy bypassing the obstruction. (By permission of SW Gray, LJ Skandalakis, JS Rowe, et al. In: Nyhus LM, Baker, RJ. *Mastery of Surgery*, 2nd ed. Boston: Little, Brown, 1992, pp 764–772.)

9

Pancreas

ANATOMY

■ GENERAL DESCRIPTION OF THE PANCREAS

The pancreas lies transversely in the retroperitoneal area between the
duodenum on the right and the spleen on the left. It is related to the
omental bursa above, the transverse mesocolon anteriorly, and the
greater sac below, and it is a fixed organ.

Anteriorly, the pancreas is related to other organs from right to left as
follows (Fig. 9.1):

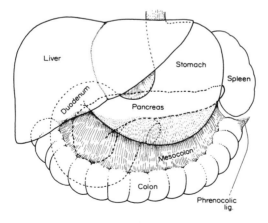

Figure 9.1. Anterior relationships of the pancreas. (By permission of JE Skandalakis, SW Gray, JS Rowe, et al., *Contemp Surg* 15(5):17–40, 1979.)

ABOVE: Duodenum, pylorus, liver, stomach, spleen

BELOW: Duodenum, jejunum, transverse colon, spleen

INTERMEDIATE: Transverse colon, mesocolon, transverse mesocolon, spleen

On the anterior surface of the head and across the duodenum, the transverse mesocolon is very short, so that the colon itself is attached to the underlying organ.

The second and third parts of the duodenum are overlapped by the head of the pancreas, so that there is a pancreatic "bare area" of the duodenum that is not covered by peritoneum. A second bare area exists on the anterior surface of the second portion of the duodenum, where the transverse colon is attached (Fig. 9.2). With pancreatic cancer or pancreatitis, the pancreas and the mesocolon with its middle colic artery become firmly fixed.

Posteriorly the pancreatic bed in the retroperitoneal space consists of an area between the hilum of the right kidney, the hilum of the spleen, the celiac artery, and the inferior mesenteric artery. From right to left, the area contains the hilum of the right kidney, the inferior vena cava, the portal vein, the superior mesenteric vein, the aorta, the left kidney, and the hilum of the spleen (Fig. 9.3).

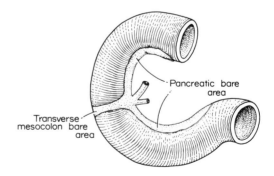

Figure 9.2. Bare areas of the duodenum. The whole of the concave surface is in intimate contact with the pancreas; the attachment of the transverse mesocolon crosses the anterior surface of the second portion. (By permission of JE Skandalakis, SW Gray, JS Rowe, et al., *Contemp Surg* 15(5):17–40, 1979.)

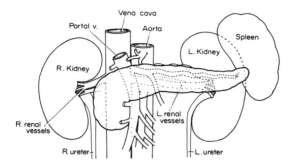

Figure 9.3. Posterior relationships of the pancreas. Anterior view. (By permission of JE Skandalakis, SW Gray, JS Rowe, et al, *Contemp Surg* 15(5)17–40, 1979.)

■ PARTS OF THE PANCREAS

The pancreas may be arbitrarily divided into five parts: head, uncinate process, neck, body, and tail (Fig. 9.4).

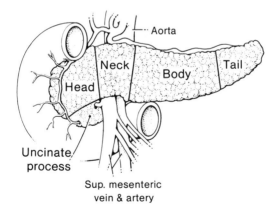

Figure 9.4. The five parts of the pancreas. The line between the body and the tail is arbitrary. (By permission of JE Skandalakis, SW Gray, and JR Rowe, *Anatomical Complications in General Surgery*, New York: McGraw-Hill, 1983.)

Head

The head of the pancreas is that portion lying to the right of the superior mesenteric artery and vein. It is firmly fixed to the medial aspect of the second and third parts of the duodenum. Its junction with the neck is marked anteriorly by an imaginary line from the portal vein above to the superior mesenteric vein below.

The anterior pancreaticoduodenal arcade parallels the duodenal curvature, but it must be considered to be related to the anterior pancreatic surface rather than to the duodenum.

Posteriorly, the surface is related to the hilum and medial border of the right kidney, the right renal vessels, the inferior vena cava with the entrance of the left renal vein into it, the right crus of the diaphragm, the posterior pancreaticoduodenal arcade, the right gonadal vein, and the distal portion of the common bile duct.

Uncinate Process

The uncinate process of the pancreas is an extension of the lower left part of the posterior surface of the head, usually passing behind the portal vein and the superior mesenteric vessels and in front of the aorta and inferior vena cava. In sagittal section, the uncinate process is located between the superior mesenteric artery and the aorta, having the left renal vein above and the third or fourth part of the duodenum below (see Fig. 8.14).

The uncinate process may be absent or it may completely encircle the superior mesenteric vessels (Fig. 9.5). If the process is well developed, sectioning of the neck of the pancreas must be done from the front to avoid injury to the superior mesenteric vessels or the portal veins.

Very short vessels from the superior mesenteric artery and vein provide the blood supply to the uncinate process. They must be ligated with extreme care.

Neck

The neck, from 1.5 to 2 cm in length, is fixed between the celiac trunk above and the superior mesenteric vessels below. It is roughly that portion of the pancreas lying over the superior mesenteric vessels.

At the right, the gastroduodenal artery gives off the anterosuperior pancreaticoduodenal artery, its origin being at the upper part of the neck near its junction with the head.

Posteriorly, the portal vein is formed by the confluence of the superior mesenteric and splenic veins. One or two small veins may enter the portal

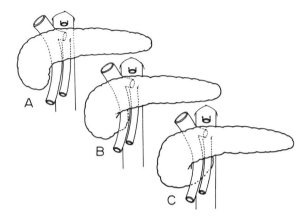

Figure 9.5. Variations in the extent of the uncinate process of the pancreas. (By permission of JE Skandalakis, SW Gray, JS Rowe, et al., *Contemp Surg* 15(5):17–40, 1979.)

vein, and four or five may enter the superior mesenteric vein. Careful elevation of the neck and ligation of these short vessels, if they are present, may be necessary to avoid bleeding that will make it difficult to evaluate the structures lying beneath the neck.

Entering the portal vein from the right are a few small, short lateral veins; from the left are the left gastric, the splenic, and rarely, the inferior mesenteric vein.

Body

The body of the pancreas lies to the left of the superior mesenteric vessels and is related to the fourth part of the duodenum, the suspensory muscle (of Treitz), some jejunal loops, and the left side of the transverse colon. The superior mesenteric artery on the left and the superior mesenteric vein on the right emerge from under the inferior border and pass over the uncinate process of the head (Fig. 9.5). Superiorly, the border is related to the celiac axis and the hepatic artery on the right and to the splenic vessels on the left.

Anteriorly, the body of the pancreas is covered by the double peritoneal layer of the posterior wall of the omental bursa, which separates the pancreas from the stomach. It is also related to the transverse mesocolon, which separates into two layers, one leaf covering the anterior surface and one leaf covering the inferior surface. The middle colic artery travels between the leaves of the mesocolon (see Fig. 8.14). The paraduodenal fossae and the inferior mesenteric vein are close to the distal portion of the inferior border of the pancreatic body.

Posteriorly, the surface is related to the aorta, the origin of the superior mesenteric artery, the left crus of the diaphragm, the left adrenal gland, the perirenal fascia, the left renal vessels, the left kidney, and the splenic vein (Fig. 9.3). The splenic vein, the most superficial of all the vessels, accepts numerous small veins from the pancreas. These must be ligated carefully in order to avoid injury to the splenic vein if the spleen is to be preserved.

Tail

The tail is relatively mobile, and its tip reaches the visceral surface of the spleen. Together with the splenic artery and the beginning of the splenic vein, it is enveloped by the two layers of the splenorenal ligament.

The outer layer of this ligament forms the posterior layer of the gastrosplenic ligament, so careless division may injure the short gastric vessels. The ligament itself is nearly avascular, but digital excavation should stop at the pedicle.

■ PANCREATIC DUCTS

The main pancreatic duct (of Wirsung) and the accessory duct lie anterior to the major pancreatic vessels. Pathological ducts are readily palpated and opened from the anterior surface.

Because of the developmental origin of the two pancreatic ducts, a number of variations are encountered. The relative frequency of the ductal patterns is as follows:

- In 60 percent, both ducts open into the duodenum (Fig. 9.6A).
- In 30 percent, the duct of Wirsung carries the entire secretion. The duct of Santorini ends blindly (Fig. 9.6B).
- In 10 percent, the duct of Santorini carries the entire secretion. The duct of Wirsung is small or absent (Fig. 9.6C).
- Other configurations are rare.

The greatest diameter of the pancreatic duct is in the head of the pancreas, just before the duct enters the duodenal wall.

Two to 3 ml of contrast medium will fill the main pancreatic duct in the living patient, and 7 to 10 ml will fill the branches and the smaller ducts.

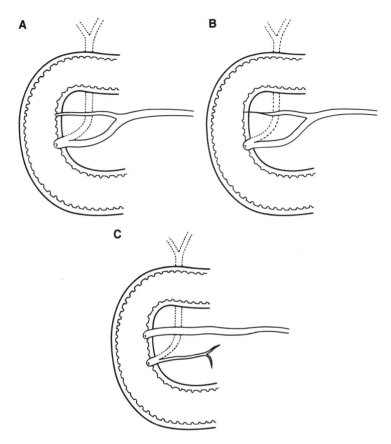

Figure 9.6. Variations of the pancreatic ducts. Degrees of suppression of the accessory duct: (A) both ducts open into the duodenum; (B) the accessory duct ends blindly in the duodenal wall; (C) the main duct is smaller than the accessory duct and they are not connected. (Modified by permission of JE Skandalakis, SW Gray, JS Rowe, et al., *Contemp Surg* 15(5):17–40, 1979.)

Duodenal Papilla

The duodenal papilla (of Vater) lies at the end of the intramural portion of the common bile duct. It is on the posteromedial wall of the second part of the duodenum, to the right of the 2nd or 3rd lumbar vertebra in most cases. On endoscopy, the papilla was found to the right of the spine at the level of the 2nd lumbar vertebra in most patients. The distance of the papilla from the pylorus is highly variable, ranging from 1.5 to 12 cm. Inflammation of the proximal duodenum may shorten the distance; the pylorus is not a useful landmark.

The present concept of musculature is that there is a complex of four sphincters composed of circular or spiral smooth muscle fibers surrounding the intramural portion of the common bile and pancreatic ducts. The complex may be broken into four separate sphincters, as shown in Fig. 9.7.

The sphincteric complex varies from 6 to 30 mm in length, depending on the obliquity of the ducts. In some individuals, the complex may extend into the pancreatic portion of the common bile duct. This is important to know when complete anatomical transection of all elements of the complex may not be necessary for satisfactory function. Incision by 5-mm steps while testing with a suitable dilator will help limit the incision to the shortest length necessary to obtain the desired results. On the mucosal surface of the duodenum, the duodenal papilla of Vater is found where a longitudinal mucosal fold meets a transverse fold to form a T (Fig. 9.8).

These are some practical considerations:

■ Too much lateral or distal traction on the opened duodenum may erase the folds and distort the T.

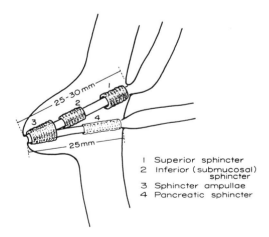

Figure 9.7. Diagram of the four sphincters making up the sphincter of Boyden. (By permission of JE Skandalakis, SW Gray, JS Rowe, et al., *Contemp Surg* 15(5):17–40, 1979.)

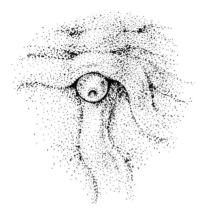

Figure 9.8. The T arrangement of mucosal folds of the duodenum indicating the site of the major duodenal papilla. The papilla is sometimes covered by these folds. (By permission of JE Skandalakis, SW Gray, JS Rowe, et al., *Contemp Surg* 15(5):17–40, 1979.)

- The papilla is often covered by a transverse fold. One must gently elevate the folds in the assumed location.
- If the T is not apparent and the papilla cannot be palpated, the common bile duct must be probed from above.
- A duodenal diverticulum lying close to the papilla may present difficulties for the surgeon or the endoscopist. The papilla has been found in a diverticulum. It separated from the duodenal wall and was immediately reimplanted.

The ampulla is the common pancreaticobiliary channel below the junction of the ducts within the papilla (Fig. 9.9A). If the septum between the ducts extends to the orifice of the papilla, there is no ampulla.

The most useful classification is as follows:

Type 1. The pancreatic duct opens into the common bile duct at a variable distance from the orifice of the major duodenal papilla. The common channel may or may not be dilated (85 percent) (Figs. 9.9A and B).

Type 2. The pancreatic and common bile ducts open separately on the major duodenal papilla (5 percent) (Fig. 9.9C).

Type 3. The pancreatic and common bile ducts open into the duodenum at separate points (9 percent).

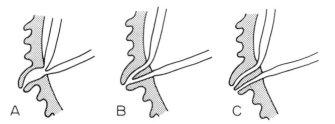

Figure 9.9. Diagram of the relations of the pancreatic and common bile ducts. (A) Minimal embryonic absorption of the ducts into the duodenal wall; an ampulla is present. (B) Partial embryonic resorption of the ducts; no true ampulla is present. (C) Maximum embryonic resorption of the ducts; two separate orifices open on the papilla. (By permission of JE Skandalakis, SW Gray, JS Rowe, et al., *Contemp Surg* 15(5):17–40, 1979.)

■ ARTERIAL SUPPLY TO THE PANCREAS

The pancreas is supplied with blood from both the celiac trunk and the superior mesenteric artery. The general plan is shown in Figs. 8.4 and 8.5, but variations are common.

In general, it appears that the blood supply is greatest to the head of the pancreas, less to the body and tail, and least to the neck.

The head of the pancreas and the concave surface of the duodenum are supplied by two pancreaticoduodenal arterial arcades (anterior and posterior). Ligation of both vessels will result in duodenal ischemia and necrosis. All major arteries lie posterior to the ducts.

Pancreatic Arcades

The gastroduodenal artery divides to form the anterosuperior and posterosuperior pancreaticoduodenal arteries.

The anteroinferior pancreaticoduodenal artery arises from the superior mesenteric artery at or above the inferior margin of the pancreatic neck. It may form a common trunk with the posteroinferior artery. Ligation of the jejunal branch itself will endanger the blood supply to the fourth part of the duodenum.

Dorsal Pancreatic Arcade

The dorsal pancreatic arcade lies posterior to the neck of the pancreas and, often, posterior to the splenic vein.

Transverse Pancreatic Artery

The transverse (inferior) pancreatic artery is the left branch of the dorsal pancreatic artery, and it supplies the body and tail of the pancreas.

Branches of the Splenic Artery

The splenic artery is located on the posterior surface of the body and tail of the pancreas (see Fig. 8.5). From 2 to 10 branches of the splenic artery anastomose with the transverse pancreatic artery. The largest of these, the great pancreatic artery (of von Haller), is the main blood supply to the tail of the pancreas. Ligation of the splenic artery does not require splenectomy, but ligation of the splenic vein does.

Caudal Pancreatic Artery

The caudal pancreatic artery arises from the left gastroepiploic artery or from a splenic branch at the hilum of the spleen.

■ VENOUS DRAINAGE OF THE PANCREAS

In general, the veins of the pancreas parallel the arteries and lie superficial to them. Both lie posterior to the ducts. The drainage is to the portal vein, the splenic vein, and the superior and inferior mesenteric veins (see Figs. 8.6 and 8.7).

The hepatic portal vein is formed behind the neck of the pancreas by the union of the superior mesenteric and the splenic veins (see Fig. 8.7).

The portal vein lies in front of the inferior vena cava, with the common bile duct to the right and the hepatic artery to the left.

■ LYMPHATIC DRAINAGE OF THE PANCREAS

Fig. 9.10, from the studies of Cubilla et al., shows the chief groups of lymph nodes receiving lymphatic vessels from the pancreas. Lymphatic drainage may prove to be as frustrating a problem as is arterial supply.

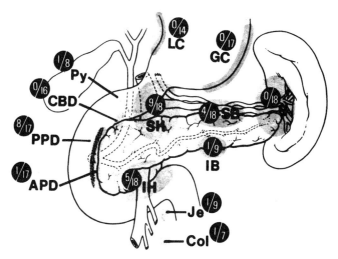

Figure 9.10. Distribution of lymph nodes in 18 pancreatectomy resection specimens. Numerator of fraction of each group indicates number of patients with metastasis in that lymph node group; denominator indicates number of patients in which group nodes were examined. Thirteen cases were pancreas duct cancer, five were other cancers in the head of the pancreas area. SH = superior head; SB = superior body; IH = inferior head; IB = inferior body; APD = anterior pancreaticoduodenal; PPD = posterior pancreaticoduodenal; CBD = common bile duct; Py = pyloric; LC = lesser curvature; GC = greater curvature; S = tail of pancreas and splenic; Je = jejunal; Col = midcolic. (By permission of AL Cubilla, J Fortner, and PJ Fitzgerald, *Cancer* 41(3):880–887, 1978.)

■ NERVE SUPPLY OF THE PANCREAS

The pancreas is innervated by sympathetic and parasympathetic divisions. In general, these nerves follow blood vessels to their destination.

The celiac ganglion is the central station of both sympathetic and parasympathetic innervation. Extirpation, surgical or chemical, of the celiac ganglion should interrupt afferent fibers of both sympathetic and parasympathetic systems. Tetraethyl ammonium chloride, phenol, and alcohol have been used to destroy the ganglion. Such treatment is effective for only a few months.

■ ECTOPIC AND ACCESSORY PANCREAS

Pancreatic tissue in the stomach, duodenal, or ileal wall, in Meckel's diverticulum, or at the umbilicus is not unusual. Less common sites are the colon, the appendix, the gallbladder, the omentum or mesentery, and in an anomalous bronchoesophageal fistula. Most such pancreatic tissue is functional. Islet tissue is often present in gastric and duodenal heterotopia, but it is usually absent in accessory pancreatic tissue elsewhere in the body. Fig. 9.11 shows the possible sites of ectopic pancreatic tissue.

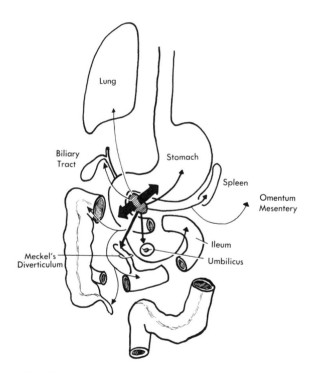

Figure 9.11. Sites of pancreatic heterotopia. The relative frequency is indicated by the width of the arrows. The stomach and duodenum are by far the most common sites. (By permission of JE Skandalakis, SW Gray, RR Ricketts, et al. The pancreas. In: Skandalakis, JE and Gray, SW. *Embryology for Surgeons*. 2nd ed. Baltimore: Williams & Wilkins, 1994.)

■ EVALUATION OF RESECTABILITY OF THE PANCREAS

The authors strongly advise angiograms prior to surgery. Also, we suggest the following steps in the operating room:

1. Good general exploration of the abdomen with special attention to the pancreas.

2. Attention to specific areas of lymph node drainage that are accessible without further incision. These are the pyloric and pancreaticoduodenal nodes and the nodes at the root of the mesentery (Fig. 9.10).

3. Further investigation of lymph nodes, which requires some incision of the gastrohepatic omenta. This will also require a Kocher maneuver. Pancreaticoduodenal, celiac, and left gastric nodes, together with nodes of the superior and inferior pancreatic borders, should be inspected.

4. Final steps in evaluation may now be taken, assuming that the diagnosis of cancer has been determined and that the exploration just outlined has indicated a resectable lesion. These final steps should be undertaken before the start of the actual resection:

    a. Further exploration of the area of the muscle of Treitz to ensure mobility of the fourth part of the duodenum and the first portion of the jejunum.

    b. Evaluation of the posterior surface of the head of the pancreas and the distal common bile duct to ensure that there is no fixation to underlying structures, including the inferior vena cava.

    c. Gentle examination of the uncinate process and elevation of the neck of the pancreas with one or two fingers to ensure that they are not fixed to the superior mesenteric vessels or to the portal vein.

    d. Final review of the local anatomy to identify any previously undetected vascular anomalies. Any available angiograms should be studied.

95 Percent Distal Pancreatectomy for Chronic Pancreatitis

Orientation: Fig. 9.20

Note: The authors question whether "95 percent" is an accurate number. The size of the head and the presence or lack of the uncinate process play an important role. Our sixth sense tells us that the remaining pancreas is far more than 5 percent.

Procedure:

Step 1. Explore and intubate the common bile duct and perform cholecystectomy.

Step 2. Mobilize the head, uncinate process, body, and tail of the pancreas. The uncinate process should be treated carefully if present. Care must also be taken with the following vessels: splenic artery, splenic vein, superior mesenteric vein, tributaries. Using 4–0 silk, carefully ligate small veins without traction. Mobilize the neck by dissecting bluntly with the index fingers between the posterior surface of the pancreas and the underlying superior mesenteric vessels (Fig. 9.21).

Step 3. Using electrocautery, divide the head of the pancreas from the remaining gland very close to the duodenal loop (Fig. 9.22). For the duodenum and thin pancreatic rim to survive, it is very important to protect the superior and inferior pancreaticoduodenal arteries. One of these vessels can provide enough blood,

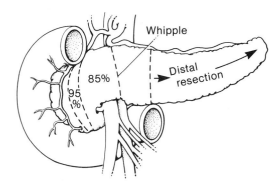

Figure 9.20. Partial pancreatectomy: (1) 95 percent pancreatectomy; (2) 85 percent pancreatectomy; (3) Whipple procedure; (4 and 5) distal pancreatectomy. Distal pancreatectomy includes resection from any point between 4 and 5 to the tip of the tail. (By permission of JE Skandalakis, SW Gray, and JR Rowe, *Anatomical Complications in General Surgery*, New York: McGraw-Hill, 1983.)

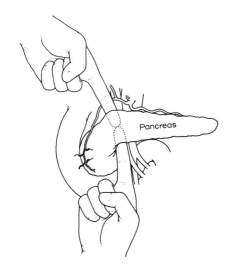

Figure 9.21. Exploration of the pancreas. The surgeon's index fingers are passed behind the neck of the pancreas. The neck should be separated easily from the underlying vessels. (By permission of JE Skandalakis, SW Gray, JS Rowe, et al., *Contemp Surg* 15(6):21–50, 1979.)

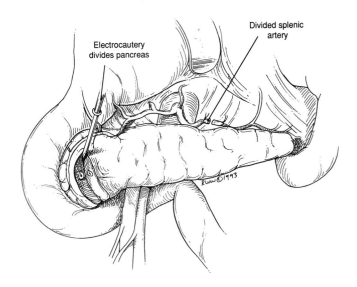

Figure 9.22

so if the other is accidentally injured and ligated, no harm results; but *do not ligate both*. Palpate and preserve the third and fourth portions of the common bile duct.

Step 4. Identify the divided pancreatic duct and close it with a mattress suture of 4-0 synthetic absorbable material. Doubly ligate the splenic artery, the splenic vein, and their tributaries, and perform splenectomy (Figs. 9.23–9.26). Remove specimen consisting of distal pancreas and spleen.

Step 5. Insert T-tube and Jackson–Pratt drain, and close the abdominal wall in layers.

Distal Pancreatectomy (With or Without Splenectomy)

Orientation: Fig. 9.12

Keeping in mind all the technical steps of the previously discussed pancreatic procedures, we present the following:

Procedure:

Step 1. Transect the pancreas approximately where it crosses the portal vein (Fig. 9.27).

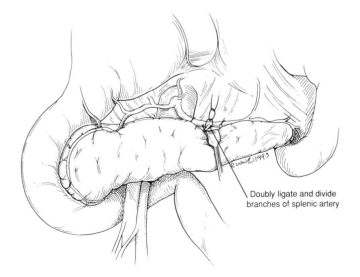

Doubly ligate and divide
branches of splenic artery

Figure 9.23

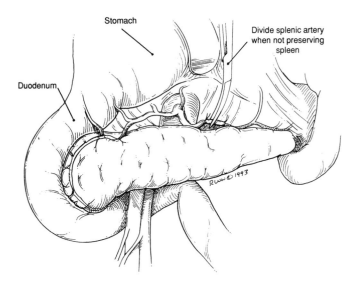

Stomach

Divide splenic artery
when not preserving
spleen

Duodenum

Figure 9.24

Step 2. Create a Roux-en-Y loop by anastomosing the pancreatic head
or part of the remaining body by invagination to a divided
jejunal loop approximately 45 cm from the ligament of Treitz
(as described in step 11 of the procedure for Pancreaticoduodenectomy with Pyloric Preservation, below) using an end-to-
end pancreaticojejunostomy. Fashion an end-to-side jejuno-

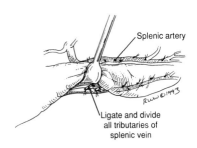

Splenic artery

Ligate and divide
all tributaries of
splenic vein

Figure 9.25

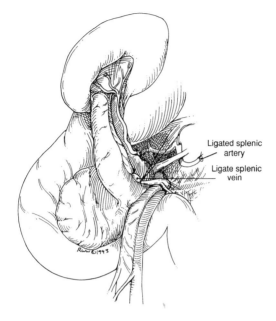

Figure 9.26

jejunostomy (Fig. 9.28), producing continuity of the gastro-intestinal tract plus a defunctionalized limb of approximately 60 cm.

Note: An alternative method is to oversew the pancreas and drain the area.

Total Pancreatectomy (With or Without Splenectomy)

Procedure:

Step 1. The pancreas is not divided; therefore there is no pancreatico-jejunostomy. Remove both the spleen and the pancreaticoduo-denal duo in continuity.

Step 2. With 3-0 silk, carefully ligate all arterial or venous branches connecting the spleen, pancreas, and duodenum. These vascu-lar collections are totally unpredictable and the surgeon should be careful to avoid traction. Occasionally a splenopancreatic ligament is present and should be ligated close to the pancreas.

Step 8. The pancreaticoduodenectomy steps
After total exposure of the superior mesenteric vein, and with the left index finger under the neck of the pancreas, divide the pancreatic parenchyma using electrocautery (Fig. 9.31). Ligate the small veins and arteries. Shave the remaining distal pancreas and send the specimen to the lab for frozen section.

Step 9. Localize the ligament of Treitz in the paraduodenal fossae. Using the GIA stapler, divide the jejunum approximately 10–12.5 cm distal to the ligament of Treitz. Be careful not to injure the inferior mesenteric vein, which is located to the left of the paraduodenal fossae. Clamp, divide, and ligate the mesentery at the mesenteric border of the proximal jejunal limb. With careful digital elevation of the proximal jejunum and fourth and third portions of the duodenum, push the jejunal loop gently under the vessels and to the right (Fig. 9.32).

Step 10. If the uncinate process is still attached and if the uncinate process ligament is present, it should be divided between

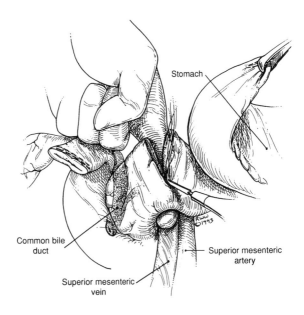

Figure 9.31

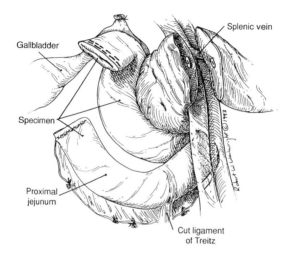

Gallbladder

Splenic vein

Specimen

Proximal jejunum

Cut ligament of Treitz

Figure 9.32

clamps and the distal part should be ligated (Fig. 9.33). Carefully dissect the uncinate process from the portal vein and the superior mesenteric vein. Send the specimen to the lab for more frozen sections.

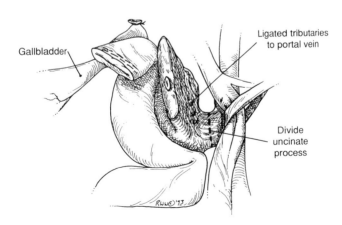

Gallbladder

Ligated tributaries to portal vein

Divide uncinate process

Figure 9.33

may bifurcate to supply each side, or they may pass singly to alternate sides of the intestine (Fig. 10.4). They branch, but do not anastomose beneath the serosa before piercing the muscularis externa. There is no collateral circulation between the vasa recta or their branches at the surface of the intestines. This configuration provides the best supply of oxygenated blood to the mesenteric side of the intestine and the poorest supply to the antimesenteric border.

Venous Drainage

The veins travel with the arteries in the mesentery to reach the superior mesenteric vein.

■ LYMPHATIC DRAINAGE

The lymphatic flow is to nodes lying between the leaves of the mesentery. Over 200 small mesenteric nodes lie near the vasa recta and along the

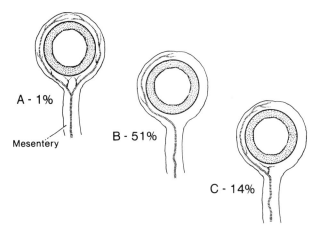

Figure 10.4. (A) The vasa recta may divide into two short vessels to the mesenteric side of the intestine and two long vessels supplying the rest of the intestinal wall. (B) More frequently, a single, long vessel supplies one side of the intestine, alternating with a vessel supplying the other side. (C) A single long and a single short vessel serving one side only. The remaining 34 percent are various combinations of paired, single, long, and short vessels. (By permission of JE Skandalakis, SW Gray, and JR Rowe, *Anatomical Complications in General Surgery*, New York: McGraw-Hill, 1983.)

intestinal arteries. Drainage from these is finally to the large superior mesenteric lymph nodes at the root of the mesentery. Efferent vessels from these and the celiac nodes form the intestinal lymphatic trunk, which passes beneath the left renal artery and ends in the left lumbar lymphatic trunk (70 percent) or the cisterna chyli (25 percent).

■ ABNORMAL DEVELOPMENT OF THE SMALL INTESTINE

Meckel's Diverticulum

When present, Meckel's diverticulum arises from the antimesenteric surface of the ileum about 40 cm from the ileocecal valve in infants and about 50 cm from the valve in adults. It may be less than 15 cm or as much as 167 cm from the valve (Fig. 10.5). Not less than 1.5 m of ileum should be inspected to be sure that the diverticulum has not been overlooked. The length of the diverticulum may be as little as 1 cm or as long as 26 cm: in 75 percent of individuals it will be from 1 to 5 cm; the rest will be longer.

The diverticulum may be free and mobile or its tip may be attached to

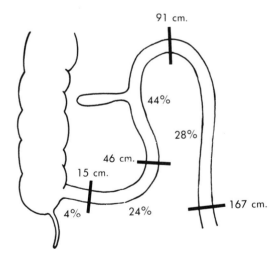

Figure 10.5. Location on the ileum and frequency of occurrence of Meckel's diverticulum. (By permission of JE Skandalakis, SW Gray, RR Ricketts, et al. The small intestines. In: Skandalakis JE and Gray SW. *Embryology for Surgeons*. 2nd ed. Baltimore: Williams & Wilkins, 1994.)

the anterior body wall at the umbilicus. In a few cases, the structure is patent to the outside (omphaloileal fistula), a solid cord, or a cystic remnant (Fig. 10.6).

The mucosa of the diverticulum is largely ileal, but gastric, pancreatic, or duodenal mucosa may also be present.

■ SURGICAL ANATOMY OF INTUSSUSCEPTION

An intussusception is created when a proximal segment of intestine (the intussusceptum) invaginates into the portion of intestine immediately distal to it (the intussuscipiens) (Fig. 10.7).

Meckel's diverticulum is the most common identifiable cause of intussusception in children. Other known causes are intestinal polyps, duplications, atresias, and tumors of the intestine, but 85 percent of our cases of intussusceptions in children could not be assigned to any cause.

In adults, our "⅔ rule" may be applied: ⅔ of adult intussusceptions are from known causes. Of these, ⅔ are due to neoplasms. Of the neoplasms, ⅔ will be malignant. (All numbers are approximate.)

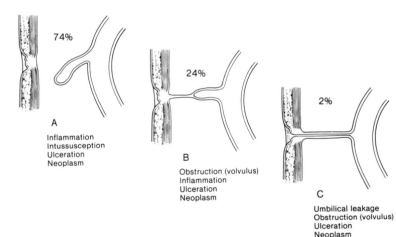

74%

A
Inflammation
Intussusception
Ulceration
Neoplasm

24%

B
Obstruction (volvulus)
Inflammation
Ulceration
Neoplasm

2%

C
Umbilical leakage
Obstruction (volvulus)
Ulceration
Neoplasm

Figure 10.6. Three major types of Meckel's diverticulum. (A) Diverticulum with free end not attached to the body wall. (B) Diverticulum connected to the anterior body wall by a fibrous cord. (C) Fistula opening through the umbilicus. (By permission of JE Skandalakis, SW Gray, and JR Rowe, *Anatomical Complications in General Surgery*, New York: McGraw-Hill, 1983.)

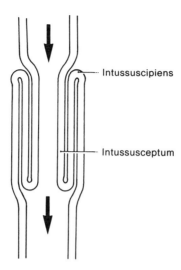

Figure 10.7. Diagram of the anatomy of an intestinal intussusception. Such a formation can enlarge distally until the leading edge reaches the anus. (By permission of JE Skandalakis, SW Gray, and JR Rowe, *Anatomical Complications in General Surgery*, New York: McGraw-Hill, 1983.)

Reduction of the intussusception may be spontaneous, or it may be achieved by barium enema or by operation.

For children, we recommend reduction with resection if necessary; for adults, we recommend resection without reduction.

■ ANATOMICAL GUIDELINES FOR SURGERY

There is no good way to identify an isolated loop of small intestine without following it in one direction to the duodenojejunal junction or in the other direction to the ileocecal junction.

Exposure and Mobilization

Few organs are more easily exposed and mobilized than are loops of small intestine. Adhesions from previous surgery are the chief obstacles to good mobilization.

About the only procedures we perform in this part of the gastrointestinal tract are resection and anastomosis of the small bowel. In benign disease, we make every effort to save the ileocecal valve, but when malignancy is present, resection is a must. When dealing with resection of the small bowel, the surgeon should always be conservative. The decision in the operating room should be based on pathology, such as tumor (benign or malignant), mesenteric thrombosis of arterial or venous type, and inflammatory processes, such as regional enteritis, tumors of the mesentery, Meckel's diverticulum, etc.

TECHNIQUE

■ RESECTION OF SMALL BOWEL FOR TUMOR

Procedure:

Step 1. Isolate the small bowel approximately 10 cm proximal and 10 cm distal to the mass. In benign and malignant tumors, we prefer to remove a triangle of mesentery reaching as deep as possible, since occasionally a frozen section will not give the correct diagnosis (e.g., leiomyoma) (Figs. 10.8–10.10).

Step 2. Use two clamps for each intestinal side, proximal and distal. For the specimen, use a straight Kocher; for the areas where the anastomosis will take place, use a noncrushing enteric straight clamp. To minimize the risk of hematoma, ligate the mesenteric vessels very carefully one at a time (Figs. 10.9 and 10.11).

Step 3. Establish good alignment of proximal and distal ends of the bowel. Place the corner sutures first (Fig. 10.12).

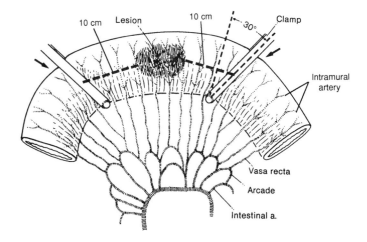

Figure 10.8. Recommended position of noncrushing clamps for segmental resection of intestine. The 30-degree angle from a vertical transection preserves as much of the antimesenteric blood supply as possible (arrows) and slightly increases the functional diameter of the anastomosis. (Modified by permission of JE Skandalakis, SW Gray, and JR Rowe, *Anatomical Complications in General Surgery*, New York: McGraw-Hill, 1983.)

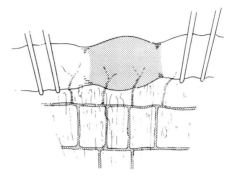

Figure 10.9

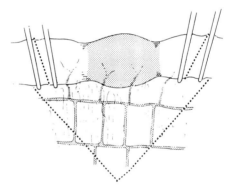

Figure 10.10

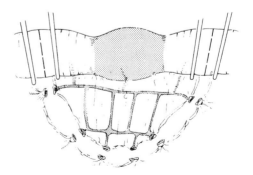

Figure 10.11

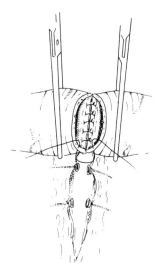

Figure 10.12

Step 4. We prefer two-layer anastomosis, using interrupted 4–0 silk and a continuous 3–0 chromic.

Step 5. Check patency with thumb and index finger.

Notes:

✓ One-layer anastomosis through-and-through is acceptable as well as mechanical sutures.

✓ A side-to-side anastomosis bypassing the nonresectable tumor may be done.

✓ A side-to-side staple anastomosis also can be done (see Chapter 12, Colon and Anorectum).

■ MECKEL'S DIVERTICULUM

Orientation (Fig. 10.5)

We prefer a wedge resection of the diverticulum with extension to the mesenteric wall or a segmental resection of the ileum and end-to-end anastomosis in one or two layers (Fig. 10.13).

A side-to-side anastomosis may be done, but to avoid the blind loop syndrome, take care in constructing it (Figs. 10.14–10.16).

11

Appendix

ANATOMY

■ RELATIONS AND POSITIONS OF THE APPENDIX

The cecum from which the appendix arises is related posteriorly to the iliopsoas muscle and the femoral nerve, and anteriorly to the abdominal wall, the greater omentum, or the coils of the ileum.

The five typical locations of the appendix, in order of frequency, are: (1) retrocecal-retrocolic, free or fixed; (2) pelvic or descending; (3) subcecal, passing downward and to the right; (4) ileocecal, passing upward and to the left anterior to the ileum; and (5) ileocecal, posterior to the ileum. Studies have found that the first two positions are the most common, but there is significant variation.

The vermiform appendix originates from the posteromedial side of the cecum about 1.7 cm from the end of the ileum. The base of the appendix is located at the union of the teniae. For all practical purposes, the anterior tenia will end at the appendiceal origin.

■ MESENTERY

The mesentery of the appendix is derived from the posterior side of the mesentery of the terminal ileum. It attaches to the cecum as well as to the proximal appendix and contains the appendiceal artery.

■ BLOOD SUPPLY

The appendiceal artery arises from the ileocolic artery, from the ileal branch of the ileocolic artery, or from a cecal artery. The artery is usually

TECHNIQUE

■ APPENDECTOMY

The incision for appendectomy is usually made over McBurney's point. It is made at right angles to a line between the anterosuperior spine of the ilium and the umbilicus at ⅔ the distance from the umbilicus; ⅓ of the incision should be above the line, and ⅔ should be below.

The cecum should be identified first. It can be distinguished from the transverse colon by the absence of attachments of the omentum. If the cecum cannot be located, malrotation of the intestines or undescended cecum should be considered.

When the cecum has been identified, one of the teniae coli can be traced downward to the base of the appendix. In spite of the great mobility of the tip, the base of the appendix always arises from the cecum at the convergence of the teniae. In exposing a deeply buried retrocecal appendix, it may be necessary to incise the posterior peritoneum lateral to the cecum. Congenital absence of the appendix is too rare to be considered seriously, but its apparent absence may be the result of intussusception. In such a case, there should be an obvious dimple at the normal site of the appendix. Of course, the surgeon should inspect the abdomen for signs of previous operation.

Procedure:

Step 1. Choice of incision is up to the surgeon. We prefer McBurney (Fig. 11.3).

Step 2. Incise the aponeurosis of the external oblique along the lines of its fibers (Fig. 11.4).

Step 3. Use a curved Kelly clamp to make an opening on both the internal oblique and the transversus abdominis muscles. Enlarge the opening with the Kelly clamp and insert two Richardson's retractors.

Step 4. If the transversalis fascia was divided together with the flat muscles, occasionally there will be a thick stroma of preperitoneal fat which can be pushed laterally or, sometimes, medially, revealing the peritoneum.

Step 5. Elevate the peritoneum and, if applicable, the transversalis fascia. Make a small opening in the peritoneum with a knife or scissors, then enlarge it with both index fingers and insert the retractors of your choice (Fig. 11.5).

Step 6. Take cultures of the free peritoneal fluid and, using moist

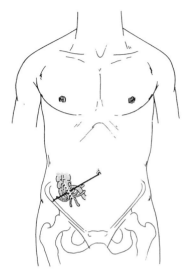

Figure 11.3

gauze, pull the cecum out of the wound. In most cases, the appendix is delivered with the cecum or may be seen.

Step 7. Grasp and study the mesentery of the appendix and reinsert the cecum into the peritoneal cavity. Divide the mesoappendix between clamps (Fig. 11.6).

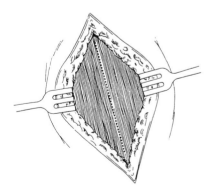

Figure 11.4

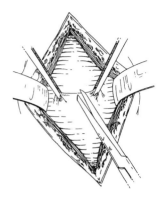

Figure 11.5

Step 8. Ligate the mesoappendix with 2-0 silk. Occasionally, a transfixing suture is necessary, especially when the appendix can not be delivered well out of the wound or when the mesoappendix is fatty and friable (Fig. 11.7).

Step 9. With hemostasis completed, lift the appendix straight up and attach two clamps to its base. Remove the clamp close to the cecum and ligate the appendiceal base doubly with 0 chromic catgut. The surgeon can either invert the appendiceal stump

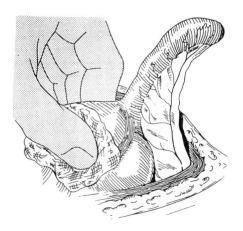

Figure 11.6

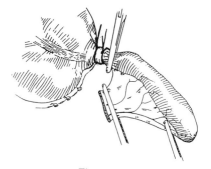

Figure 11.7

or not. If inverted, this is done using a 3-0 silk purse string (Fig. 11.8).

Step 10. Divide the appendix between the clamp and the catgut ligatures using a knife with phenol and alcohol or electrocautery. Invert the appendiceal stump and tie the purse string. If necessary to further invert the stump, a figure-of-eight 4-0 silk may be used (Figs. 11.9–11.12).

Step 11. Irrigate. Close in layers using catgut or absorbable synthetic suture. If peritonitis is present, close the muscle, but not the

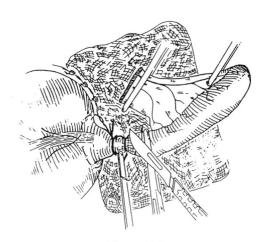

Figure 11.8

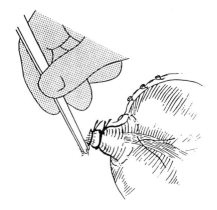

Figure 11.9

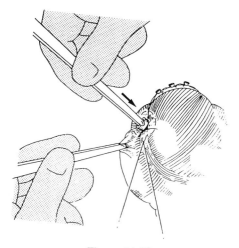

Figure 11.10

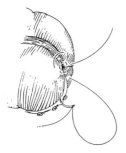

Figure 11.11

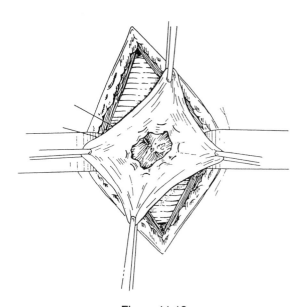

Figure 11.12

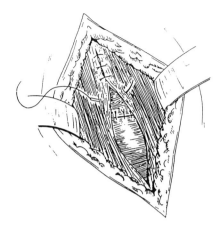

Figure 11.13

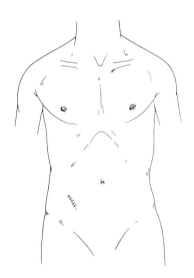

Figure 11.14

skin. The authors use iodoform gauze to pack the wound. We also insert 3–0 vertical mattress sutures, which will be tied a few days later when infection is controlled (Figs. 11.13 and 11.14).

12

Colon and Anorectum

ANATOMY

■ RELATIONS

The large intestine, or colon, about 150 cm long, extends from the terminal ileum to the rectum. The classic divisions are the cecum, colon proper, rectum, and anal canal. The cecum, the first 6 cm of the large bowel just below the ileocolic valve, together with the ascending and hepatic flexures, forms a surgical unit, the right colon.

Cecum

The cecum lies in the right iliac fossa, and in about 60 percent of living, erect individuals, it lies partly in the true pelvis. In approximately 20 percent, almost the entire posterior surface of the cecum is attached to the abdominal wall, and, at the other extreme, the cecum is wholly unattached in approximately 25 percent. Among the latter are cases of true "mobile cecum," in which the cecum and the lower part of the ascending colon are unattached.

Folds from the mesentery of the terminal ileum may be attached to the lower colon and cecum, forming a superior ileocecal fossa and an inferior ileocecal fossa. Both these folds are inconstant, and the associated fossae may be shallow or absent (Fig. 12.1). Occasionally, a retrocecal fossa is present. A fixed terminal ileum may be present and, rarely, a common ileocecal mesentery.

Colon Proper

The ascending limb of the colon proper is normally fused to the posterior body wall and covered anteriorly, partially laterally, and medially by the

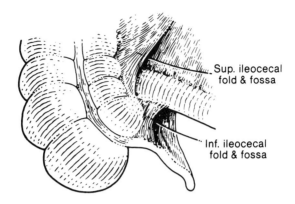

Sup. ileocecal
fold & fossa

Inf. ileocecal
fold & fossa

Figure 12.1. Superior and inferior ileocecal folds forming fossae. (By permission of JE Skandalakis, SW Gray, and JR Rowe, *Anatomical Complications in General Surgery*, New York: McGraw-Hill, 1983.)

peritoneum. There are variations of incomplete fusion ranging from a deep lateral paracolic groove to the persistence of an entire ascending mesocolon (Fig. 12.2). A mesocolon long enough to permit volvulus occurs in approximately 11 percent. In cadavers, the ascending colon may be mobile in approximately 37 percent of cases. A mobile cecum, together with a mobile right colon, may be present.

Where the mesocolon is present, the cecum and the proximal ascending colon are unusually mobile. It is this condition that is termed mobile cecum and which can result in volvulus of the cecum and the right colon (Fig. 12.3).

Two conditions must be present for right colon volvulus to occur: (1) an abnormally mobile segment of colon, and (2) a fixed point around which the mobile segment can twist.

Decreased mobility of the colon may be produced by abnormal connective tissue bands that pass across the ascending colon beneath the peritoneum (Jackson's membrane or veil) (Fig. 12.4). It may or may not be vascularized.

The transverse colon begins where the colon turns sharply to the left (the hepatic flexure) just beneath the inferior surface of the right lobe of the liver. It ends at a sharp downward bend (the splenic flexure) in relation to the posterolateral surface of the spleen, the tail of the pancreas above, and the anterior surface of the left kidney medially.

The transverse colon has a mesentery that has secondarily fused with

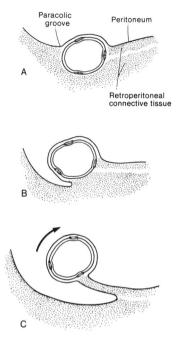

Figure 12.2. Degrees of attachment of the right colon to the abdominal wall. (A) Normal retroperitoneal location of the colon. (B) Paracolic gutter. (C) Mobile colon with mesentery. (By permission of JE Skandalakis, SW Gray, and JR Rowe, *Anatomical Complications in General Surgery*, New York: McGraw-Hill, 1983.)

the posterior wall of the omental bursa (see Fig. 8.1). At the splenic flexure, the colon is supported by the renocolic ligament, a part of the left side of the transverse mesocolon.

The descending colon is covered anteriorly by peritoneum; normally it has no mesentery lateromedially. When a mesentery exists, it is rarely long enough to permit volvulus of the left colon. The surgical unit of the left colon consists of the splenic flexure and the descending and sigmoid colon.

At the level of the iliac crest, the descending colon becomes the sigmoid colon, which has two parts: iliac (fixed) and pelvic (with mesentery). The average length of the attachment and the average breadth of the mesentery are shown in Fig. 12.5A. The left ureter passes through the base of the sigmoid mesocolon through the intersigmoid recess (Fig. 12.5B).

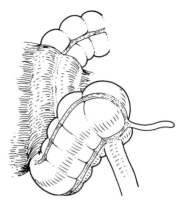

Figure 12.3. Mobile cecum, distal ileum, and proximal right colon. This configuration is subject to volvulus. (By permission of JE Skandalakis, SW Gray, and JR Rowe, *Anatomical Complications in General Surgery*, New York: McGraw-Hill, 1983.)

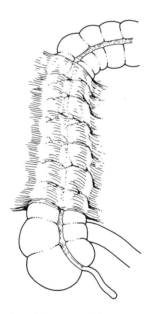

Figure 12.4. "Jackson's veil" may contain many small blood vessels from the second lumbar or renal arteries. The extent of the "veil" is variable. (By permission of JE Skandalakis, SW Gray, and JR Rowe, *Anatomical Complications in General Surgery*, New York: McGraw-Hill, 1983.)

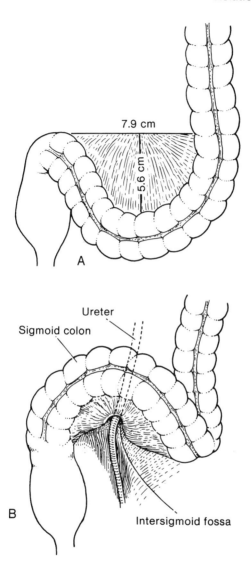

Figure 12.5. (A) Average measurements of the sigmoid mesocolon. (B) The relation of the base of the sigmoid mesocolon to the left ureter. (By permission of JE Skandalakis, SW Gray, and JR Rowe, *Anatomical Complications in General Surgery*, New York: McGraw-Hill, 1983.)

Rectum and Anal Canal

The junction between the sigmoid colon and the rectum has been variously described:

1. The level at which the sigmoid mesentery disappears, sacculations and epiploic appendages disappear, and the teniae broaden to form a complete muscle layer (long transition)

2. The level at which the superior rectal artery divides into right and left branches

The surgeon considers the anal canal to be the region lying distal to the insertion of the levator ani muscle. The surgical anal canal has a length of 4 cm, 2 cm above the pectinate line and 2 cm below.

■ PERITONEAL REFLECTIONS

The entire upper third of the rectum is covered by peritoneum (Fig. 12.6). The peritoneum leaves the rectum and passes anteriorly and superiorly over the uterus in females or over the bladder in males. This creates a depression, the rectouterine or rectovesical pouch.

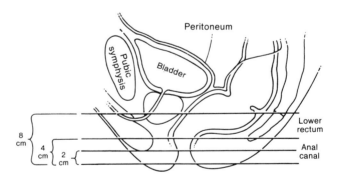

Figure 12.6. The line of peritoneal reflection on the rectum; lateral view in the male. More of the rectum is covered anteriorly than posteriorly. The measurements of the anal canal and lower rectum from the anal verge are approximate. (By permission of JE Skandalakis, SW Gray, and JR Rowe, *Anatomical Complications in General Surgery*, New York: McGraw-Hill, 1983.)

■ PELVIC DIAPHRAGM AND CONTINENCE

The floor of the pelvis is the pelvic diaphragm (Fig. 12.7), which is composed of two paired muscles, the levator ani and the coccygeus. The levator ani may be considered to be made up of three muscles: the ileococcygeus, the pubococcygeus, and the puborectalis. The puborectalis is essential to maintaining rectal continence, and is considered by some authors to be part of the external sphincter and not a part of the levator ani. The puborectalis is attached to the lower back surface of the symphysis pubis and the superior layer of the deep perineal pouch (urogenital diaphragm). Fibers from each side of the muscle pass posteriorly and then join posterior to the rectum, forming a well-defined sling (Fig. 12.7). The puborectalis, with the superficial and deep parts of the external sphincter and the proximal part of the internal sphincter, forms the so-called anorectal ring. This ring can be palpated; and since cutting through it will produce incontinence, it must be identified and protected during surgical procedures.

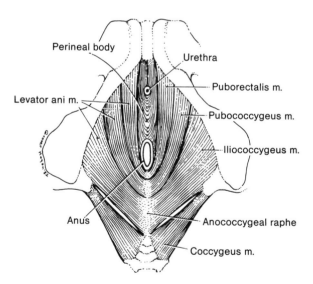

Figure 12.7. Diagram of the pelvic diaphragm from below. Note that the levator ani is composed of three muscles: puborectalis, pubococcygeus, and iliococcygeus. Some authors would exclude the puborectalis from the levator ani. (By permission of JE Skandalakis, SW Gray, and JR Rowe, *Anatomical Complications in General Surgery*, New York: McGraw-Hill, 1983.)

■ FASCIAL RELATIONS AND TISSUE SPACES

Six potential spaces around the rectum are recognized. They are important because they may become sites of infection. The fascial layers that bound these spaces help limit the spread both of infection and of neoplastic disease, although all are potentially confluent with one another (Figs. 12.8 and 12.9).

■ GENERAL ANATOMY

Colon

The layers of the wall of the large intestine are essentially similar to those of the wall of the small intestine. The chief differences are: (1) the absence of mucosal villi, (2) longitudinal muscularis externa in three discrete bands (teniae) rather than in a continuous cylinder, and (3) the presence of epiploic appendages.

The epiploic appendages are of interest to the surgeon because they may be the sites of diverticula (Fig. 12.10A). The fat may conceal the presence of the diverticula on inspection, but fecoliths in the diverticula are frequently palpable. The appendages are also subject to infarction and torsion; both produce symptoms of acute abdomen. Epiploic ap-

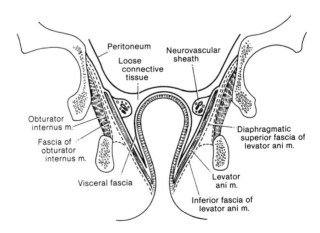

Figure 12.8. Diagram of some of the fasciae of the pelvis seen in coronal section. (By permission of JE Skandalakis, SW Gray, and JR Rowe, *Anatomical Complications in General Surgery*, New York: McGraw-Hill, 1983.)

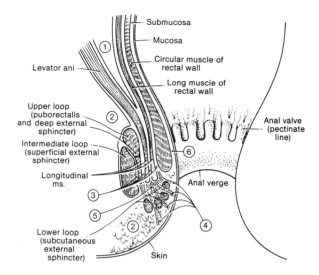

Figure 12.9. The spaces of the anus and rectum: (1) pelvirectal space; (2) ischiorectal space; (3) intersphincteric spaces; (4) subcutaneous space; (5) central space; (6) submucous space. (By permission of JE Skandalakis, SW Gray, and JR Rowe, *Anatomical Complications in General Surgery*, New York: McGraw-Hill, 1983.)

pendages should be ligated without traction to prevent pulling a loop of a long colic artery into the appendiceal neck and being included in the ligation (Fig. 12.10B).

Rectum

The upper rectum contains three folds: left superior, right middle, and left inferior (valves of Houston). They are encountered by the sigmoidoscope at 4–7 cm, 8–10 cm, and 10–12 cm from the anal verge.

Anal Canal

The Musculature of the Wall of the Anal Canal

Two layers of smooth muscle surround the anal canal. The innermost layer is formed by a circular coat. This is the internal sphincter of the anal canal (Fig. 12.9). The second smooth muscle layer is composed of longitudinal fibers continuous with the fibers of the teniae coli.

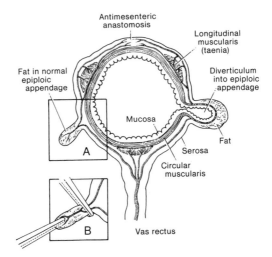

Figure 12.10. Diagram of the transverse colon showing long and short branches of the vasa recta. On the left is a normal epiploic appendage; on the right, a diverticulum extending into an epiploic appendage. *Inset:* Effect of too much traction on an epiploic appendage resulting in injury to a long branch of a vas rectus followed by antimesenteric ischemia. (By permission of JE Skandalakis, SW Gray, and JR Rowe, *Anatomical Complications in General Surgery*, New York: McGraw-Hill, 1983.)

The longitudinal muscle fibers prevent separation of the sphincteric elements from each other and also permit a telescopic movement between internal and external sphincters. We witness this in the operating room when the external sphincter rolls back and the internal sphincter rolls forward.

Composed of striated muscle, the external sphincter has three separate loops: subcutaneous, superficial, and deep. It is useful to consider the three parts separately (Figs. 12.11 and 12.12), but the three loops together form an efficient anal closure. Any single one of the loops is capable of maintaining continence to solid stools, but not to fluid or gas. The subcutaneous portion surrounds the outlet of the anus, attaching to the perianal skin anteriorly. Some fibers completely encircle the anus.

The superficial portion surrounds the anus and joins the anococcygeal ligament, which attaches posteriorly to the coccyx. This creates the small triangular space of Minor behind the anus. Anteriorly, some fibers insert into the transverse perineal muscles at the peritoneal body, creating a potential space toward which anterior midline fistulas may point.

The deep portion surrounds the canal and is closely related to the puborectalis sling.

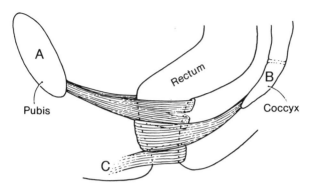

Figure 12.11. The three loops of the external anal sphincter. Continence depends on the preservation of at least one of the three. Some subcutaneous muscle fibers encircle the anus; some attach to the perianal skin anteriorly at C. (By permission of JE Skandalakis, SW Gray, and JR Rowe, *Anatomical Complications in General Surgery*, New York: McGraw-Hill, 1983.)

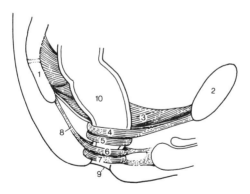

Figure 12.12. Diagram of the extrinsic muscles of the surgical anal canal. (1) Coccyx; (2) pubis; (3) levator ani muscle; (4) puborectalis muscle; (5) deep external sphincter; (6) superficial external sphincter; (7) subcutaneous external sphincter; (8) anococcygeal ligament; (9) anal verge; (10) rectum. (By permission of JE Skandalakis, SW Gray, and JR Rowe, *Anatomical Complications in General Surgery*, New York: McGraw-Hill, 1983.)

The Lining of the Surgical Anal Canal

There are three histologic regions of the anal canal. The cutaneous zone, up to the anal verge (anocutaneous line), is covered by pigmented skin that has hair follicles and sebaceous glands. Above the anal verge is the transitional zone, which consists of modified skin that has sebaceous glands without hair. It extends to the pectinate line defined by the free edges of the anal valves. Above the line begins the true mucosa of the anal canal (Fig. 12.13).

The pectinate line is formed by the margins of the anal valves, small mucosal pockets between the five to ten vertical folds of the mucosa known as the anal columns of Morgagni. These columns extend upward from the pectinate line to the upper end of the surgical anal canal, at the level of the puborectalis sling. They are formed by underlying parallel bundles of the muscularis mucosae. The actual junction of stratified squamous and columnar epithelia is usually just above the pectinate line; hence the mucocutaneous line is not precisely equivalent to the pectinate line.

The pectinate line is the most important landmark in the anal canal. It marks the transition between the visceral area above and the somatic area below. The arterial supply, the venous and lymphatic drainage, the nerve supply, and the character of the lining all change at or very near the pectinate line (see Table 12.1).

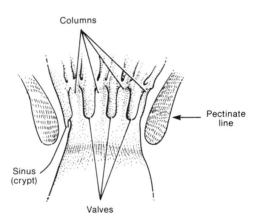

Figure 12.13. The interior of the anal canal showing the rectal columns, anal valves, and anal sinuses (crypts). They form the pectinate line. (By permission of JE Skandalakis, SW Gray, and JR Rowe, *Anatomical Complications in General Surgery*, New York: McGraw-Hill, 1983.)

Table 12.1 The Pectinate Line and Changes in the Surgical Anal Canal

	Below the pectinate line	Above the pectinate line
Embryonic origin	Ectoderm	Endoderm
Anatomy		
Lining	Stratified squamous	Simple columnar
Arterial supply	Inferior rectal artery	Superior rectal artery
Venous drainage	Systemic, by way of inferior rectal vein	Portal, by way of superior rectal vein
Lymphatic drainage	To inguinal nodes	To pelvic and lumbar nodes
Nerve supply	Inferior rectal nerves (somatic)	Autonomic fibers (visceral)
Physiology	Excellent sensation	Sensation quickly diminishes
Pathology		
Cancer	Squamous cell carcinoma	Adenocarcinoma
Varices	External hemorrhoids	Internal hemorrhoids

(By permission of JE Skandalakis, SW Gray, and JR Rowe, *Anatomical Complications in General Surgery*, New York: McGraw-Hill, 1983.)

Anal Glands and Anal Papillae

Anal glands and anal papillae may be appreciated from Fig. 12.13.

■ BLOOD SUPPLY OF THE COLON AND RECTUM

Arterial Supply

Superior Mesenteric Artery

The cecum and the ascending colon receive blood from two arterial branches of the superior mesenteric artery: the ileocolic and right colic arteries (Fig. 12.14). These arteries form arcades from which vasa recta pass to the medial colon wall.

As the vasa recta reach the surface of the colon, they divide into short and long branches, the former serving the medial or mesenteric side of the colon and the latter serving the lateral and antimesenteric side. The long branches send twigs into the epiploic appendages (Fig. 12.10).

The transverse colon is similarly supplied by the middle colic artery from the superior mesenteric artery. The left portion of the transverse colon is supplied by the left colic artery, a branch of the inferior mesenteric artery.

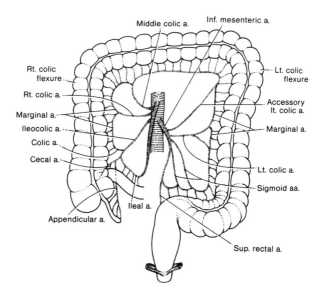

Figure 12.14. Schema of the blood supply to the large intestine. There are many variations of this basic pattern. (By permission of JE Skandalakis, SW Gray, and JR Rowe, *Anatomical Complications in General Surgery*, New York: McGraw-Hill, 1983.)

Middle Colic Artery

The middle colic artery supplies the transverse colon and bifurcates from 3 to 11 cm from the colonic wall. It may be absent in 5–8 percent of individuals.

The origin of the middle colic artery is from the superior mesenteric artery in most cases, the inferior pancreaticoduodenal artery in a few, or from various other arteries. It may be absent.

Inferior Mesenteric Artery

The inferior mesenteric artery arises from the aorta above its bifurcation opposite the lower portion of the 3rd lumbar vertebra. The length of the artery before its first branch varies from 1.5 to 9.0 cm.

The branches of the inferior mesenteric artery are the left (ascending) colic artery, one to nine sigmoid arteries, and the superior rectal (hemorrhoidal) artery (Figs. 12.14 and 12.15C).

Marginal Artery (of Drummond)

The marginal artery is composed of a series of arcades forming a single vessel that parallels the mesenteric border of the large intestine from 1 to 8 cm from the intestinal wall (Figs. 12.15A–C). It may or may not terminate at the superior rectal artery (Fig. 12.15C). Occasionally, however, the continuity of this artery is disrupted in one or more points.

Arteries of the Rectum and Anal Canal

These are the superior, middle, inferior, and median sacral rectal arteries. One unpaired and two paired arteries supply the rectum and anal canal (Fig. 12.16). The superior rectal (hemorrhoidal) artery arises from the inferior mesenteric artery and descends to the posterior wall of the upper rectum. Supplying the posterior wall, it divides and sends right and left branches to the lateral walls of the middle portion of the rectum down to the pectinate line.

The main trunk of the middle rectal artery is inferior to the rectal stalk and could be endangered when the rectum is separated from the seminal vesicle, prostate, or vagina. These findings may explain why some surgeons feel that the lateral ligaments may be cut with impunity.

The middle rectal artery is usually absent in the female. It is probably replaced by the uterine artery. In the male, the chief beneficiaries of the artery are the rectal musculature and the prostate gland.

The inferior rectal (hemorrhoidal) arteries arise from the internal pudendal arteries and proceed ventrally and medially to supply the anal canal distal to the pectinate line.

The median sacral artery arises just above the bifurcation of the aorta and descends beneath the peritoneum on the anterior surface of the lower lumbar vertebrae, the sacrum, and the coccyx. It sends several very small branches to the posterior wall of the rectum.

Venous Drainage

The veins of the colon follow the arteries. On the right, the veins join to form the superior mesenteric vein. The superior rectal vein drains the descending and sigmoid colon; it passes upward to form the inferior mesenteric veins.

The rectum is drained by the superior rectal veins, which enter the inferior mesenteric veins. This drainage is to the portal system. The middle and inferior rectal veins enter the internal iliac and thus the systemic circulation (Fig. 12.17).

Remember that anastomoses occur between the superior rectal vein

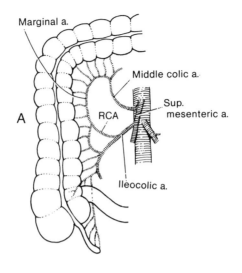

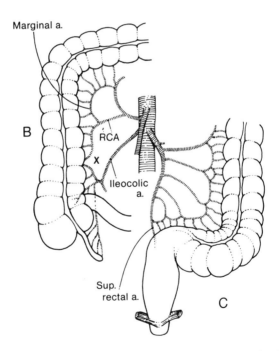

Figure 12.15. Variations of the arteries to the right colon. (A) Usual pattern. (B) The marginal artery is incomplete at "X." (C) Arteries to the left colon. There may be fewer sigmoid arteries than shown here. (By permission of JE Skandalakis, SW Gray, and JR Rowe, *Anatomical Complications in General Surgery*, New York: McGraw-Hill, 1983.)

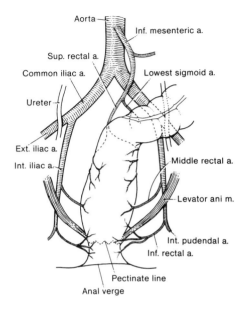

Figure 12.16. Diagram of the arterial supply to the rectum and anus. The median sacral artery supplying a few small branches to the posterior wall of the rectum is not shown in this figure. (By permission of JE Skandalakis, SW Gray, and JR Rowe, *Anatomical Complications in General Surgery*, New York: Mc-Graw-Hill, 1983.)

(portal) and the middle and inferior rectal veins (systemic). These constitute a portosystemic shunt.

■ LYMPHATIC DRAINAGE

The lymph nodes of the large intestine have been divided into four groups: epicolic, under the serosa of the wall of the intestine; paracolic, on the marginal artery; intermediate, along the large arteries (superior and inferior mesenteric arteries); and principal, at the root of the superior and inferior mesenteric arteries (Fig. 12.18). This last group includes mesenteric root nodes (which also receive lymph from the small intestine), aortic nodes, and left lumbar nodes.

Wide resection of the colon should include the entire segment supplied by a major artery. This also will remove most, but not all, of the lymphatic drainage of the segment (Fig. 12.19).

The lymph channels of the rectum and anal canal form two extramural

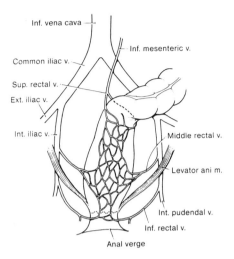

Figure 12.17. Diagram of the venous drainage of the rectum and anus. The superior rectal vein drains to the portal system, and the middle and inferior rectal veins drain to the systemic veins. The venous plexus between the veins forms a portacaval shunt. (By permission of JE Skandalakis, SW Gray, and JR Rowe, *Anatomical Complications in General Surgery*, New York: McGraw-Hill, 1983.)

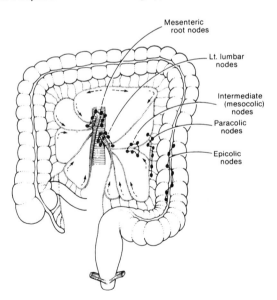

Figure 12.18. The lymphatics of the colon follow the arteries and drain to the principal nodes at the root of the mesentery. The path is by way of the epiploic, paracolic, and mesocolic lymph nodes. (By permission of JE Skandalakis, SW Gray, and JR Rowe, *Anatomical Complications in General Surgery*, New York: McGraw-Hill, 1983.)

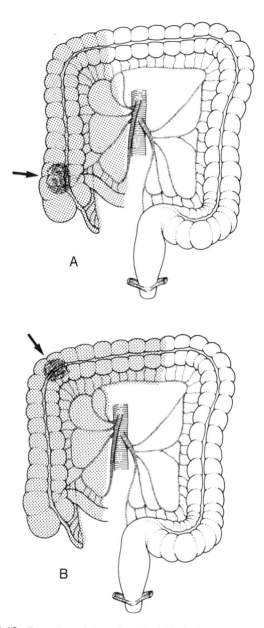

A

B

Figure 12.19. Resection of the colon should include the entire area served by a major artery, as well as the lesion itself. Most of the lymphatic drainage will be included. Areas of resection (shaded) for lesions in various segments of the colon are shown in A–F. An arrow indicates the site of the lesion. (By permission of JE Skandalakis, SW Gray, and JR Rowe, *Anatomical Complications in General Surgery*, New York: McGraw-Hill, 1983.)

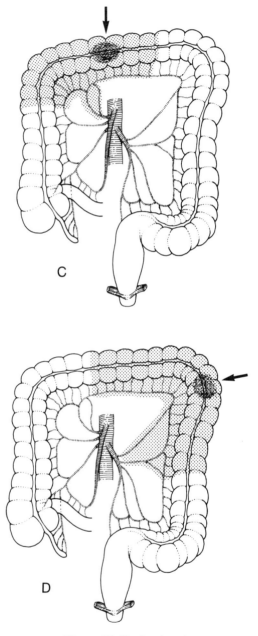

C

D

Figure 12.19. Continued

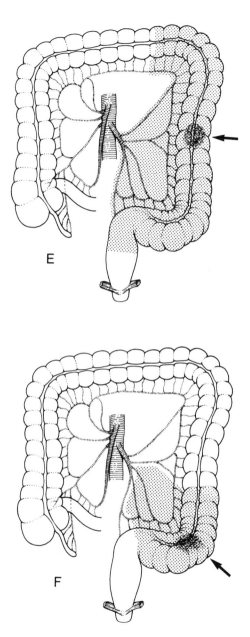

E

F

Figure 12.19. Continued

plexuses, one above and one below the pectinate line. The upper plexus drains through the posterior rectal nodes to a chain of nodes along the superior rectal artery to the pelvic nodes (Fig. 12.20). Some drainage follows the middle and inferior rectal arteries to the hypogastric nodes. Below the pectinate line, the plexus drains to the inguinal nodes.

The "watershed" of the extramural lymphatic vessels is at the pectinate line. The watershed for the intramural lymphatics is higher, at the level of the middle rectal valve (Fig. 12.21). These two landmarks may be kept in mind by the mnemonic "two, four, eight," meaning:

- 2 cm = anal verge to pectinate line
- 4 cm = surgical anal canal (above and below the pectinate line)
- 8 cm = anal verge to middle rectal valve

Downward spread of lesions of the rectum is similarly rare. Perhaps only 2 percent may spread downward. A margin of 2–3 cm distal to the tumor should be allowed in anterior resection.

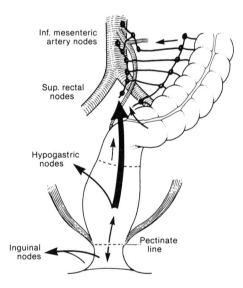

Figure 12.20. Lymphatic drainage of the sigmoid colon, rectum, and anus. Above the pectinate line, drainage is to the inferior mesenteric nodes. Below the line, drainage is to the inguinal nodes. (By permission of JE Skandalakis, SW Gray, and JR Rowe, *Anatomical Complications in General Surgery*, New York: McGraw-Hill, 1983.)

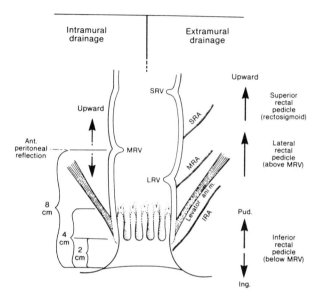

Figure 12.21. Diagram of lymph drainage of the anus and rectum. The watershed for extramural drainage is at the pectinate line (Fig. 12.20). The watershed for intramural drainage is at the level of the middle rectal valve, about 8 cm above the anal verge. IRA = inferior rectal artery; MRA = middle rectal artery; SRA = superior rectal artery; LRV = lower rectal valve; MRV = middle rectal valve; SRV = superior rectal valve. (By permission of JE Skandalakis, SW Gray, and JR Rowe, *Anatomical Complications in General Surgery*, New York: McGraw-Hill, 1983.)

■ NERVE SUPPLY TO THE RECTUM AND ANUS

Motor innervation of the internal rectal sphincter is supplied by sympathetic fibers that cause contraction and by parasympathetic fibers that inhibit contraction. Parasympathetic sacral afferent nerves mediate sensation of rectal distention. The external rectal sphincter is innervated by the inferior hemorrhoidal branch of the internal pudendal nerve and by the perineal branch of the 4th sacral nerve.

The pelvic splanchnic nerve (parasympathetic) and the hypogastric nerve (sympathetic) supply the lower rectal wall. Together these two nerves form the rectal plexus. The levator ani muscles are controlled by the 3rd and 4th sacral nerves.

The inferior rectal branches of the internal pudendal nerve follow the inferior rectal arteries and supply the sensory innervation of the perianal skin.

Remember that the pudendal nerve innervates the external sphincter and the puborectalis muscle. The sympathetic nerves have no influence on the muscular wall of the rectum. Evacuation is accomplished by the pelvic splanchnic nerve; continence is maintained by the pudendal and the pelvic splanchnic nerves.

TECHNIQUE

■ THE DECALOGUE OF GOOD COLON SURGERY

1. Prepare bowel with Golytely and Nichol's preparation (erythromycin and neomycin).

2. Administer intravenous antibiotics during the surgery and for 24–48 hours afterward.

3. Use nasogastric tube and Foley catheter when appropriate.

4. Understand anatomy of blood supply and lymphatics. When doing cancer surgery, ligate vessels at their origins.

5. Good technique for performing anastomosis includes:

   a. Observing whether the cut edges of the intestinal segments to be anastomosed have good color and are bleeding slightly. Avoid formation of hematomata at the anastomotic area.

   b. Clearing all fatty tissue from the anastomotic area by removing, without traction, the mesenteric border and the epiploic appendages.

6. Avoid tension of the anastomosis.

7. Use the omentum for wrap, if possible.

8. Be familiar with all surgical procedures and their modifications.

9. Identify the ureter to avoid injury.

10. Reapproximate the mesentery to avoid internal hernias.

■ CECOPEXY

Occasionally, the cecum and ascending colon are very mobile (Fig. 12.22). To avoid volvulus of the right colon and, therefore, intestinal obstruction, a cecopexy extending up to the ascending colon is performed. Suture the cecal and ascending tenia to the lateral peritoneum with interrrupted 3–0 synthetic absorbable material or silk, and perform an appendectomy (Fig. 12.23).

Occasionally a cecostomy is necessary, using a Foley catheter (Fig. 12.24).

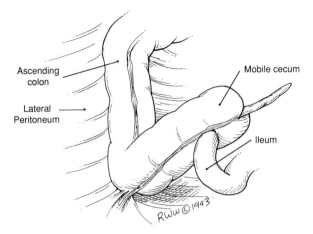

Ascending colon

Mobile cecum

Lateral Peritoneum

Ileum

Figure 12.22

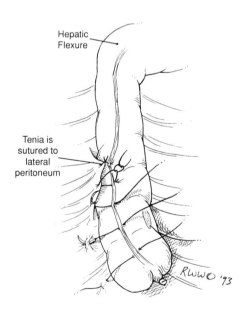

Hepatic Flexure

Tenia is sutured to lateral peritoneum

Figure 12.23

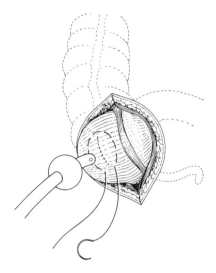

Figure 12.24. Cecostomy. The broken line surrounded by the purse-string suture indicates the incision for the insertion of the Foley catheter. (By permission of JE Skandalakis, SW Gray, and JR Rowe, *Anatomical Complications in General Surgery*, New York: McGraw-Hill, 1983.)

■ CECOSTOMY

Although cecostomy is less popular than it once was, we have used the procedure successfully several times for decompression and for suture-line protection. With a short transverse mesocolon in an obese patient, cecostomy is the ideal operation.

Loop Colostomy

A loop colostomy (Fig. 12.25) is feasible only in the transverse or sigmoid colon because a mesentery is required. If the transverse mesocolon is short, mobilization of the hepatic and splenic flexures will provide a more mobile loop.

Sigmoid loop colostomy is, for practical purposes, left colon colostomy. The stoma should be located at the junction of the descending and the sigmoid colon so that the peritoneal fixation of the descending colon will protect the proximal stoma from prolapse.

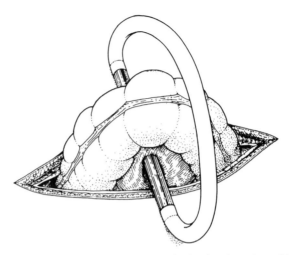

Figure 12.25. Loop colostomy. The loop of colon has been brought through the incision, held in place by a glass tube with rubber tubing connecting its ends. (By permission of JE Skandalakis, SW Gray, and JR Rowe, *Anatomical Complications in General Surgery*, New York: McGraw-Hill, 1983.)

Loop Transverse Colostomy

Procedure:

Step 1. Make a 4 to 6-cm transverse incision at the right, or occasionally at the left, lateral border of the rectus abdominis muscle (Fig. 12.26).

Step 2. Divide the anterior rectus sheath, rectus abdominis muscle, and posterior sheath.

Step 3. Deliver the transverse colon into the wound outside the peritoneal cavity and form a small hole at the omentum and the mesenteric border of the colon to permit the entrance of a plastic rod (Fig. 12.27).

Step 4. Open the colon as shown and mature to the skin with 4-0 Vicryl sutures (Fig. 12.28). However, maturation of the colostomy in the operating room depends on the philosophy of the surgeon (Fig. 12.29).

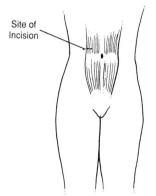

Site of
Incision

Figure 12.26

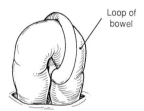

Loop of
bowel

Figure 12.27

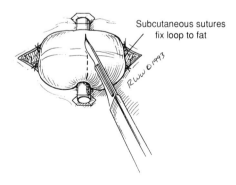

Subcutaneous sutures
fix loop to fat

Figure 12.28

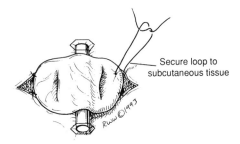

Secure loop to
subcutaneous tissue

Figure 12.29

End Colostomy (Figs. 12.30–12.32)

The stoma is located at the lower descending colon or at a loop of the upper sigmoid colon. Good mobilization is a must, especially when the stoma is at the lower descending colon or at the iliac part of the sigmoid colon. The mesenteric root should be incised very carefully to avoid bleeding, which would jeopardize the vitality of the bowel. The procedures of end colostomy are the same as in left colectomy, except that the proximal loop is secured to a special skin opening and the distal loop is reinserted into the peritoneal cavity.

Procedure:

Step 1. In the vicinity of the left lower quadrant, excise a round piece of skin the size of a half-dollar. Use electrocoagulation for the division and separation of fat. Expose the fascia and make a cruciate incision (Fig. 12.30).

Step 2. Divide the muscles and expose the peritoneum as in appendectomy (Fig. 12.30). Direct two fingers from the orignal incision to the new, round one (Fig. 12.31). Open the peritoneum and insert a Babcock clamp through the skin opening into the peritoneal cavity and grasp the proximal end of the colon. Gently manipulate the end through the skin. The authors prefer a length of 4–5 cm of proximal colon to hang outside the skin. Attach the colonic wall to the fat, using four sutures of 3-0 catgut, approximately 2–3 cm from the colonic edge (Fig. 12.32).

Step 3. If the surgeon prefers operating room maturation, then the closed end of the proximal colon should be excised and the full thickness of the colonic wall sutured to the edges of the skin using 4-0 Vicryl absorbable sutures.

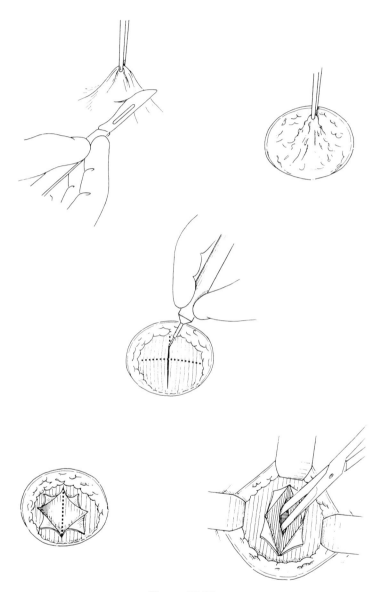

Figure 12.30

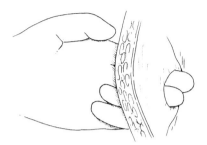

Figure 12.31

Prasad End Loop Colostomy

Procedure:

Step 1. Prior to surgery, place a mark for the stoma close to the obstruction (Fig. 12.33).

Step 2. Using a GIA stapler, perform a typical segmental colectomy appropriate to the disease.

Step 3. Bring the proximal end of the colon through the abdominal wall. Then deliver the antimesenteric corner of the distal colonic staple line through the skin incision (Fig. 12.34).

Step 4. Mature the proximal colon by removing the staple line and suturing the edges to the skin. The distal colon is then matured by removing the stapled corner and fixing it to the proximal colon and to the skin (Figs. 12.35 and 12.36).

Closure of Colostomy

Procedure:

Step 1. Insert moist gauze at both colostomy stomata.

Step 2. Carefully mobilize the colostomy by inserting the index finger into the stoma and cutting the skin and subcutaneous fat, being sure not to incise the colonic wall or to go deep into the peritoneal cavity (Fig. 12.37).

Step 3. Use 3-0 chromic suture for full-thickness interrupted or running closure of the bowel wall. Follow with silk Lembert seromuscular suture as a second layer (Fig. 12.38).

Step 4. With clean instruments, close the wound in layers.

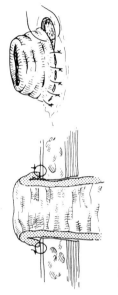

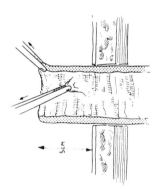

Figure 12.32

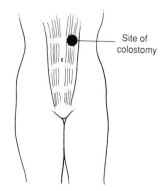

Site of
colostomy

Figure 12.33

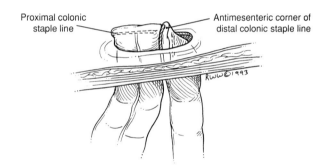

Proximal colonic
staple line

Antimesenteric corner of
distal colonic staple line

Figure 12.34

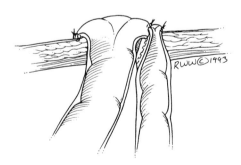

Figure 12.35

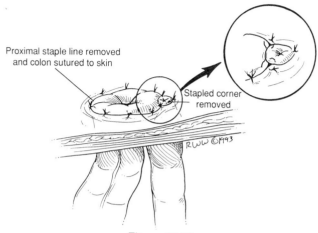

Proximal staple line removed
and colon sutured to skin

Stapled corner
removed

Figure 12.36

■ COLON RESECTION

Fig. 12.19 shows the extent of colectomy recommended for cancer at various sites in the colon. A standard right colectomy is essentially a midline resection, including a few centimeters of the terminal ileum, the cecum, and the right colon and proximal half of the transverse colon.

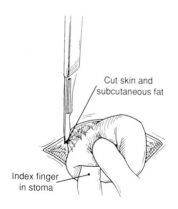

Cut skin and
subcutaneous fat

Index finger
in stoma

Figure 12.37

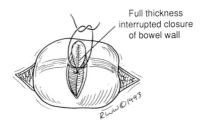

Full thickness
interrupted closure
of bowel wall

Figure 12.38

These are the segments served by the ileocolic, right colic, and right branches of the middle colic arteries (Fig. 12.19B).

In left colectomy, the lowest sigmoid artery may be too short for adequate sigmoid resection.

Benign and malignant pathologic processes require different colon resection techniques. We will discuss briefly step-by-step technique for the following conditions:

1. Malignant process: right colectomy, left colectomy, low resection for rectal cancer, abdominoperineal sigmoidoprostectomy

2. Benign process: abdominoperineal prostectomy, colectomy for obstruction cecostomy, sigmoid colectomy, colectomy for diverticulitis, rectal prolapse

PREOPERATIVE PREPARATION:

- barium enema
- colonoscopy and biopsy
- intravenous pyelogram
- nasogastric tube and Foley catheter in the operating room
- bowel preparation, including Golytely preparation, oral neomycin and erythromycin base, and intravenous antibiotics prior to incision

POSITION: Supine

ANESTHESIA: General

INCISION: Up to the surgeon

Right Colectomy (Fig. 12.19A)

Procedure:

Step 1. As soon as the abdomen is open, decide whether to use the routine or no-touch technique. With the no-touch technique that we prefer, we proceed as follows:

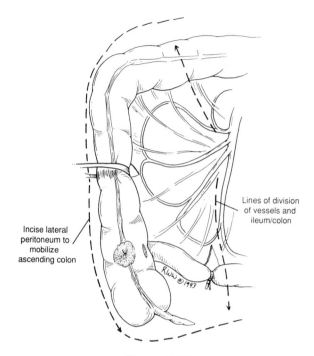

Incise lateral peritoneum to mobilize ascending colon

Lines of division of vessels and ileum/colon

Figure 12.39

a. Lumina of terminal ileum and transverse colon are occluded with umbilical tape proximally and distally to the tumor (Fig. 12.39).

b. Vessels are ligated at their origin (at the superior mesenteric artery or superior mesenteric vein) for complete isolation of the lymphovascular tree (Figs. 12.39 and 12.40).

Step 2. Explore the peritoneal cavity, saving until last the vicinity of pathology, i.e., the cecum, ascending colon, or right transverse colon.

Step 3. Make a very superficial incision at the mesentery indicating the line of resection, which should be lateral to the umbilical tape ligatures (Figs. 12.39 and 12.40).

Step 4. Carefully mobilize the right colon (cecum, ascending, right transverse) by incising the peritoneal reflection of the paracolic area. Elevate the colon with the index finger, protecting

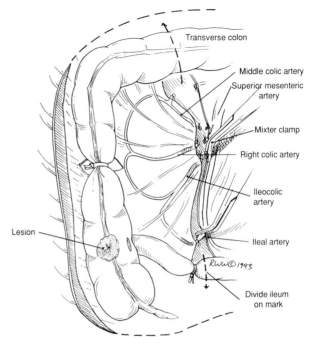

Figure 12.40

the duodenum, right ureter (over the right common iliac artery), and superior mesenteric vessels (Fig. 12.40).

Step 5. Carry out partial omentectomy, removing the right ¾ of the greater omentum, including the corresponding part of the gastrocolic ligament, if necessary (Fig. 12.41).

Step 6. Keeping in mind that occasionally the right colic artery springs directly from the superior mesenteric artery, ligate the two lymphovascular pedicles (ileocolic and middle colic). These ligations should be done carefully to avoid injury to the superior mesenteric vessels as well as to branches of the middle colic supplying the left transverse colon.

Remember:

✓ There are several variations to the anatomy here. Ligate the vessels twice using Mixter clamps.

Step 7. Be sure that both colon and ileum have a good blood supply.

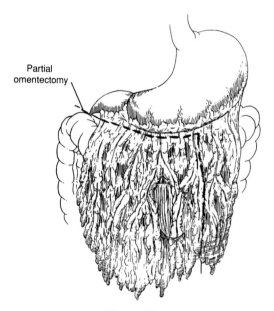

Partial
omentectomy

Figure 12.41

We prefer a side-to-side ileotransverse anastomosis using the stapling device.

Step 8. This is done as follows:

    a. Division of the ileum by GIA stapler (Fig. 12.42).

    b. Division of the colon by TA-55 stapler (Fig. 12.42).

    c. Align colon and ileum side by side (Fig. 12.43).

    d. Partial triangular excision of the antimesenteric corner of the stapled ileal and colonic edges.

    e. At the triangular defect, insert the two parts of the GIA stapler, one into the ileal lumen and the other into the colonic lumen. Be sure that the ends of the two parts are at the same point and fire the instrument. Remove the GIA stapler, inspect the lumina for bleeding, and use the TA-55 stapler to close the triangular areas (Fig. 12.44).

The authors like to reinforce the staple line with a few interrupted 3-0 silk Lembert sutures. The mesenteric defect is closed with interrupted 3-0 catgut.

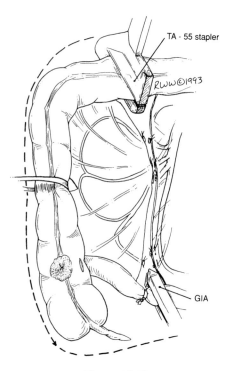

Figure 12.42

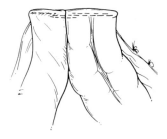

Figure 12.43

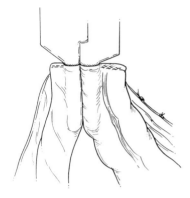

Figure 12.44

Step 9. We wrap the anastomosis with the remaining omentum before we close the mesenteric defect.

Step 10. Insert Jackson–Pratt drain and close.

Note: Alternatively, a two-layer end-to-end anastomosis can be done using a running 3-0 chromic for the mucosal layer and interrupted 3-0 silk Lembert sutures for the seromuscular layer (Fig. 12.45).

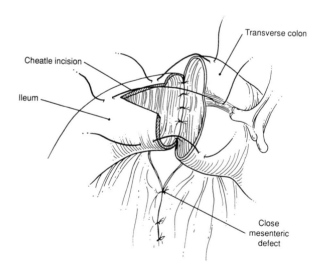

Figure 12.45

Left Colectomy (Fig. 12.19E)

Many steps for this procedure are similar to the right colectomy. There are three dangerous points, from above downward (from the left upper quadrant to the pelvis):

1. The splenocolic, phrenicocolic, and pancreaticocolic ligaments should be divided carefully to avoid rupture of the splenic capsule or injury to the pancreas (Fig. 12.46).

2. Identify the left ureter, which may be found crossing the left common iliac vessels. Knowing its location minimizes the possibility it will be injured (Fig. 12.47).

3. Avoid injury to the third portion of the duodenum, which almost always covers the origin of the inferior mesenteric artery and its downward continuation, the superior rectal artery. The third part of the duodenum is especially vulnerable if it is located low.

Remember:

✓ With good mobilization, you avoid tension.

Low Anterior Resection, Triple Staple Procedure (Fig. 12.19F)

Study previous information on left colectomy (Figs. 12.19E, 12.46, and 12.47). Ligate the inferior mesenteric artery and some sigmoidal branches (Fig. 12.48).

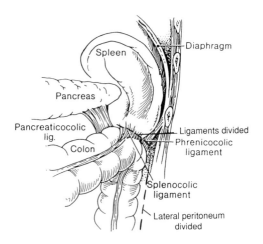

Figure 12.46. (By permission of JE Skandalakis, GL Colborn, LB Pemberton, et al., *Prob Gen Surg* 7(1):1–17, 1990.)

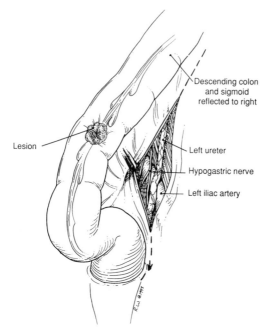

Descending colon
and sigmoid
reflected to right

Lesion

Left ureter

Hypogastric nerve

Left iliac artery

Figure 12.47

Procedure:

Step 1. Mobilize the rectosigmoid colon by incising the lateral peritoneal reflection upward to the splenic flexure and downward
to the sacral promontory and the presacral area. The downward incision should be gentle. Blunt dissection by the surgeon's hand is advisable (Fig. 12.49).

  Remember:

  ✓ The presacral fascia is part of the endopelvic fascia,
  without lymphatics, and it is not necessary to remove
  it. Invasion of the fascia by cancer means it is not cur-
  able (Fig. 12.49).

  ✓ Between the fascia and the presacral periosteum, there
  is a network of veins that drain into the sacral foramina. Dissect very close to the posterior colonic wall to
  avoid bleeding and injury to the fascia. It is extremely
  difficult to stop bleeding, even with ligation of both

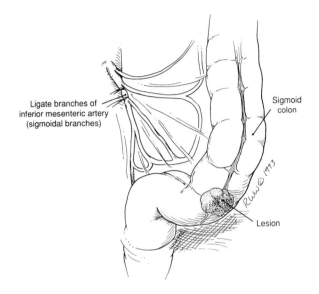

Ligate branches of
inferior mesenteric artery
(sigmoidal branches)

Sigmoid
colon

Lesion

Figure 12.48

hypogastric arteries. Tack insertion at the bleeding point is helpful (Fig. 12.50).

✓ To avoid dysfunction of the urinary bladder, as well as impotence in the male, dissect the left ureter carefully because it travels together with the left hypogastric nerve. Topographicoanatomically, both are located at the posterolateral pelvic wall and hypogastric artery, and the nerve is medial to the ureter (Fig. 12.49).

Step 2. In males, dissect at the prostatic area by dividing Denonvilliers fascia. In females, divide the cul-de-sac and further separate the urinary bladder and vaginal wall from the rectum.

Step 3. After satisfactory mobilization of the rectosigmoid, ligate the lymphovascular elements as described in the left colon resection and proceed downward for further vascular ligation and further careful rectal detachment, as described above. (Steps may vary depending on sex, local topographical anatomy, and obesity of the patient.)

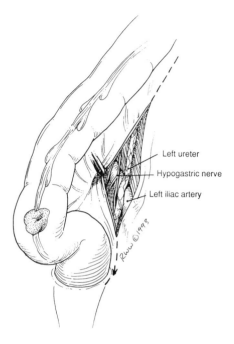

Left ureter

Hypogastric nerve

Left iliac artery

Figure 12.49

Step 4. Place a TA-55 stapler approximately 2–4 cm below the tumor and fire, thus placing a double row of staples across the rectosigmoid. Place an angled bowel clamp proximal to the staple line and divide the colon between the staple line and the bowel clamp (Fig. 12.51).

Step 5. Place a bowel clamp where the proximal line of excision is to be, divide the colon, and remove the specimen.

Step 6. *The triple staple technique.* This is accomplished by inserting the anvil of the EEA into the proximal colon and then stapling the colon closed with the anvil inside (Fig. 12.52). The anvil-connecting end, which is cone-shaped and sharp, can then be pushed through the line of staples.

Step 7. Next insert the EEA into the rectum, and when up against the staple line, begin to turn the knob on the device so that the connector end (also sharp and cone-shaped) will slide through the staple line (Fig. 12.53).

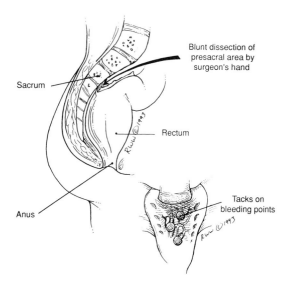

Sacrum

Blunt dissection of
presacral area by
surgeon's hand

Rectum

Anus

Tacks on
bleeding points

Figure 12.50

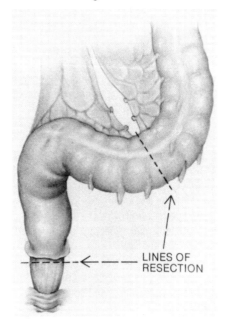

LINES OF
RESECTION

Figure 12.51. (Copyright 1980, 1994, United States Surgical Corporation. All rights reserved. Reprinted with the permission of the United States Surgical Corporation.)

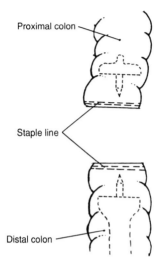

Proximal colon

Staple line

Distal colon

Figure 12.52

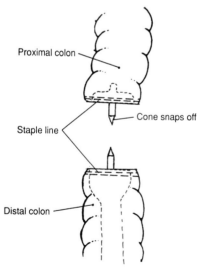

Proximal colon

Staple line

Cone snaps off

Distal colon

Figure 12.53

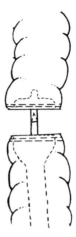

Figure 12.54

Step 8. Next the connectors from the anvil and the EEA snap together (Fig. 12.54). The knob at the end of the EEA is then
slowly turned, thus approximating the proximal colon and
distal rectum (Fig. 12.55).

Step 9. When they are correctly approximated as indicated on the
dial of the EEA, the device can be fired. The knob on the

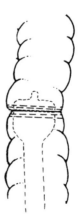

Figure 12.55

EEA is then opened one turn and the EEA is then rotated gently and removed from the rectum.

Note: There should be a complete doughnut of tissue present in the EEA indicating a satisfactory anastomosis. (If the surgeon has any doubt about the anastomosis, a temporary colostomy may be done. One month following the colostomy, a low-pressure Gastrografin enema may be done and, if no leakage occurs, the colostomy may be closed.)

Step 10. Jackson-Pratt drainage is up to the surgeon. Close in layers.

Total Colectomy and Ileoanal Anastomosis with Mucocectomy

POSITION: Lithotomy

Procedure, Part A:

Step 1. Expose the anal canal with Hill–Ferguson and Pratt retractors. Identify the dentate line (2 cm above the anal verge) (Fig. 12.56).

Step 2. Make a circumferential mucosal incision just above the den-

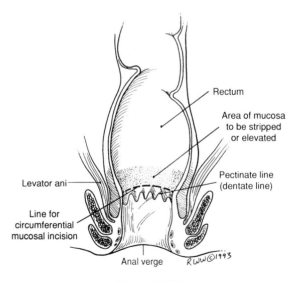

Figure 12.56

tate line. Carefully elevate the rectal mucosa (which is the end of the surgical anal canal) approximately 2 cm upward, separating it from the internal sphincter (Fig. 12.57).

Step 3. Oversew the cut edge of the mucosa with 3-0 chromic catgut (Fig. 12.58).

Procedure, Part B:

Step 4. Perform a typical total colectomy from the ileocecal junction (terminal ileum) to the levator ani level. Be careful to include the dissected distal mucosa of Part A (Fig. 12.59).

Step 5. With the specimen out of the peritoneal cavity, prepare a J-pouch construction using the terminal ileum, which may be mobilized carefully. Make the loop approximately 15-20 cm long. Approximate the parts of the loop using 4-0 silk interrupted sutures four or five times. Be sure to have the distal part of the terminal ileum facing upward (Fig. 12.60).

Step 6. Use the GIA stapler to anastomose both limbs, forming a common ileoileal pouch (Fig. 12.61).

Step 7. Anastomose the apex of the pouch to the vicinity of the dentate line with deep bites of 3-0 synthetic absorbable suture in an interrupted fashion (Fig. 12.62).

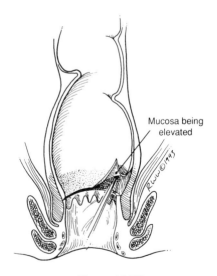

Mucosa being elevated

Figure 12.57

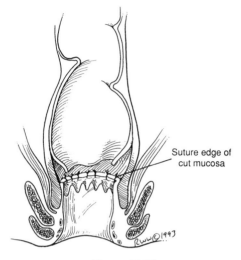

Suture edge of
cut mucosa

Figure 12.58

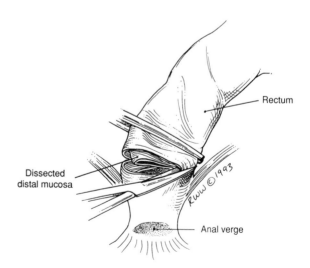

Rectum

Dissected
distal mucosa

Anal verge

Figure 12.59

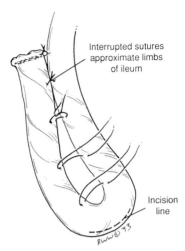

Interrupted sutures
approximate limbs
of ileum

Incision
line

Figure 12.60

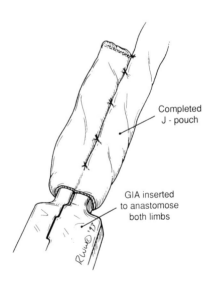

Completed
J - pouch

GIA inserted
to anastomose
both limbs

Figure 12.61

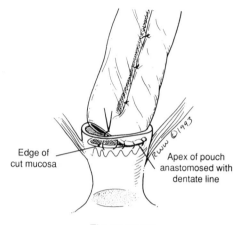

Edge of
cut mucosa

Apex of pouch
anastomosed with
dentate line

Figure 12.62

Step 8. To protect the anastomosis, the authors advise a diverting ileostomy.

Step 9. Two months postoperatively, a Gastrografin study should be done to check the function of the anastomotic pouch to the last 2 cm of the rectum. If the condition is satisfactory, the ileostomy can be closed.

An alternative procedure is the total colectomy and ileoanal anastomosis without mucocectomy. This procedure may be done by performing the J-pouch and anal anastomosis using the double staple technique, which eliminates the need for the mucocectomy and allows the anastomosis to be done almost at the dentate line.

Abdominoperineal Resection

The abdominal phase of an abdominoperineal resection is an extended left colectomy with a presacral dissection to mobilize the rectum, which will be removed by the perineal phase.

The left colon has been mobilized down to the rectovesical or rectouterine fossa by medial and lateral incision of the peritoneal ligaments of the sigmoid colon. The left ureter and left gonadal vessels are visualized; the inferior mesenteric artery and its downward continuation as the superior rectal artery are identified, the duodenum is pushed upward, and the surgeon is ready to enter the presacral area by the bloody presacral dissection.

Most of the bleeding is from the presacral veins which lie beneath the endopelvic fascia. The fascia should not be removed. Use clips for hemostasis; warm packs with Gelfoam will reduce the bleeding. Thumbtacks may be used.

Use long scissors for the perirectal tissues and the fascia of Waldeyer which bridges the sacrum and coccyx to the lower rectum. Blunt dissection with the surgeon's hand may be used to complete the procedure.

The tip of the prostate, with Denonvilliers fascia, or the tip of the uterine cervix as well as the tip of the coccyx may now be palpated; the hypogastric nerve and hypogastric (pelvic) plexus must be preserved lest there be problems with ejaculation or a neurogenic bladder.

The ureter (and the lateral ligaments of the rectum) must be traced deep into the pelvis by careful dissection without elevation. Division of the colon and formation of the colostomy may now be done. The pelvic peritoneum should be closed to avoid herniation and obstruction of the small bowel.

The perineal phase of the abdominoperineal resection encounters the following structures: the pudendal vessels, which should be ligated, the levator sling, which should be excised widely, and the membranous urethra of the male in which a Foley catheter has been placed prior to surgery. Use sharp dissection to separate the prostate from the lower rectum. The perineum should be partially or completely closed; a suction drain is advisable.

Abdominoperineal Resection Procedure

This resection is composed of two parts: abdominal and perineal. The abdominal portion is simply a low, anterior resection without anastomosis, and formation of a permanent colostomy.

The perineal portion is a separation of the surgical anal canal (the last 4 cm of the anorectum) from the pelvic diaphragm by dissection and sacrifice of the sphincteric apparatus and by removing the specimen and all perineal tissues related to the spaces around the anus (ischiorectal, fossae–retrorectal, etc.)

Procedure:

Step 1. Close the anal orifice by using a subcutaneous continuous purse-string suture of 0 silk at the skin of the anal verge. Make a circumferential perianal incision approximately 3 cm from the closed anus (Fig. 12.63).

Step 2. Use chromic catgut to ligate the inferior and middle rectal vessels and all vessels at the lateral aspect of the wound. End the procedure with blunt and sharp dissection, and remove the

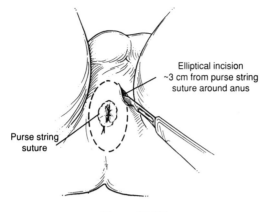

Figure 12.63

specimen by division of the pelvic diaphragm with cautery or knife (Figs. 12.64 and 12.65).

Step 3. Tailor end colostomy according to the body and size of the abdomen.

Step 4. If it is possible, approximate the right and left pelvic diaphragms with synthetic absorbable suture.

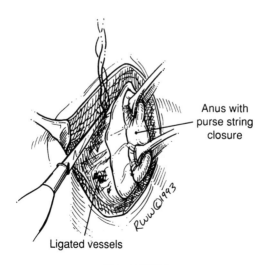

Figure 12.64

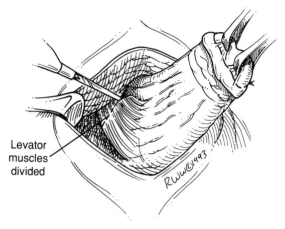

Levator muscles divided

Figure 12.65

Step 5. Close the perineal wound with chromic catgut or 3-0 Vicryl sutures. Place two 10 mm Jackson-Pratt drains exiting from the perineum and draining the presacral space and area of the pelvic diaphragm. Close the skin with a stapler.

■ PROCEDURES OF THE SURGICAL ANAL CANAL AND PERIANAL REGIONS

No anorectal procedure should be undertaken without digital and sigmoidoscopic examination. The following is the anatomy as encountered by the examiner's finger or as seen in the sigmoidoscope. Digital examination should always precede sigmoidoscopy. It relaxes the sphincters and reveals any obstruction that might be injured by the sigmoidoscope.

The anal verge separates the pigmented perianal skin from the pink transition zone. The verge is the reference line for the position of all other structures encountered (Fig. 12.66).

When the gloved and lubricated index finger is inserted so that the distal interphalangeal joint is at the anal verge, the subcutaneous portion of the external (voluntary) sphincter is felt as a tight ring around the distal half of the distal phalanx (Fig. 12.67A). The fingertip should detect the pectinate line of anal valves that lies about 2 cm above the anal verge. The anal columns (Morgagni) above the valves also may be felt. External

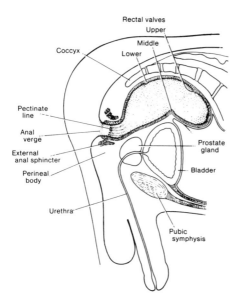

Figure 12.66. Diagram of anorectal landmarks for sigmoidoscopic examination: patient in knee/chest or knee/elbow position. (By permission of JE Skandalakis, SW Gray, and JR Rowe, *Anatomical Complications in General Surgery*, New York: McGraw-Hill, 1983.)

hemorrhoids, polyps, and hypertrophied anal papillae in this region are readily detected. Good palpation of the prostate in males is paramount.

Further insertion of the finger to the level of the middle interphalangeal joint brings the first joint to the anorectal ring formed by the deep component of the external sphincter, the puborectalis loop, and the upper margin of the internal sphincter. The ring is felt posteriorly and laterally, but not anteriorly (Fig. 12.67B).

Still further penetration of the finger to the level of the metacarpophalangeal joint allows the distal phalanx to enter the rectum. The left lower rectal fold may often be touched. At this point the pelvirectal space lies lateral and the rectovesical or rectovaginal space lies anterior. Further anterior to the rectum one can palpate the prostate gland in men and the upper vagina and cervix in women (Fig. 12.67C).

The sigmoidoscope should be inserted, aimed at the patient's umbilicus. At 5 cm from the anal verge, the tip will be at the anorectal ring (Fig. 12.68A). With the obturator removed, the left lower rectal fold should be visible. At about 8 cm from the verge, the middle rectal fold may be seen. This is the level of the peritoneal reflection. The superior

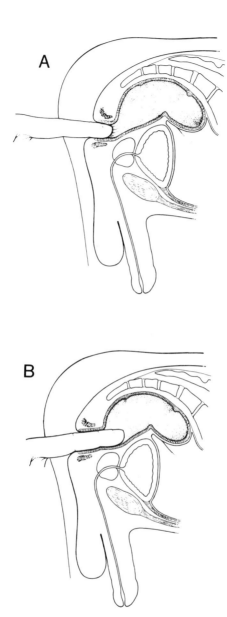

Figure 12.67. Digital examination. (A) Distal interphalangeal joint at the anal verge. Hemorrhoids can be detected at this stage. (B) Middle interphalangeal joint at the anal verge. (C) Metacarpophalangeal joint at the anal verge. The tip of the finger is at or just above the inferior rectal valve. (By permission of JE Skandalakis, SW Gray, and JR Rowe, *Anatomical Complications in General Surgery*, New York: McGraw-Hill, 1983.)

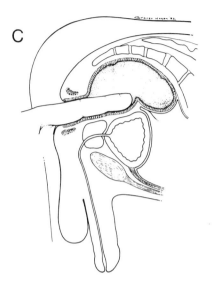

Figure 12.67. Continued

rectal fold is reached at 10–12 cm, and beyond this, passage of the instrument is easy (Fig. 12.68B).

The most dangerous area is between the middle and superior rectal folds, just above the peritoneal reflection. This is the area in which perforation by the sigmoidoscope may occur.

Ischiorectal Abscess: Incision and Drainage (Fig. 12.69)

POSITION: Prone

ANESTHESIA: Local; in most cases, as an office procedure

PROCEDURE: Make an incision (radial or parallel, and long enough to drain the cavity) close to the anus if possible, depending, of course, on the localized maximum swelling and tenderness (Fig. 12.69). Perform intracavital digital examination to break possible septa. Light packing with petrolatum and iodoform gauze should be removed in 24 hours (Figs. 12.70 and 12.71).

   Remember:

   ✓ Later, if fistulas requiring excision develop, they will be close to the anal verge.

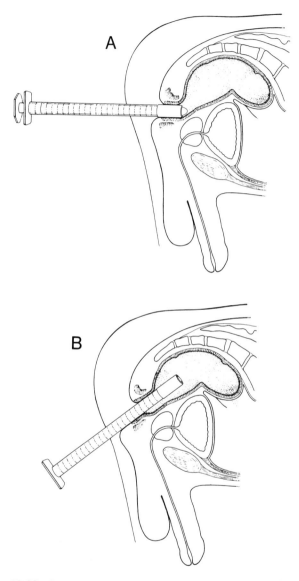

Figure 12.68. Sigmoidoscopic examination. (A) The instrument is directed toward the umbilicus. The tip is just past the anorectal ring. (B) With obturator removed, the instrument is passed by direct observation. The tip shown here is almost up to the middle rectal valve. (By permission of JE Skandalakis, SW Gray, and JR Rowe, *Anatomical Complications in General Surgery*, New York: McGraw-Hill, 1983.)

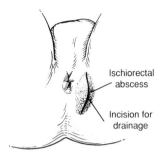

Figure 12.69

Anal Fistulectomy (Figs. 12.72–12.75)

PREOPERATIVE PREPARATION: 1–2 enemas

POSITION: Prone

ANESTHESIA: General or spinal

EXAMINATION: Digital, dilatation, retractor of choice and very careful external and internal probing. Methylene blue staining may be of great help.

Remember:

✔ Most of the fistulas in ano are midline posterior.

✔ Goodsall's rule must be learned.

PROCEDURE: If the fistula is simple and not deep, the fistulous tract may be excised in toto, leaving the wound open.

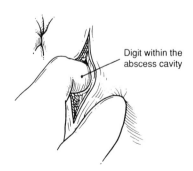

Figure 12.70

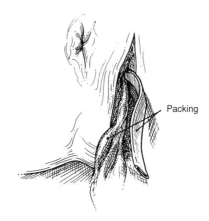

Packing

Figure 12.71

Remember:

✓ The subcutaneous and the superficial external sphincter may be divided with impunity, but be very careful with the deep external sphincter and the puborectalis.

✓ If the fistula is deep, the seton procedure is the treatment of choice (Figs. 12.74 and 12.75).

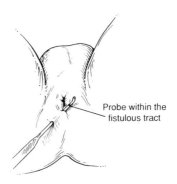

Probe within the fistulous tract

Figure 12.72

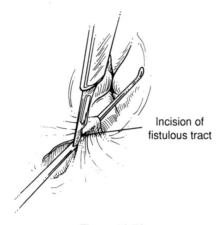

Incision of
fistulous tract

Figure 12.73

Anal Fissure

ANESTHESIA: Up to the surgeon

PROCEDURE: Lateral internal sphincterotomy. The fissure is left alone. The surgeon palpates the intersphincteric groove with the finger, and at the lateral position the internal sphincter is transected distally to the groove.

Hemorrhoidectomy (Fig. 12.76)

PREPARATION: Repeated enemas

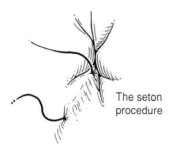

The seton
procedure

Figure 12.74

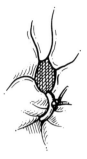

Figure 12.75

POSITION: As described previously

ANESTHESIA: Spinal or general

Procedure:

Step 1. Perform sigmoidoscopy, if not done prior to surgery.

Step 2. Perform anal dilatation and anoscopic evaluation. Insert a gauze sponge into the lower rectum to prevent downward fecal leakage. Withdraw sponge and identify hemorrhoids (Fig. 12.77).

Step 3. With a clamp of your choice, grasp hemorrhoids at the 3, 7, and 11 o'clock positions (Fig. 12.78).

Step 4. Make a triangular-shaped incision, including the skin of the anal verge up to the pectinate line or to the base of the hemorrhoid (Fig. 12.78).

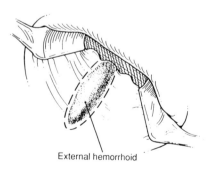

External hemorrhoid

Figure 12.76

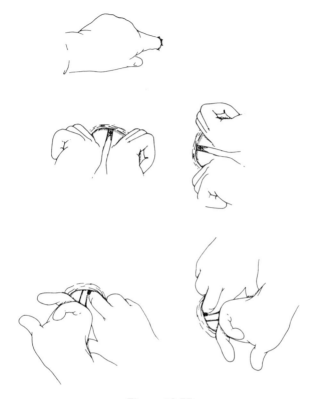

Figure 12.77

Step 5. Clamp the dissected hemorrhoid. Excise it using knife and 0 chromic catgut for an over-and-over continuous suture, including the mucosa but not the skin of the anal verge. Be sure to save enough mucosa between the excised hemorrhoids to prevent anal stenosis (Figs. 12.78 and 12.79).

Step 6. Occasionally an internal hemorrhoid has a polyp-like formation and may be excised in toto. The floor should be sutured with continuous 3–0 chromic (Fig. 12.80).

Incision and Drainage of External Thrombosed Hemorrhoids

POSITION AND PREPARATION: As described for hemorrhoids

ANESTHESIA: Local around the thrombosed hemorrhoid

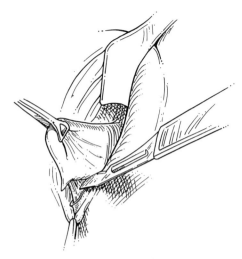

Figure 12.78

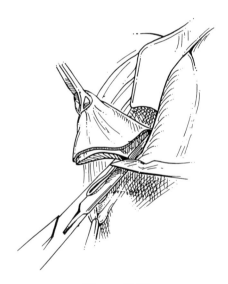

Figure 12.79

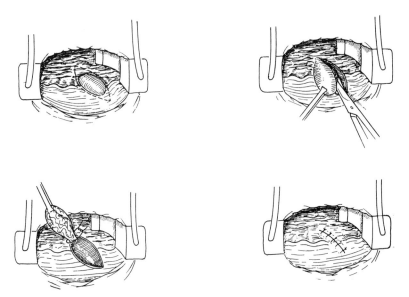

Figure 12.80

PROCEDURE: Incise at the hemorrhoidal apex and evacuate the thrombus by pressure at the base of the hemorrhoid or by instrument (curette or curved hemostat).

Excision of Pilonidal Cyst

POSITION, PREPARATION, AND ANESTHESIA: As previously described

Procedure:

Step 1. Fix extra-large adhesive tape to both lower gluteal areas and perineum. Anchor the tape to the operating room table, separating the intergluteal fold (Fig. 12.81).

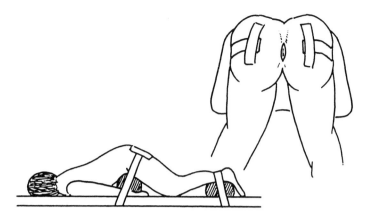

Figure 12.81

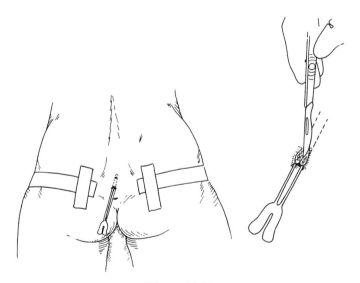

Figure 12.82

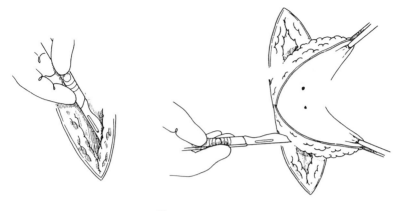

Figure 12.83

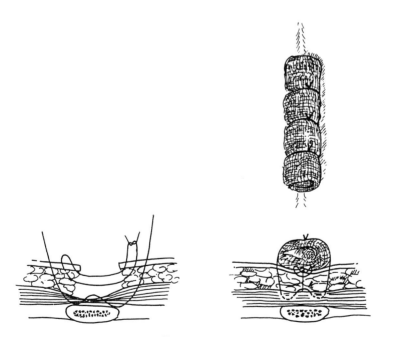

Figure 12.84

Step 2. Probe the sinus gently, since occasionally it may travel laterally (Fig. 12.82). With an ovoid incision down to the fascia,
remove the cyst and the sinuses en bloc and in toto, including
subcutaneous tissue (Fig. 12.83).

Step 3. After good hemostasis is established, pack the wound with
iodoform gauze, or, if there is no infection, close the wound
in one layer using 3–0 nylon with interrupted vertical mattress
sutures, including the fascia, as demonstrated in Fig. 12.84.

13

Liver

ANATOMY

■ TOPOGRAPHIC ANATOMY OF THE LIVER

Diaphragmatic Surface Relations

For descriptive purposes, the diaphragmatic surface is divided into superior, posterior, anterior, and right portions:

1. The superior portion is related to the diaphragm and, from right to left, the right pleura and lung, the pericardium and heart, and the left pleura and lung.

2. The posterior portion is related to the diaphragm and the lower ribs. The sulcus for the inferior vena cava and most of the bare area of the liver and diaphragm are located here.

3. Anteriorly the liver is related to the diaphragm, the costal margins, the xiphoid process of the sternum, and the anterior abdominal wall.

4. The right portion is a continuation of the posterior surface and is related to the diaphragm, the right pleura and lung, and the 7th to the 11th ribs.

Anteriorly, the inferior border of the liver is marked by two notches. A deep notch indicates the site of the round ligament (ligamentum teres); a shallower notch marks the presence of the gallbladder.

Visceral Surface Relations

The visceral surface of the liver is related to the following organs from right to left:

1. The hepatic flexure and part of the right transverse colon. The colonic impression extends from the right lobe to the medial segment of the left lobe.

2. Behind the colonic impression is the peritoneum of the hepatorenal pouch, the right kidney, and the right adrenal gland. Here the right adrenal gland is in direct contact with the liver at the bare area.

3. The gallbladder.

4. The first and second parts of the duodenum lie medial to the gallbladder.

5. The esophagus is to the left of the ligamentum venosum.

6. The remainder of the left lobe is in contact with the stomach.

■ PERITONEAL REFLECTIONS AND LIGAMENTS OF THE LIVER

The liver is attached to the anterior abdominal wall and to the inferior surface of the diaphragm by the falciform, round, and coronary ligaments. The peritoneum covering the liver is reflected onto the diaphragm as two separate leaves, the anterior and posterior coronary ligaments. Between these is an area in which the diaphragm and the liver are in contact without peritoneum. This is the "bare area." On the left, the two leaves of the coronary ligament approach and join to form the left triangular ligament; on the right, their apposition forms the right triangular ligament (Fig. 13.1).

Anteriorly, the anterior layer of the coronary ligament forms a fold that extends over the superior surface of the liver and is reflected over the anterior abdominal wall. This fold is the falciform ligament. Between the two layers of the fold, the remnant of the embryonic left umbilical vein forms the round ligament (ligamentum teres) of the liver. The falciform and round ligaments extend into the liver to form the obvious fissure that separates the apparent left and right "lobes" of the liver (which in reality are the two segments of the left lobe). On the visceral surface, the fissure for the round ligament extends posteriorly on the fissure for the ligamentum venosum. Between the fissure and the bed of the gallbladder lies the quadrate "lobe." It is separated from the more posterior caudate "lobe" by the transverse fissure, or porta hepatis (Fig. 13.2).

At the porta hepatis, the peritoneum of the liver forms the lesser omentum, which extends to the lesser curvature of the stomach as the gastrohepatic ligament and to the first inch of the duodenum as the

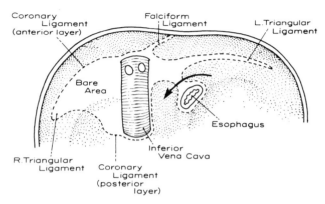

Figure 13.1. The inferior surface of the diaphragm showing the peritoneal attachments of the liver (broken lines). Within the boundaries of these attachments is the "bare area" of the liver and the diaphragm. The arrow passes through the posterior layer of the coronary ligament. (From Gray SW, Rowe JS Jr, Skandalakis JE. Surgical anatomy of the gastroesophageal junction. Am Surg 1979; 45(9): 575-587. Redrawn from Hollingshead WH. Anatomy for Surgeons. Harper & Row, 1956. Reprinted by permission of JB Lippincott Co.)

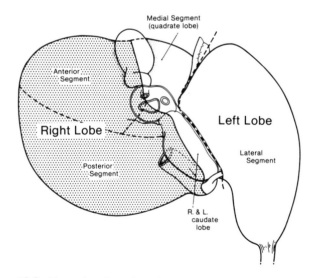

Figure 13.2. Visceral surface of the liver. The plane between the left medial and left lateral segments is variously referred to as the umbilical fissure, the fissure of the ligamentum teres, or the fissure of the falciform ligament. (By permission of JE Skandalakis, SW Gray, and JR Rowe, *Anatomical Complications in General Surgery*, New York: McGraw-Hill, 1983.)

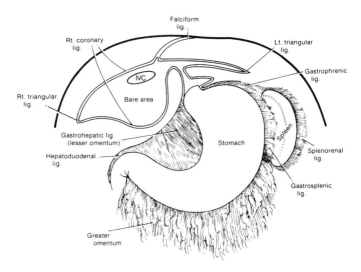

Figure 13.3. Peritoneal reflections of the liver: the lesser omentum (gastrohepatic and hepatoduodenal ligaments) and its relation to the coronary ligament of the liver and diaphragm. (By permission of JE Skandalakis, SW Gray, and JR Rowe, *Anatomical Complications in General Surgery*, New York: McGraw-Hill, 1983.)

hepatoduodenal ligament (Fig. 13.3). The right margin of the lesser omentum contains the hepatic artery, the portal vein, and the common bile duct. The bile duct is usually on the right, in the free edge of the omentum.

The surgeon should remember the approximate rib levels of the liver, lungs, and pleurae, as shown in Table 13.1.

Table 13.1 Approximate Rib Levels of Liver, Lungs, and Pleura

	At the lateral sternal line	At the midaxillary line	At the vertebral spine line
Liver	5	6	8
Lung	6	8	10
Pleura	7	10	12

(By permission of Lockhart RD, Hamilton GF, Fyfe FW. Anatomy of the Human Body. Philadelphia: JB Lippincott, 1959, p. 549.)

■ MORPHOLOGY OF THE LIVER

Injection and corrosion preparations of the bile ducts, hepatic arteries, and portal veins have shown conclusively that there are true right and left lobes of the liver, approximately equal in size (Fig. 13.4). Remember that hepatic veins do not follow this division.

On the visceral surface of the liver, the plane separating the right and left lobes passes through the bed of the gallbladder below and the fossa of the inferior vena cava above. On the diaphragmatic surface, there is no visible external mark. The line of separation is an imaginary line that passes from the notch of the gallbladder anteriorly, parallel to the fissure of the round ligament, to the inferior vena cava above (Fig. 13.2). The true left lobe thus consists of a left medial segment and a left lateral segment. The latter is the apparent left "lobe" of the older anatomists. Each of these segments may be divided into superior and inferior subsegments.

The right lobe may be similarly divided into anterior and posterior segments by imaginary lines. The intersegmental fissure, when present, indicates this separation. Each of these segments may be divided again into superior and inferior subsegments.

The caudate lobe is a separate region that lies in direct contact with the

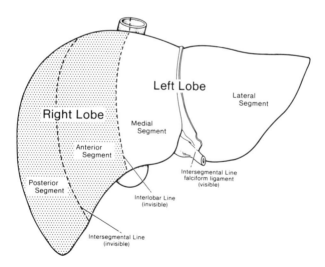

Figure 13.4. The true lobulation and segmentation of the liver: diaphragmatic surface. (By permission of JE Skandalakis, SW Gray, and JR Rowe, *Anatomical Complications in General Surgery*, New York: McGraw-Hill, 1983.)

left side of the inferior vena cava and may extend posterior to it. It may be divided into a right portion, a left portion, and the caudate process. Its bile ducts, hepatic arteries, and portal veins are supplied from both right and left main branches. The lobe is drained by two fairly constant hepatic veins that enter the vena cava on the left. The quadrate lobe is located between the gallbladder and the falciform ligament. It is a part of the median segment of the left lobe and is related to the pylorus and the first part of the duodenum.

The middle hepatic vein occupies the plane separating the true right and left lobes and does not follow the branches of the biliary tree.

At the present time, we believe that there are interlobar anastomoses between the right and left lobes. In other words, there is communication between the right and left arteries, veins, and ducts.

Clinically, hepatic artery ligation is effective and feasible, and interruption of a lobar bile duct usually produces only transitory jaundice. In spite of these findings, we must remember Michel's dictum that "the blood supply of the liver is always unpredictable." Possible collateral pathways are not always actual.

Intrahepatic Duct System

The usual pattern of intrahepatic ducts is shown in Fig. 13.5 and Table 13.2. The most frequent variations are those in which the right anterior or posterior segmental duct crosses the midline to enter the left hepatic duct (Fig. 13.6).

Notice that the caudate lobe has a right and a left drainage. Only the caudate process can be considered to be asymmetric. An aberrant biliary duct, moreover, may occasionally be found in the left triangular ligament. The ligament should always be incised between clamps and ligated.

■ ANOMALIES

The most common hepatic anomaly is diminished size of the left "lobe."

Small accessory lobes attached to the liver or to a mesentery are often reported. The most striking of these is Riedel's lobe, an elongated tongue of liver extending from the right "lobe" to or below the umbilicus (Fig. 13.7).

■ BLOOD SUPPLY TO THE LIVER

The liver receives blood from two sources: the hepatic artery and the portal vein. The hepatic artery provides about 25 percent of the hepatic

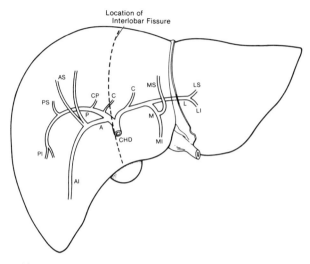

Figure 13.5. Diagram of the intrahepatic distribution of the bile ducts. The segmental branches are labeled: A = anterior; C = caudate; I = inferior; L = lateral; M = medial; P = posterior; S = superior; CHD = common hepatic duct; CP = caudate process. (By permission of JE Skandalakis, SW Gray, and JR Rowe, *Anatomical Complications in General Surgery*, New York: McGraw-Hill, 1983.)

blood supply and 50 percent of the oxygen. The hepatic portal vein contributes about 75 percent of the blood flow and 50 percent of the oxygen.

Hepatic Artery

In the usual pattern, the hepatic artery arises from the celiac trunk and divides into right and left hepatic arteries just before it enters the liver. An aberrant hepatic artery is one that arises from some other vessel than the celiac trunk and reaches the liver by an abnormal course.

Such an aberrant artery is *accessory* if it supplies a segment of the liver that also receives blood from a normal hepatic artery (Fig. 13.8A). It is *replacing* if it is the only blood supply to such a segment (Fig. 13.8B).

At the porta hepatis, the right hepatic artery passes behind the common bile duct in 85–95 percent of individuals. The left hepatic artery usually supplies the entire left lobe of the liver (Fig. 13.9A), but in some individuals, the left artery supplies only the left lateral segment, the left

Table 13.2 Terminology and Pattern of Intrahepatic Bile Ducts

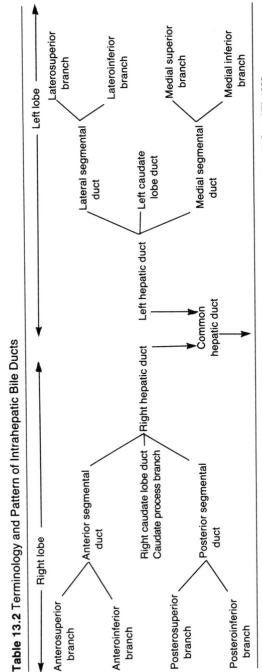

Source: By permission of JE Skandalakis, SW Gray, and JR Rowe, *Anatomical Complications in General Surgery*, New York: McGraw-Hill, 1983.

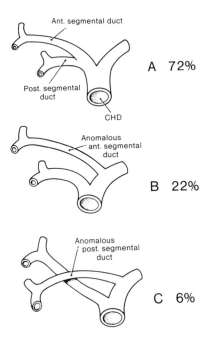

Figure 13.6. Intrahepatic segmental ducts. (A) Usual pattern. (B) Anomalous origin of right anterior duct. (C) Anomalous origin of right posterior duct. Both ducts cross the midline to reach their destinations. (By permission of JE Skandalakis, SW Gray, and JR Rowe, *Anatomical Complications in General Surgery*, New York: McGraw-Hill, 1983.)

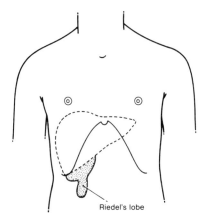

Figure 13.7. Riedel's lobe of the liver. This anomalous lobe is found usually in middle-aged women and presents as an asymptomatic but unexplained mass. (By permission of JE Skandalakis, SW Gray, and JR Rowe, *Anatomical Complications in General Surgery*, New York: McGraw-Hill, 1983.)

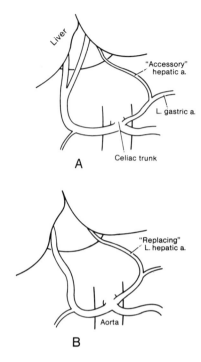

Figure 13.8. Aberrant hepatic arteries. (A) Accessory type; (B) replacing type. (By permission of JE Skandalakis, SW Gray, and JR Rowe, *Anatomical Complications in General Surgery*, New York: McGraw-Hill, 1983.)

medial segment being supplied by a branch of the right hepatic artery crossing the midline (Fig. 13.9B).

Within the liver, the arteries follow the course of the bile ducts, dividing into anterior and posterior branches in the right lobe and into lateral and medial branches in the left lobe (Fig. 13.10).

Ligation of the right or left hepatic artery results in ischemia for about 24 hours, after which translobar and transsegmental collateral vessels restore arterial blood to the deprived segment. With arteriography in patients, the existence of an interlobar arterial net following ligation of one hepatic artery has been appreciated.

Remember:

✓ Hepatic arteries are not end arteries in vivo; ligation of the right or left hepatic artery results in translobar and subcapsular collateral circulation within 24 hours.

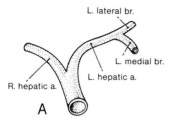

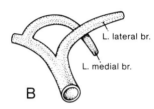

Figure 13.9. Hepatic arteries. (A) Usual pattern of segmental hepatic arteries. (B) Anomalous origin of the left medial segmental artery from the right hepatic artery, crossing the midline to reach the medial segment of the left lobe. This may be encountered in 25 percent of individuals. (By permission of JE Skandalakis, SW Gray, and JR Rowe, *Anatomical Complications in General Surgery*, New York: McGraw-Hill, 1983.)

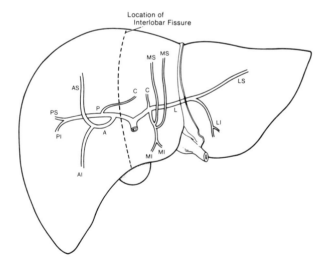

Figure 13.10. Diagram of the intrahepatic distribution of the hepatic artery. Abbreviations as in Fig. 13.5. (By permission of JE Skandalakis, SW Gray, and JR Rowe, *Anatomical Complications in General Surgery*, New York: McGraw-Hill, 1983.)

✓ After proximal ligation of the common hepatic artery, the right gastric and gastroduodenal arteries will maintain hepatic blood flow.

✓ Hepatic artery ligation is well tolerated. Death following such ligation is not usually the result of ligation.

✓ Cholecystectomy must always accompany hepatic artery ligation.

The Portal Vein

The portal vein originates with the confluence of the superior mesenteric and splenic veins behind the pancreas. In about ⅓ of individuals, the inferior mesenteric vein enters at this confluence; in the rest, it enters either the superior mesenteric vein or the splenic vein below the junction.

In its upward course, the portal vein receives the left gastric and several smaller veins before dividing into right and left branches at the porta hepatis. Here it lies beneath the hepatic duct and the hepatic artery (Fig. 13.11).

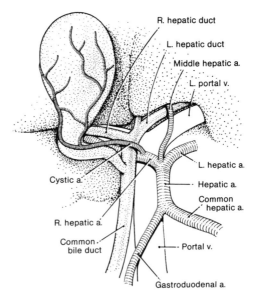

Figure 13.11. Relationship of the hepatic ducts, the hepatic artery, and the portal vein at the porta hepatis. (By permission of JE Skandalakis, SW Gray, and JR Rowe, *Anatomical Complications in General Surgery*, New York: Mc-Graw-Hill, 1983.)

On the right, the portal vessels follow the pattern of the hepatic arteries and the bile ducts. The right portal vein divides into anterior and posterior vessels, each dividing further into superior and inferior branches. Near its origin, the right vein sends a branch to the right side of the caudate lobe.

The left portal vein is smaller and longer than the right vein. It divides into medial and lateral vessels, each with superior and inferior branches, and it gives a branch to the left side of the caudate lobe. The medial vessel contains a dilatation, the pars umbilicus, which represents the orifice of the obliterated embryonic ductus venosus (Fig. 13.12).

Remember:

✓ Portal veins may be ligated without fatality. Intersegmental communication is from hepatic sinusoids of adjacent lobules. There are few true anastomoses between venous branches.

✓ Reduction in portal blood flow increases hepatic artery blood flow. The reverse is not true.

✓ Atrophy follows portal vein ligation.

✓ Ligation of both the lobar hepatic artery and the portal vein will result in atrophy without necrosis.

✓ Following a radical pancreaticoduodenal resection, the portal vein should not be ligated. Portal blood flow must be restored by a shunt or a replacement graft.

Hepatic Veins

Unlike the bile ducts, the hepatic arteries, and the portal veins, all of which serve lobes and segments of the liver, the hepatic veins lie in the planes between the lobes and segments. They are thus intersegmental and drain parts of adjacent segments. The presence of the hepatic veins requires the line of resection for a right lobectomy to be placed just to the right of the interlobar plane; for a left lobectomy, the line should be just to the left. The usual pattern of the hepatic veins is as follows (Fig. 13.13):

- The right hepatic vein drains (1) both posterior segments and (2) the anterosuperior segment. It is located in the right segmental fissure.

- The middle hepatic vein drains (1) the anteroinferior segment and (2) the medial inferior segment. It is located in the main lobar fissure.

- The left hepatic vein drains (1) the ductus venosus (in the fetus), (2) the left lateral segment, and (3) the medial superior segment. It is located in the upper portion of the left segmental fissure.

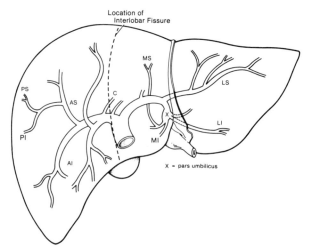

Figure 13.12. Diagram of the intrahepatic distribution of the portal vein. Abbreviations as in Fig. 13.5. (By permission of JE Skandalakis, SW Gray, and JR Rowe, *Anatomical Complications in General Surgery*, New York: McGraw-Hill, 1983.)

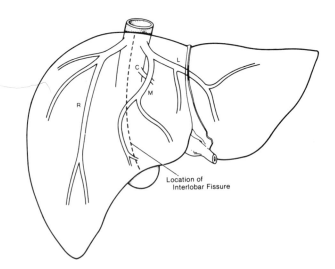

Figure 13.13. Diagram of the intrahepatic distribution of the hepatic veins. Note that they are interlobular, rather than lobular. C = caudate; L = left; M = medial; R = right. (By permission of JE Skandalakis, SW Gray, and JR Rowe, *Anatomical Complications in General Surgery*, New York: McGraw-Hill, 1983.)

- The middle and left hepatic veins approach one another and often form a common trunk as they enter the vena cava less than 1 cm below the diaphragm. In addition to three major veins, there are as many as 50 smaller veins (dorsal hepatic veins), most of which are of insignificant size. The three major veins can be divided into types based on (1) length of vein, (2) tributaries or lack of tributaries, and (3) availability for ligation; 1 cm of vein can be assumed to be adequate for successful ligation.

Remember:

✓ Lobar or segmental hepatic vein ligation is feasible.

✓ Hepatic resection following ligation of a hepatic vein is not necessary.

✓ Ligation of the right hepatic vein is possible prior to transection of the liver in the majority, but it should not be done in the middle and left hepatic veins.

■ LYMPHATICS OF THE LIVER

Superficial Lymphatics

The superficial lymphatics lie on the surface of the liver in the connective tissue beneath the peritoneal covering (Fig. 13.14).

Deep Lymphatics

The pathways of the deep lymphatics are (1) to the right middle phrenic nodes of the diaphragm; and (2) to the nodes of the porta hepatis. These trunks carry the largest quantity of hepatic lymph. There is free communication between the superficial and deep components of the liver.

The lymph nodes of the porta, in the transverse fissure of the liver, are closer to the portal vein and the hepatic artery than they are to the bile duct.

Perihepatic Spaces

The perihepatic spaces (subphrenic and subhepatic) and the collection of fluid within may be appreciated surgicoanatomically from Figs. 13.15–13.22.

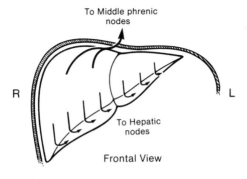

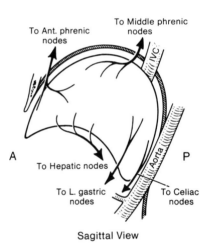

Figure 13.14. Diagram of the superficial lymphatic drainage of the liver: frontal and sagittal views. (By permission of JE Skandalakis, SW Gray, and JR Rowe, *Anatomical Complications in General Surgery*, New York: McGraw-Hill, 1983.)

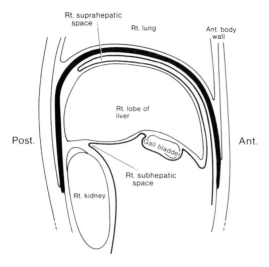

Figure 13.15. Diagrammatic parasagittal section through the upper abdomen showing the potential right suprahepatic and subhepatic spaces. The thick black line represents the diaphragm. (By permission of JE Skandalakis, SW Gray, and JR Rowe, *Anatomical Complications in General Surgery*, New York: McGraw-Hill, 1983.)

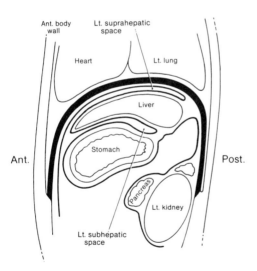

Figure 13.16. Diagrammatic parasagittal section through the trunk showing the potential left suprahepatic and subhepatic spaces. (By permission of JE Skandalakis, SW Gray, and JR Rowe, *Anatomical Complications in General Surgery*, New York: McGraw-Hill, 1983.)

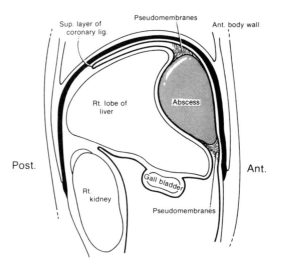

Figure 13.17. Relations of an abscess in the anterior portion of the right suprahepatic space. (By permission of JE Skandalakis, SW Gray, and JR Rowe, *Anatomical Complications in General Surgery*, New York: McGraw-Hill, 1983.)

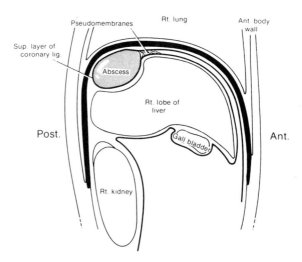

Figure 13.18. Relations of an abscess in the posterior portion of the right suprahepatic space. (By permission of JE Skandalakis, SW Gray, and JR Rowe, *Anatomical Complications in General Surgery*, New York: McGraw-Hill, 1983.)

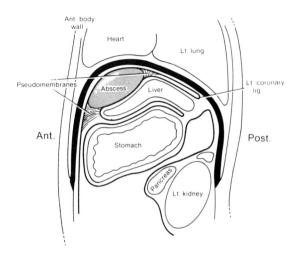

Figure 13.19. Relations of an abscess in the anterior portion of the left supra-hepatic space. (By permission of JE Skandalakis, SW Gray, and JR Rowe, *Anatomical Complications in General Surgery*, New York: McGraw-Hill, 1983.)

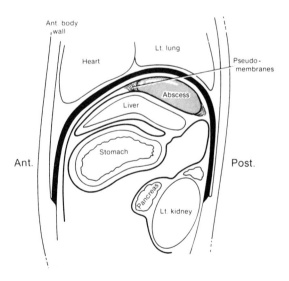

Figure 13.20. Relations of an abscess in the posterior portion of the left suprahepatic space. (By permission of JE Skandalakis, SW Gray, and JR Rowe, *Anatomical Complications in General Surgery*, New York: McGraw-Hill, 1983.)

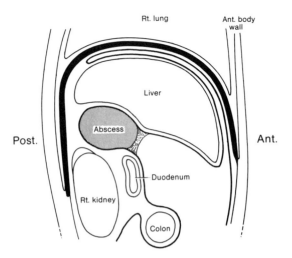

Figure 13.21. Relations of an abscess in the right infrahepatic space. (By permission of JE Skandalakis, SW Gray, and JR Rowe, *Anatomical Complications in General Surgery*, New York: McGraw-Hill, 1983.)

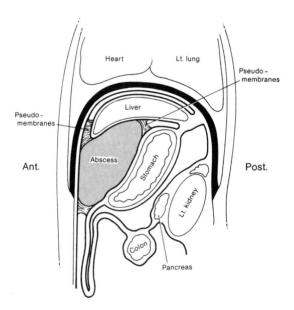

Figure 13.22. Relations of an abscess in the left infrahepatic space. (By permission of JE Skandalakis, SW Gray, and JR Rowe, *Anatomical Complications in General Surgery*, New York: McGraw-Hill, 1983.)

TECHNIQUE

■ PORTAL HYPERTENSION

Portal Shunts (Fig. 13.23)

When preparing to insert a portal shunt, expose the portal vein and ascertain whether it is long enough to reach the vena cava without undue tension. If not, a venous graft will be required.

A second obstacle to anastomosis is the presence of an aberrant right hepatic artery arising from the superior mesenteric artery.

The "surgical length" of the portal vein varies from 2 to 7 cm. In most specimens, the inferior vena cava lies beneath the distal ⅔ of the portal vein. In others, the vena cava lies under the proximal ⅔ of the portal vein or under the proximal third.

The splenic vein may be mobilized for 4–5 cm following removal of the spleen. The vein is largest where it crosses the lumbar vertebrae and may be ligated and divided at that point.

Some surgeons recommend an inframesocolic approach to the splenic and renal veins for a splenorenal shunt. The left renal vein has an average length of 8.3 cm, and 4–5 cm of this can be prepared for anastomosis. The distal splenorenal shunt developed by Warren does not require splenectomy (Fig. 13.23E).

The ideal mesocaval shunt meets the following requirements:

1. An unobstructed 2-cm-long surgical segment of the vein.

2. Absence of a large tributary vein entering the superior mesenteric vein from the left.

3. Absence of an artery crossing the surgical segment either above or below.

4. No extensive overriding of the vein by the superior mesenteric artery.

Several other portal systemic shunts have been proposed. They include left gastric caval, left gastric gonadal, left gastric adrenal, and left gastric renal shunts.

The left gastric vein terminates in the portal vein in about ⅔ of individuals and in the splenic vein in the remainder. The left gastric vein should be ligated near its termination to interrupt esophageal tributaries that join the left gastric vein.

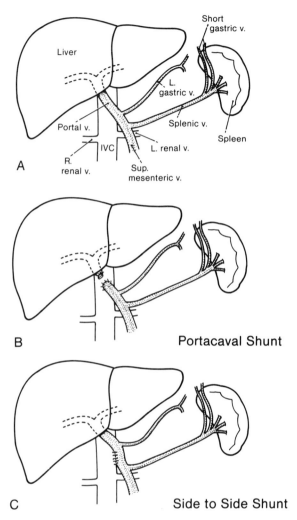

Figure 13.23. Diagrams of types of portasystemic shunts. (A) Normal configuration of the portal and systemic veins. (B) Portacaval shunt; end-to-end anastomosis of the portal vein and the inferior vena cava. (C) Portacaval shunt; side-to-side anastomosis. (D) Splenorenal shunt; anastomosis of the proximal splenic vein and the left renal vein. (E) Splenorenal (Warren) shunt; anastomosis of distal splenic vein and the left renal vein. (F) Mesocaval shunt; a vein graft connects the superior mesenteric vein to the inferior vena cava without interruption of the continuity of either vein. (By permission of JE Skandalakis, SW Gray, and JR Rowe, *Anatomical Complications in General Surgery*, New York: McGraw-Hill, 1983.)

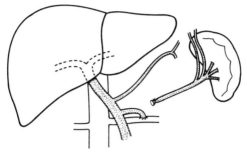

D   Proximal Splenorenal Shunt

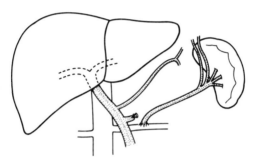

E   Distal Splenorenal Shunt
(Warren)

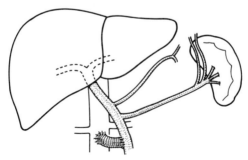

F   Mesocaval Shunt

Figure 13.23. Continued

■ DISTAL SPLENORENAL SHUNT (Figs. 13.24 and 13.25)

Procedure:

Step 1. Make a bilateral subcostal incision (rooftop) extending more laterally on the left. Avoid the dilated veins of the abdominal wall.

Step 2. Carefully explore the peritoneal cavity.

Step 3. Upwardly mobilize the transverse colon and retract the small bowel forward and to the right by division of the ligament of Treitz. Divide the greater omentum between the greater curvature of the stomach and the transverse colon to gain access to the retroperitoneum. Preserve the short gastric vessels to the hilum of the spleen.

Step 4. Incise the peritoneum and upwardly retract the body of the pancreas to locate the splenic vein. Carefully ligate small tributary veins.

Step 5. Insert catheter into the splenic vein for measurement of pressure.

Step 6. Perform careful retroperitoneal dissection for localization, isolation, and mobilization of the left renal vein from the inferior vena cava to the hilum of the kidney.

Step 7. If necessary for better mobilization of the renal vein, ligate the left gonadal and adrenal veins.

Step 8. Divide the splenic vein at the junction with the superior mesenteric vein. Approximate the splenic vein to the left renal vein without tension.

Step 9. Oversew the hepatic end of the splenic vein and anastomose its distal end end-to-side to the left renal vein using continuous 6–0 polypropylene for the posterior wall and continuous or interrupted 6–0 for the anterior wall.

Step 10. Ligate the left gastric (coronary) vein and the right gastroepiploic vein.

Step 11. Take blood pressure prior to careful closure of the abdominal wall.

■ MESOCAVAL SHUNT

Procedure:

Step 1. Make a long midline incision from the xiphoid to the symphysis pubis. Avoid the dilated veins of the abdominal wall.

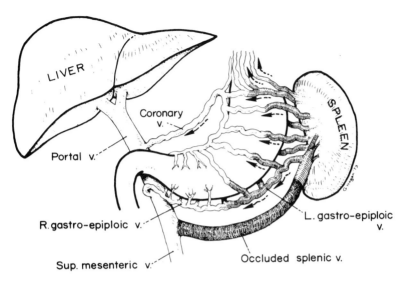

Figure 13.24. Diagrammatic representation of collateral circulation characteristic of isolated occlusion of the splenic vein. (By permission of AA Salam and WD Warren, *Surg Clin NA* 54(6):1247–1257, 1974.)

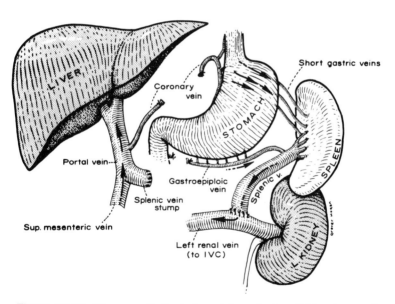

Figure 13.25. Diagrammatic illustration of the selective distal splenorenal shunt. (By permission of AA Salam and WD Warren, *Surg Clin NA* 54(6):1247–1257, 1974.)

Step 2. Carefully explore the peritoneal cavity.

Step 3. Upwardly mobilize the transverse colon and retract the small bowel forward and to the right by division of the ligament of Treitz.

Step 4. Incise the peritoneum over the superior mesenteric vessels and locate and mobilize the superior mesenteric vein at the base of the transverse mesocolon to the vicinity of the uncinate process, if the process is present.

Step 5. Continue dissection to the right of the superior mesenteric vein and expose the inferior vena cava. A duodenal mobilization in toto is a very useful procedure (see previous duodenal mobilization in Chapter 8, Duodenum).

Step 6. After carefully cleansing the designated areas of both the inferior vena cava and the superior mesenteric vein, use a graft to bridge both veins, without tension or kinking, using 5–0 continuous polypropylene suture.

■ PORTACAVAL SHUNT

Procedure:

Step 1. Make a right subcostal incision extending across the midline. Avoid the dilated veins of the abdominal wall.

Step 2. Carefully explore the peritoneal cavity.

Step 3. Explore, isolate, and carefully mobilize the portal vein by incising the peritoneum of the gastroduodenal ligament.

Step 4. Measure portal pressure through any omental vein.

Step 5. Kocherize the duodenum and expose the inferior vena cava.

Step 6. Perform a side-to-side anastomosis or end-to-side portacaval shunt. After high division of the portal vein, oversew the hepatic portal stump with 5–0 polypropylene and anastomose the portal vein to the inferior vena cava using 6-0 polypropylene continuous suture. Blood pressure should be taken prior to the portal division and after the anastomosis is completed.

■ PERCUTANEOUS NEEDLE BIOPSY

Unless a specific predetermined region of the liver is to be biopsied, the site is selected by percussion. The area of maximal dullness will usually be in the right midaxillary line beneath the 8th, 9th, or 10th intercostal spaces.

■ EXCISIONAL BIOPSY

There are two excisional biopsy procedures: wedge-type and non-wedge-type or circumferential.

Wedge-Type

Procedure:

Step 1. With 0 chromic catgut or synthetic absorbable, place mattress sutures 1½-2 cm from the periphery of the lesion (Fig. 13.26).

Step 2. Remove the lesion with at least 1 cm healthy liver tissue. Proceed using electrocautery.

Step 3. Send specimen to the lab to confirm that margins are clean.

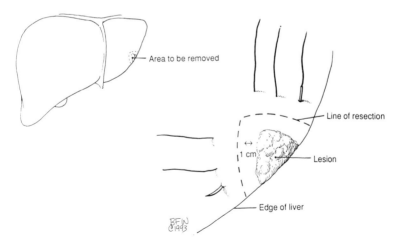

Figure 13.26

Step 4. After good hemostasis has been obtained by cautery, gently approximate with catgut sutures.

Non-Wedge- or Circumferential-Type (Figs. 13.27 and 13.28)

Procedure:

Step 1. Place deep hemostatic sutures, as in step 1 of wedge-type excisional biopsy, at least 1½–2 cm from the periphery of the lesion.

Step 2. Remove lesion by electrocautery. Suction cautery will be very helpful for controlling bleeding of liver parenchyma.

Step 3. Approximate with sutures. Occasionally a gelatin sponge within the cavity helps.

■ HEPATIC RESECTIONS

Anatomical Landmarks for Liver Resection

Except for the sulcus, which divides the lateral and medial segments of the left lobe, the diaphragmatic surface of the liver gives little indication

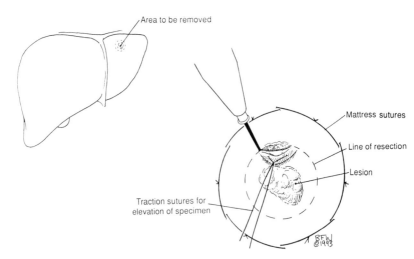

Figure 13.27

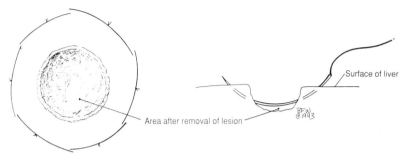

Figure 13.28

of its internal lobulation. In spite of this, at least four types of lobar and segmental resections can be performed. The four most common types are shown in Fig. 13.29.

The basic plan of the blood vessels within the liver is subject to many variations; hence preoperative aortic, celiac, or selective hepatic arteriography must be performed and the films studied carefully before any surgical procedure is attempted. The main arterial trunk to the medial segment arises from the right hepatic artery and passes to the left across the midline in about 25 percent of individuals (Fig. 13.9). Ligation of any arterial branch should be preceded by manual occlusion and observation of the limits of color change in the tissue.

Because the interlobar and intersegmental spaces are occupied by the hepatic veins (Fig. 13.13), it is necessary to transect the liver in a paralobular or parasegmental plane. This must be to the right of the vein for a right lobectomy or trisegmentectomy, or to the left of the vein for a left lobectomy or a lateral segmentectomy (Fig. 13.30). This is especially important in the true interlobar (umbilical) fissure, where vessels and bile ducts may lie in the fissure and return to the medial lobe more distally.

Note: In all hepatic resections, the Cavitron ultrasonic surgical aspirator dissector facilitates the exposure and ligation of the arteries, veins, and ducts within the liver parenchyma.

Right Lobectomy

For a right lobectomy or trisegmental lobectomy, a right subcostal incision is used. It may be continued upward into the thorax or to the right if necessary.

The right triangular and coronary ligaments are incised so that the right lobe may be retracted. The round and falciform ligaments are pre-

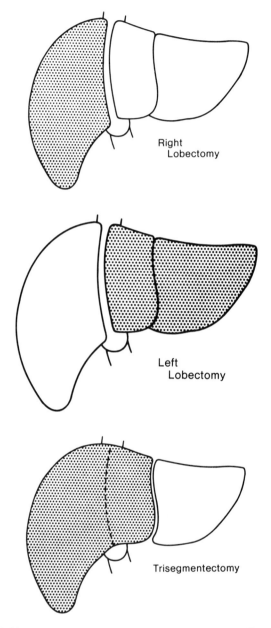

Right
Lobectomy

Left
Lobectomy

Trisegmentectomy

Figure 13.29. Types of lobar and segmental liver resections. (By permission of JE Skandalakis, SW Gray, and JR Rowe, *Anatomical Complications in General Surgery*, New York: McGraw-Hill, 1983.)

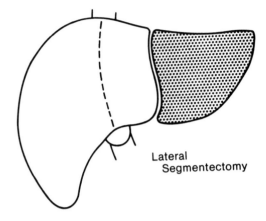

Figure 13.29. Continued

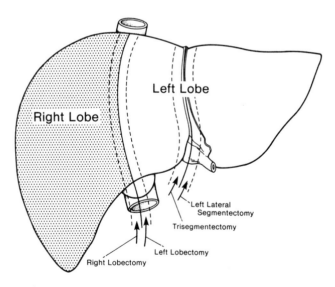

Figure 13.30. Planes of transection of the liver for lobectomy and segmentectomy. Trisegmentectomy includes the anterior and posterior segments of the right lobe and the medial segment of the left lobe. (By permission of JE Skandalakis, SW Gray, and JR Rowe, *Anatomical Complications in General Surgery*, New York: McGraw-Hill, 1983.)

served. In a "true" right or left lobectomy, the gallbladder must be sacrificed.

Dissection begins at the hilum. Branches of the hepatic artery, the portal vein, and the bile duct of the lobe to be removed are ligated, and the interlobar hepatic veins are preserved. Blunt dissection must be used throughout.

The line of the interlobar fissure extends from the gallbladder fossa below to the inferior vena cava above. The dissection must pass to the right of the middle hepatic vein to preserve drainage of the medial segment of the left lobe (Fig. 13.30). The right hepatic vein may be ligated extrahepatically before transection of the liver.

A right "extended" lobectomy (trisegmentectomy) is similar, but the liver is transected just to the right of the falciform ligament. The middle hepatic vein must be ligated, since the medial segment is to be removed.

Left Lobectomy

If the left lobe is to be resected, the left hepatic artery, the portal vein, and the bile duct should be ligated. Section of the triangular ligament will permit mobilization of the left lobe. Transection should follow a line from the left side of the fossa of the gallbladder to the left side of the fossa of the inferior vena cava (Fig. 13.30). The left and middle hepatic veins should be exposed and ligated within the liver.

In most cases, the left and middle hepatic veins form a common trunk before emerging from the liver. It is best to ligate the hepatic veins at the end of the dissection to be sure that only the veins from the resected segments are ligated. A left resection may be lobar, segmental, or even wedge-shaped for a superficially located tumor.

Liver Resection and Trauma

In contrast to elective operations on the liver, the surgeon may be faced with traumatic liver injury that does not follow segmental lines. In such cases, the surgeon must decide whether to debride and repair the wound or convert it into an anatomical segmental resection. The problem is that most injuries occur to the right lobe. The choice lies between repair and right lobectomy. If the injury is minor, lobectomy is not justified. If the injury would leave grossly devascularized areas of the liver, then formal lobectomy is necessary.

Where there is doubt about the severity of the injury and lobectomy is contemplated, operative cholangiograms and aortography can be used to further delineate the area of destruction.

In severe trauma there may be no time for angiograms or even for careful hilar dissection. The surgeon must rely on knowledge of the interlobar plane to expose vessels that must be ligated.

Two indications for formal lobectomy have been proposed:

1. Blunt or penetrating injuries resulting in extensive devitalization of a major portion of the right lobe
2. Damage to the hepatic veins or the vena cava requiring right lobectomy for visualization and repair

Left Lateral Segmentectomy (Fig. 13.4)

Procedure:

Step 1. With scissors, carefully section the right triangular and coronary ligament (Fig. 13.31). Be sure to avoid injuring the left hepatic vein.

Step 2. With the electrocautery, score the line of resection 1–1 ½ cm lateral to the falciform ligament (Fig. 13.32).

Step 3. As described in the wedge-type excisional biopsy, place mattress sutures medial to the line of resection.

Step 4. Remove the left lateral segment using electrocautery and suction cautery as required.

Step 5. Gently approximate sutures.

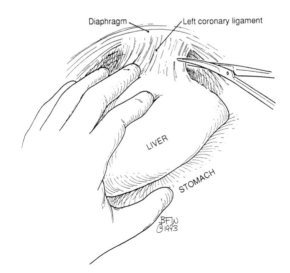

Diaphragm · Left coronary ligament

LIVER

STOMACH

BFW
© 1993

Figure 13.31

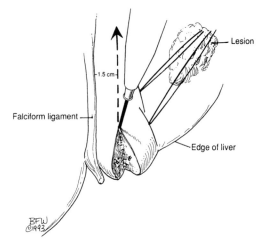

Figure 13.32

Left Hepatic Lobectomy (Fig. 13.30)

Procedure:

Step 1. Perform cholecystectomy.

Step 2. Carefully dissect and isolate the left hepatic duct, left hepatic artery, and left portal vein (Fig. 13.33).

Step 3. Divide the left triangular, left coronary, and falciform ligaments (Fig. 13.31).

Step 4. With 2–0 silk, doubly ligate the left hepatic duct and left hepatic artery. The left portal vein should be clamped proximally and distally and, after division, oversewn with 5–0 synthetic nonabsorbable suture or silk (Fig. 13.34).

Step 5. Prepare and isolate the left hepatic vein. Clamp, divide, and oversew the vein as described in step 4 for the left portal vein. If the left hepatic vein is intrahepatic, proceed with lobar division (Fig. 13.35).

Step 6. By very superficial electrocoagulation, mark the Glisson's capsule of the liver with the line of Rex. Using 0 chromic catgut, place horizontal mattress sutures at least 1–1½ cm lateral to the line of Rex. Start division of the hepatic parenchyma placing more sutures and using suction cautery or suture ligatures for additional hemostasis, as required (Figs. 13.36 and 13.37).

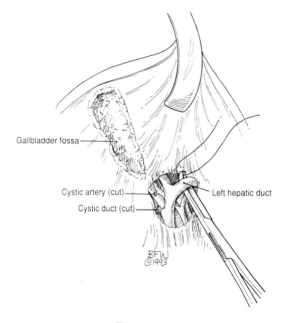

Gallbladder fossa

Cystic artery (cut)

Cystic duct (cut)

Left hepatic duct

BFW
©1993

Figure 13.33

Step 7. Insert Jackson–Pratt drains.

Step 8. Close abdominal wall in layers.

Right Hepatic Lobectomy (Fig. 13.30)

Procedure:

Step 1. Perform cholecystectomy.

Step 2. Divide the falciform, right anterior, posterior coronary, and right triangular ligaments. Be careful not to sever the right hepatic vein (Fig. 13.38).

Step 3. Rotate the right lobe medially.

Step 4. Identify, isolate, and doubly ligate the right hepatic duct and right hepatic artery. The right portal vein should be treated very carefully with the same technique used in step 5 of the left hepatic lobectomy (Fig. 13.39).

Step 5. Dissect and carefully prepare the retrohepatic inferior vena cava and its small multiple parenchymal branches, which should be ligated doubly using 4–0 or 5–0 silk (Fig. 13.40).

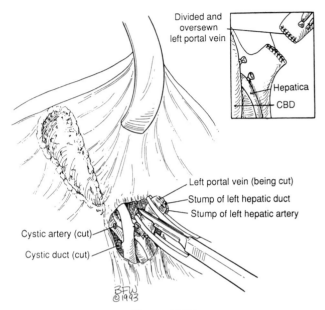

Figure 13.34

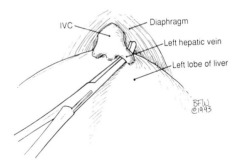

Figure 13.35

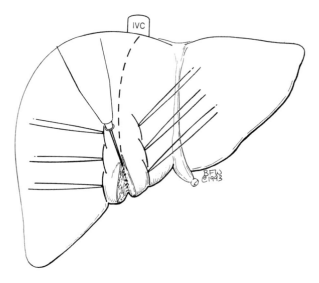

Figure 13.36

Step 6. If the right hepatic vein was not ligated previously, it should be dissected very carefully, mobilized, clamped doubly, divided, and oversewn as described in the procedure for left hepatic lobectomy.

Step 7. If discoloration and demarcation are present between the right and left lobes at this time, divide the two lobes through the

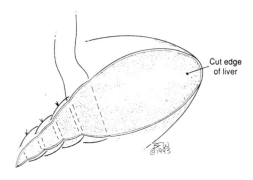

Figure 13.37

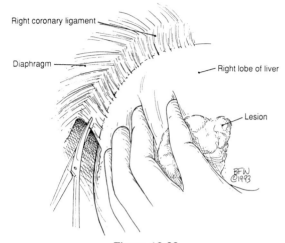

Right coronary ligament

Diaphragm

Right lobe of liver

Lesion

BFW
©1993

Figure 13.38

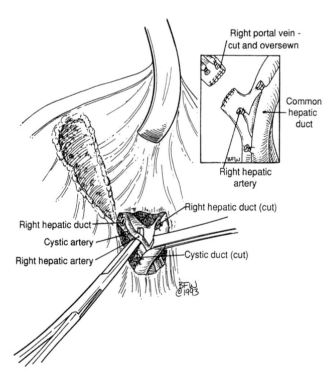

Right portal vein -
cut and oversewn

Common
hepatic
duct

Right hepatic
artery

BFW

Right hepatic duct (cut)

Right hepatic duct

Cystic artery

Right hepatic artery

Cystic duct (cut)

BFW
©1993

Figure 13.39

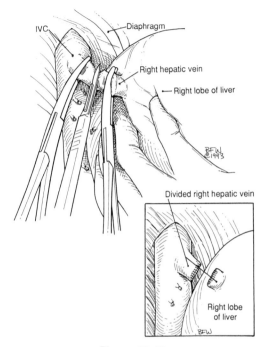

IVC

Diaphragm

Right hepatic vein

← Right lobe of liver

BFW
©1993

Divided right hepatic vein

Right lobe
of liver

BFW

Figure 13.40

previously marked area, as in step 5 of the procedure for left hepatic lobectomy.

Step 8. For hepatic stabilization, approximate the falciform ligament (Fig. 13.41).

Step 9. Insert Jackson–Pratt drain.

Liver Trauma

Procedure:

Step 1. Make a long midline incision. Suction all blood from the peritoneal cavity.

Step 2. Mobilize the liver by incising the falciform, triangular, and coronary ligaments on both lobes (Fig. 13.31).

Step 3. Explore the hepatic wound for evaluation and hemostasis. Debride and remove devascularized liver parenchyma. To control

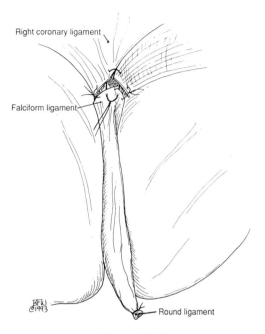

Right coronary ligament

Falciform ligament

Round ligament

Figure 13.41

bleeding, it is very helpful to use high electrocautery simultaneously with high suction (Fig. 13.42).

Step 4. If required, clamp the hepatic triad with a noncrushing clamp (Fig. 13.43).

Step 5. If bleeding cannot be controlled, ligate the right or left hepatic artery. Perform a cholecystectomy if the right hepatic artery is ligated.

Options or alternatives (use only if absolutely necessary):

1. Pack the hepatic wound for hemostasis and re-operate in 48 hours.

2. Clamp the aorta just below the diaphragm.

3. Isolate the inferior vena cava using Cameron "keepers" (umbilical tape) above the renal veins and within the pericardium. With both ends of the tape threaded into an 18 French catheter, pull them taut by clamping with a Kelly clamp. If this procedure is necessary, a median sternostomy should be performed (Fig. 13.44).

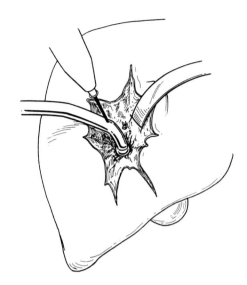

Figure 13.42

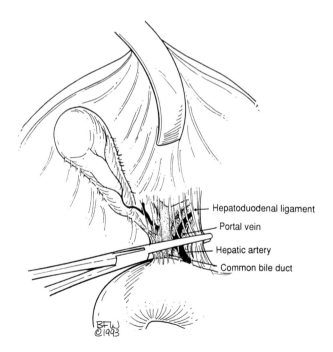

Hepatoduodenal ligament

Portal vein

Hepatic artery

Common bile duct

Figure 13.43

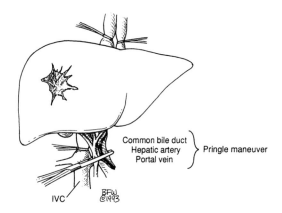

Figure 13.44

4. Occasionally, it is necessary to place a shunt into the inferior vena cava.

For more details, read the excellent book of John L. Cameron, *Atlas of Surgery, Volume I.* Philadelphia: B. C. Decker, 1990.

Extrahepatic Biliary Tract

ANATOMY

■ VASCULAR RELATIONS OF THE EXTRAHEPATIC BILIARY TRACT

In general, the major blood vessels in the area of the extrahepatic biliary tree are posterior to the ducts, but in a number of cases they may lie anterior. The surgeon must recognize and preserve these arteries. Table 14.1 shows the frequency with which specific arteries are found anterior to segments of the biliary tract.

■ RIGHT, LEFT, AND COMMON HEPATIC DUCTS

The right and left hepatic ducts join soon after emerging from the liver to form the common hepatic duct (Fig. 14.1B). The junction lies 0.25–2.5 cm from the surface of the liver. The left duct is longer (1.7 cm, average) than the right duct (0.9 cm, average). In some case, intrahepatic junction of the hepatic ducts is the result of liver enlargement (Fig. 14.1A); retraction of the liver may then be necessary to expose the junction.

Measurements of the common hepatic duct are highly variable. The duct is said to be absent if the cystic duct enters at the junction of the right and left hepatic ducts (Fig. 14.1C). In most individuals, the duct is between 1.5 and 3.5 cm long.

Three type of cystohepatic junction have been described: angular (64 percent) (Figs. 14.1A and B), parallel (23 percent) (Fig. 14.2A), and spiral (13 percent) (Figs. 14.2B and C).

Table 14.1 Segments of the Biliary Tract and the Frequency of Arteries Lying Anterior to Them

Segment	Artery anterior	Percent frequency
Right and left hepatic ducts	Right hepatic artery	12–15
	Cystic artery	<5
Common hepatic duct	Cystic artery	15–24
	Right hepatic artery	11–19
	Common hepatic artery	<5
Supraduodenal com-mon bile duct	Anterior artery to common bile duct	50
	Posterosuperior pancreatico-duodenal artery	12.5
	Gastroduodenal artery	5.7–20[a]
	Right gastric artery	<5
	Common hepatic artery	<5
	Cystic artery	<5
	Right hepatic artery	<5
Retroduodenal com-mon bile duct	Posterosuperior pancreati-coduodenal artery	76–87.5
	Supraduodenal artery	11.4

[a]In another 36 percent, the gastroduodenal artery lay on the left border of the common bile duct.
Source: Data from Johnson and Anson. *Surg Gynecol Obstet* 94:669, 1952 and Maingot (ed), *Abdominal Operations*, 6th ed. Norwalk, CT: Appleton & Lange, 1974.

■ ANOMALOUS HEPATIC DUCTS: SURGICALLY SIGNIFICANT SOURCES OF BILE LEAKAGE (Fig. 14.3)

An aberrant hepatic duct is a normal segmental duct that joins the biliary tract just outside the liver instead of just within; it drains a normal portion of the liver. Such a duct passing through the hepatocystic triangle is important because it is subject to inadvertent section with subsequent bile leakage (Fig. 14.3).

Subvesicular bile ducts, found in approximately 35 percent of individuals, are small blind ducts emerging from the right lobe of the liver and lying in the bed of the gallbladder. They do not communicate with the gallbladder.

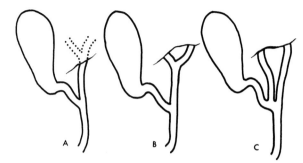

Figure 14.1. Variations of the hepatic ducts. (A) Intrahepatic union of left and right hepatic ducts; (B) usual extrahepatic union of left and right hepatic ducts; (C) distal union of hepatic ducts producing absence of the common hepatic duct. (By permission of JE Skandalakis, SW Gray, RR Ricketts, et al. The extrahepatic biliary ducts and the gallbladder. In: Skandalakis JE, Gray SW. *Embryology for Surgeons*, 2nd ed. Baltimore: Williams & Wilkins, 1994.)

Hepatocystic ducts drain bile from the liver directly into the body of the gallbladder or into the cystic duct.

Occasionally, the right, left, or even both hepatic ducts enter the gallbladder. This is an argument in favor of removing the gallbladder at the fundus, from above downward.

■ CYSTIC DUCT

The cystic duct is about 3 mm in diameter and about 2–4 cm long. If surgeons are unprepared for a short duct (Fig. 14.2E), they may find themselves inadvertently entering the common bile duct. If they underestimate the length, they may leave too long a stump, predisposing to the cystic duct remnant syndrome.

Very rarely, the cystic duct is absent and the gallbladder opens directly into the common bile duct (Fig. 14.2E). In such a case, the common bile duct might be mistaken for the cystic duct.

■ GALLBLADDER

The gallbladder lies at the junction of the right lobe and the medial segment of the left lobe on the visceral surface of the liver. The hepatic

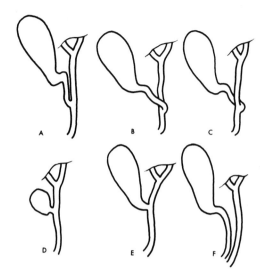

Figure 14.2. Types of cystohepatic junction. (A) Parallel type found in 20 percent; (B and C) spiral types found in 5 percent (the angular type shown in Fig. 14.1B is found in 75 percent); (D and E) short cystic ducts; (F) a long cystic duct ending in the duodenum. This may also be called "absence of the common bile duct." (By permission of JE Skandalakis, SW Gray, RR Ricketts, et al. The extrahepatic biliary ducts and the gallbladder. In: Skandalakis JE, Gray SW. *Embryology for Surgeons*, 2nd ed. Baltimore: Williams & Wilkins, 1994.)

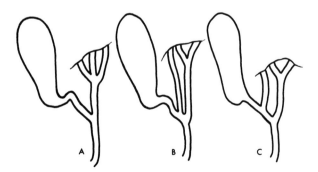

Figure 14.3. Accessory hepatic ducts. Additional, minute hepatic ducts are not unusual. (By permission of JE Skandalakis, SW Gray, RR Ricketts, et al. The extrahepatic biliary ducts and the gallbladder. In: Skandalakis JE, Gray SW. *Embryology for Surgeons*, 2nd ed. Baltimore: Williams & Wilkins, 1994.)

surface is attached to the liver by connective tissue of the liver capsule. Both the nonhepatic surface and the fundus are completely covered with peritoneum.

The body of the gallbladder is closely related to the transverse colon and to the first and proximal part of the second portions of the duodenum. The body is completely covered by peritoneum and has its own mesentery in about 4 percent of cadavers. Such gallbladders (floating or roving) are subject to torsion and infarction. Several other anomalous peritoneal folds connected with the body of the gallbladder, the cholecystogastric, cholecystoduodenal, and cholecystocolic folds, are redundancies of the lesser omentum.

The neck of the gallbladder is S-shaped and lies in the free border of the hepatoduodenal ligament (lesser omentum). The mucosa at the neck is elevated into folds that form the spiral valve (of Heister).

A deformity of the gallbladder seen in 2–6 percent of individuals is the Phrygian cap (Fig. 14.4A). Hartmann's pouch (Fig. 14.4B), at the neck of the gallbladder, is probably a normal variation rather than a true deformity.

■ COMMON BILE DUCT

The length of the common bile duct varies from 5 to 15 cm depending on the position of the entrance of the cystic duct. The duct may be divided arbitrarily into four portions (Fig. 14.5):

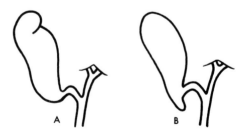

Figure 14.4. Deformities of the gallbladder. (A) "Phrygian cap" deformity; (B) Hartmann's pouch. (By permission of JE Skandalakis, SW Gray, RR Ricketts, et al. The extrahepatic biliary ducts and the gallbladder. In: Skandalakis JE, Gray SW. *Embryology for Surgeons*, 2nd ed. Baltimore: Williams & Wilkins, 1994.)

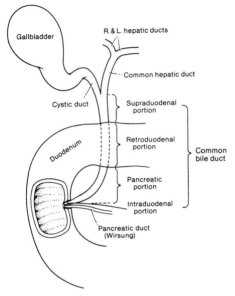

Figure 14.5. The extrahepatic biliary tract and the four portions of the common bile duct. (By permission of JE Skandalakis, SW Gray, and JR Rowe, *Anatomical Complications in General Surgery*, New York: McGraw-Hill, 1983.)

1. Supraduodenal: Average length 2 cm, range 0–4 cm

2. Retroduodenal: Average length 1.5 cm, range 1.0–3.5 cm

3. Pancreatic: average length 3.0 cm, range 1.5–6.0 cm

4. Intramural: average length 1.1 cm, range 0.8–2.4 cm

The supraduodenal portion lies between the two leaves of the hepatoduodenal ligament, in front of the foramen of Winslow, to the right of the hepatic artery, and anterior to the portal vein.

The retroduodenal portion lies between the superior margin of the first part of the duodenum and the superior margin of the head of the pancreas. The gastroduodenal artery is to the left and the posterosuperior pancreaticoduodenal artery crosses first anterior to the bile duct and then posterior to the duct just before it enters the duodenum.

The common bile duct may be partly covered by a tongue of pancreas (44 percent) (Figs. 14.6A and B), completely within the pancreatic substance (30 percent) (Fig. 14.6C), uncovered on the pancreatic surface (16.5 percent) (Fig. 14.6D), or completely covered by two tongues of pancreas (9 percent) (Fig. 14.6E). Even when completely covered, the

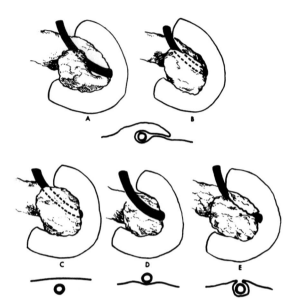

Figure 14.6. Relation of the pancreas and the common bile duct. (A and B) The duct is partially covered by a tongue of pancreas (44 percent); (C) the duct is completely covered by the pancreas (30 percent); (D) the duct lies free on the surface of the pancreas (16.5 percent); (E) the duct is covered by two tongues of pancreas with a cleavage plane between. (By permission of JE Skandalakis, SW Gray, JS Rowe, et al., *Contemp Surg* 15(5): 17–40, 1979.)

groove or tunnel occupied by the duct may be palpated by passing the fingers of the left hand behind the second part of the duodenum after mobilization with the Kocher maneuver.

The normal outside diameter of the first three regions of the common bile duct is variable (Table 14.2), but a common bile duct more than 8 mm in diameter is definitely enlarged and, therefore, pathologic.

The fourth, or intramural (sometimes called intraduodenal), portion of the common bile duct (see Fig. 9.8) passes obliquely through the duodenal wall together with the main pancreatic duct. Within the wall, the length averages 15 mm. As it enters the wall, the common duct decreases in diameter from about 5.7 to 3.3 mm. The two ducts lie side by side with a common adventitia for several millimeters. The dividing septum becomes reduced to a mucosal membrane just before the confluence of the ducts (see Chapter 9, Pancreas).

Table 14.2 Measurements of the Diameter of the Common Bile Duct (Not Including the Intramural Portion)

Material	Diameter, mm (average)	Diameter, mm (range)	Number measured
Autopsy specimens:			
Mahour et al., 1967	7.39	4–12	100
Dowdy, 1969	6.6	4–13	100
Surgical Specimens:			
Hicken and McAllister, 1952	5	<4–10	225
Surgical and autopsy:			
Leichtling et al., 1959	12	5–17	47[a]
Ferris and Vibert, 1959	8.85	4–17	98[a]
Leslie, 1968 (correction applied)	7.6	3.2–10.8	153[a]
Cholangiograms:			
Jonson, 1960	5.9	—	39
Lundström and Holm, 1979	11–15	—	110[a]
Deitch, 1981	8.1	4–14	90[b]

[a]"Without disease of common bile duct"
[b]"With cholecystitis."
Source: By permission of JE Skandalakis, SW Gray, and JR Rowe, *Anatomical Complications in General Surgery*, New York: McGraw-Hill, 1983.

■ HEPATOCYSTIC TRIANGLE OF CALOT

The hepatocystic triangle is formed by the cystic duct and the gallbladder below, the right lobe of the liver above, and the common hepatic duct medially (Fig. 14.7). Within the boundaries of the triangle are a number of structures that must be identified before they are ligated or sectioned.

The hepatocystic triangle contains the right hepatic artery (and sometimes an aberrant right hepatic artery), the cystic artery, and sometimes an aberrant (accessory) bile duct.

In 87 percent of individuals, the right hepatic artery enters the triangle posterior to the common hepatic duct, and in 13 percent it enters anterior to it. In one study of cadavers, the right hepatic artery could have been mistaken for the cystic artery 20 percent of the time. As a rule of thumb, any artery more than 3 mm in diameter within the triangle will probably not be a cystic artery.

In 18 percent, there was an aberrant right hepatic artery. In 83 percent of these specimens, the cystic artery arose from the aberrant artery within

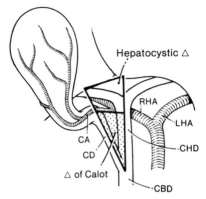

Figure 14.7. The hepatocystic triangle and the triangle of Calot. The upper boundary of the hepatocystic triangle is the margin of the liver; that of the triangle of Calot is the cystic artery; the triangle of Calot is stippled. CA = cystic artery; CD = cystic duct; CBD = common bile duct; RHA = right hepatic artery; LHA = left hepatic artery; CHD = common hepatic duct. (By permission of JE Skandalakis, SW Gray, RR Ricketts, et al. The extrahepatic biliary ducts and the gallbladder. In: Skandalakis JE, Gray SW. *Embryology for Surgeons*, 2nd ed. Baltimore: Williams & Wilkins, 1994.)

the triangle. In 4 percent, the aberrant artery was accessory to a normal right hepatic artery, and in 14 percent, it was a replacing artery, the only blood supply to the right lobe of the liver (see Fig. 13.8).

The cystic artery usually arises from the right hepatic artery or an aberrant right hepatic artery within the hepatocystic triangle. At the neck of the gallbladder, the cystic artery divides into a superficial and a deep branch (Table 14.3).

In 16 percent, there were aberrant (accessory) bile ducts within the hepatocystic triangle that may cause bile to leak into the abdominal cavity.

■ BLOOD SUPPLY OF THE BILIARY TRACT

Arterial Supply

The gallbladder is supplied by the cystic artery. The bile ducts are supplied by branches of the posterosuperior pancreaticoduodenal, retroduodenal, and right and left hepatic arteries. Do not devascularize more than 2–3 cm of the upper surface of the duct (Fig. 14.8).

Table 14.3 Origin of the Cystic Artery

Origin	Percent
Right hepatic artery	
Normal	61.4
Aberrant (accessory)	10.2
Aberrant (replacing)	3.1
Left hepatic artery	5.9
Bifurcation of common hepatic artery	11.5
	92.1
Common hepatic artery	3.8
	95.9
Gastroduodenal artery	2.5
Superior pancreaticoduodenal artery	0.15
Right gastric artery	0.15
Celiac trunk	0.3
Superior mesenteric artery	0.9
Right gastroepiploic artery	Rare
Aorta	Rare
	99.9

Source: Anson BJ. Anatomical considerations in surgery of gall-bladder. Q Bull Northwest Univ Med School 1956; 30:250.

The blood supply of the supraduodenal bile duct is essentially axial. The major supply comes from below (60 percent from the retroduodenal artery), and 38 percent comes from above (from the right hepatic artery).

The bile ducts in the hilum and the retropancreatic bile duct have an excellent blood supply.

Ischemia of the bile duct may be avoided with a high or low transection, but bleeding of the edges should be checked prior to anastomosis.

Venous Drainage

Several cystic veins, rather than one, enter the hepatic parenchyma (Fig. 14.9).

An epicholodochal venous plexus helps the surgeon identify the common bile duct. Remember that stripping of the common bile duct is not permissible.

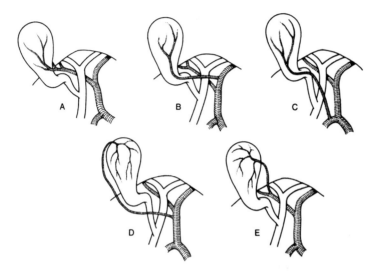

Figure 14.8. Some possible origins of the cystic artery. (A) Usual pattern (74.7 percent) from the right normal or aberrant hepatic artery; (B) origin from the common hepatic artery, its bifurcation, or from the left hepatic artery and crossing in front of the common hepatic duct (20.5 percent); (C) origin from the gastroduodenal artery (2.5 percent). The remainder arise from a variety of sources. (D and E) Very rarely the cystic artery reaches the gallbladder at the fundus or body ("recurrent" cystic artery). (By permission of JE Skandalakis, SW Gray, RR Ricketts, et al., The extrahepatic biliary ducts and the gallbladder. In: Skandalakis JE, Gray SW. *Embryology for Surgeons*, 2nd edition, Baltimore: Williams and Wilkins, 1994.)

Lymphatic Drainage

Collecting lymphatic trunks from the gallbladder drain into the cystic node in the crotch of the junction of the cystic and common hepatic ducts to the "node of the hiatus" and posterior pancreaticoduodenal nodes (Fig. 14.10).

The pericholedochal nodes receive lymphatics from the extrahepatic bile ducts and from the right lobe of the liver.

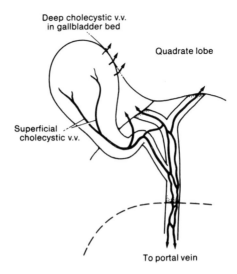

Figure 14.9. Venous drainage of the biliary tract. Most of the drainage is from the gallbladder bed into the quadrate lobe of the liver. Veins of the duct system drain upward to the liver and downward to the portal vein. (By permission of JE Skandalakis, SW Gray, and JR Rowe, *Anatomical Complications in General Surgery*, New York: McGraw-Hill, 1983.)

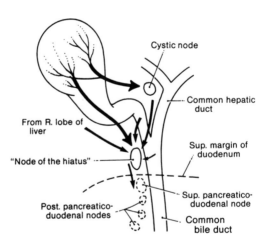

Figure 14.10. Lymphatic drainage of the biliary tract. The cystic node and the node of the hiatus are relatively constant. Drainage from the gallbladder, the cystic duct, and the right lobe of the liver reaches the posterior pancreaticoduodenal nodes. (By permission of RB Fahim et al. *Ann Surg* 156(1): 114–124, 1962.)

TECHNIQUE

■ CHOLECYSTECTOMY

Notes:

The anterior leaf of the hepatoduodenal ligament is routinely incised over the cystohepatic triangle and the underlying structures are revealed. In more difficult cases, where adhesions from inflammation or previous surgery have obscured normal relationships, greater efforts are required:

✓ The hepatic flexure of the colon and the duodenum may be mobilized to the left.

✓ The liver may be retracted to the right. This will put slight tension on the biliary ducts and open the epiploic foramen (Winslow's foramen), providing better orientation of the field.

✓ In dissecting the gallbladder away from the liver bed, the cystic artery may be exposed by the rotation of the gallbladder to the left. This will also expose the common hepatic duct, the right and left hepatic ducts, and the cystic duct. Being able to perform this maneuver is one of the advantages of removing the gallbladder from the fundus downward.

✓ Use suction and diathermy for the bleeding bed. The gallbladder bed may be filled with omentum and a drain placed over the omentum (not between the bed and the omentum).

✓ The subserous excision of the gallbladder uses the lamina propria of loose connective tissue as the plane of dissection.

✓ Another approach is to identify the cystic artery and duct, and then ligate and transect them. The gallbladder may then be dissected from its bed from below upward.

✓ Another option is to begin at the fundus of the gallbladder and dissect downward toward the neck with the following steps: (1) dissection of the gallbladder, (2) exposure of the cystic duct and its union with the common bile duct, (3) an operating room cholangiogram, and (4) dissection and ligation of the cystic duct and removal of the gallbladder.

✓ Regardless of the direction of the procedure, the junction of the cystic and common hepatic ducts should be identified.

Three procedures for cholecystectomy are presented: (1) removal of the gallbladder from above downward, (2) removal of the gallbladder from below up, and (3) laparoscopic cholecystectomy.

ANESTHESIA: General

POSITION: Supine on a special x-ray operating room table

Remember:

✓ Prior to surgery, the right upper quadrant should be x-rayed for future comparison with the cholangiogram.

✓ Intravenous antibiotic of choice should be given prior to incision.

INCISION: Right subcostal or other incision of choice

From Above Downward

Procedure:

Step 1. Dissect the area of the cystic duct and the common duct. Identify the cystic duct and double pass a 2-0 silk around it. Identify the cystic artery. Ligate proximally and distally with 2-0 silk and divide. If there is any doubt about the identity of the cystic artery, do not divide yet.

Step 2. Carefully free the gallbladder from above downward until you reach the hepatoduodenal ligament. Inspect and treat the gallbladder fossa for leakage of bile or bleeding using electrocautery (Fig. 14.11).

Step 3. If the cystic artery has not yet been divided, do so now. It should be located near and parallel to the cystic duct (Fig. 14.12).

Step 4. Isolate the cystic duct. Decide whether to perform a cholangiogram. If not, clamp the cystic duct very carefully between two clamps proximally and distally. Divide the cystic duct between the clamps and transfix the cystic duct remnant with silk. The remnant should be very short (Fig. 14.13).

Step 5. Remove the specimen and irrigate the gallbladder fossa and right upper quadrant.

Step 6. Decide whether to drain the area. If so, use a Jackson–Pratt drain, bringing it out through a stab wound. Close in layers.

From Below Up

Procedure:

Step 1. Dissect the area of the cystic and common ducts and identify these structures, as well as the cystic arteries (Figs. 14.14 and 14.15).

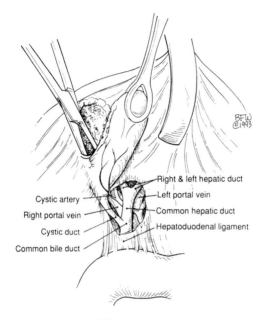

Right & left hepatic duct
Left portal vein
Cystic artery
Common hepatic duct
Right portal vein
Cystic duct
Hepatoduodenal ligament
Common bile duct

Figure 14.11

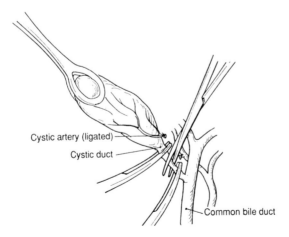

Cystic artery (ligated)
Cystic duct
Common bile duct

Figure 14.12

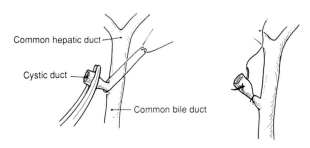

Figure 14.13

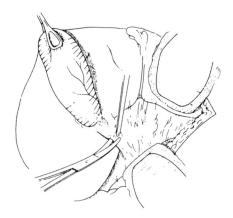

Figure 14.14

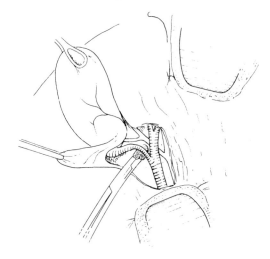

Figure 14.15

Step 2. Doubly ligate the cystic duct and cystic artery with 2–0 silk. Incise all around the serosa of the gallbladder approximately 1–1 ½ cm from the liver edge. Using the bovie and right-angle clamp, dissect the gallbladder from the liver. Upward traction by placing a clamp near the cystic duct (on the gallbladder) is helpful.

Step 3. Remove the gallbladder and electrocoagulate the gallbladder fossa to stop bleeding or bile leakage. Closure of the fossa is up to the surgeon (Fig. 14.16).

■ OPERATING ROOM CHOLANGIOGRAM

To perform an adequate operative cholangiogram, the volume of the biliary tract is more important than the length or the diameter. The capacity is between 12 and 20 ml. Obviously, the presence of stones will markedly reduce the capacity.

If a cholangiogram is performed, the patient should be rotated slightly to the right so that the common bile duct is rotated off the spine and becomes clearly visible.

An operative cholangiogram will be of great assistance to the surgeon passing a probe through the common bile duct. There is a potential

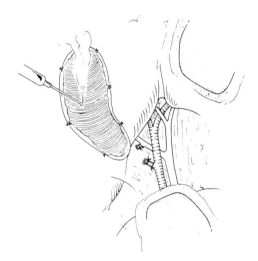

Figure 14.16

danger if the surgeon passes a probe and expects it to take a straight line to the ampulla and encounters instead a 90-degree turn as the duct enters the duodenum. If the duct is fixed by disease or prior surgery, and if the surgeon is a little too rough, catastrophe can result.

Procedure:

Step 1. For traction, use mild tension on the proximal ligation of the cystic duct (which, though ligated, is still connected to the gallbladder). Make a minute opening into the anterior wall of the cystic duct with a No. 11 blade. Through this opening, insert the special catheter and secure by tying the cystic duct and catheter with a 2–0 silk suture (Fig. 14.17).

Step 2. Take two x-rays: the first after injecting 7 cc of 30 percent Renografin, and the second using 14 cc of contrast. Have the anesthesiologist stop ventilating the patient during exposure.

Step 3. If there is no pathology, remove the catheter and doubly ligate the cystic duct. If choledocholithiasis or other pathology is found, proceed with common duct exploration. Occasionally, choledochoscopy is helpful.

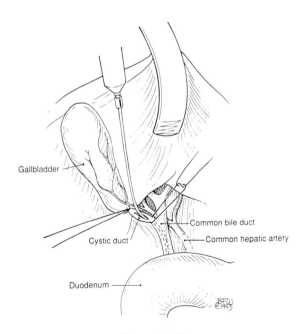

Figure 14.17

Step 4. T-tube draining is essential (Fig. 14.18).

Note: If the common bile duct is not completely filled, the patient can be placed in a little Trendelenburg position and 20 cc of 30 percent Renografin used.

■ COMMON BILE DUCT EXPLORATION

Procedure:

Step 1. Duodenal kocherization by careful incision of the lateral peritoneum and palpation of the duodenum, the head of the pancreas, and the distal common bile duct (Figs. 14.19 and 14.20).

Step 2. Dissect tissue overlying the common bile duct no more than 1–2 cm distal to the cystic stump. Skeletonization of more than 2½–3 cm is dangerous.

Step 3. Place 4-0 Vicryl stay sutures medial and lateral to the cleaned common bile duct area. Aspirate the common bile duct to make sure you are in the right place. Incise the elevated ante-

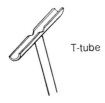

T-tube

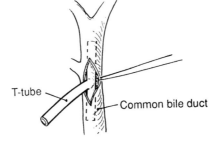

T-tube — Common bile duct

Figure 14.18

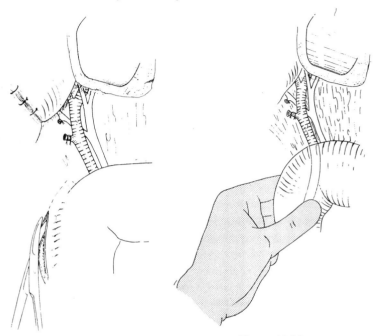

Figure 14.19   Figure 14.20

rior wall of the common bile duct to a length of 1 cm or less (Figs. 14.21–14.24).

Step 4. Remove stones by instrumentation (Randall stones forceps, scoops of several types and sizes, irrigation catheter, biliary Fogarty catheter) or extrinsic pressure by milking the stones to the upward choledochotomy (Figs. 14.25 and 14.26).

Step 5. Demonstrate ampullary patency using a small French catheter. If doubt about patency remains, use a Bakes No. 3 dilator very carefully to avoid false passage. Choledochoscopy may be helpful. Conduct repeated irrigation of the biliary ducts to remove small stones or sludge. If stones are impacted in the ampulla, papillotomy for their removal will be necessary (Figs. 14.27–14.30).

Step 6. Insert a T-tube and close the common bile duct with 4–0 interrupted Vicryl (Figs. 14.31 and 14.32).

Step 7. Carry out T-tube cholangiography and secure T-tube straight out in the abdominal wall by a minute stab wound.

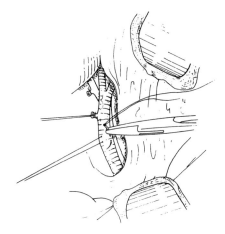

Figure 14.21

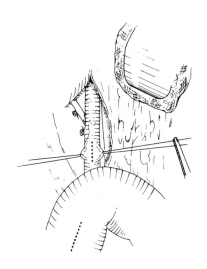

Figure 14.22

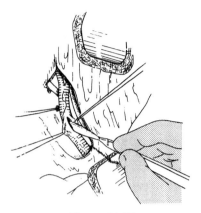

Figure 14.23.
1962.)

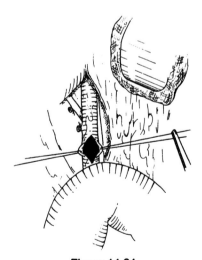

Figure 14.24

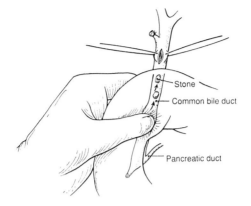

Figure 14.25

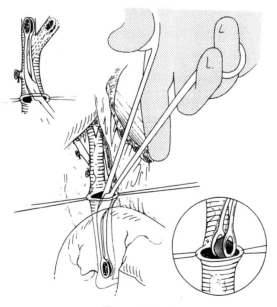

Figure 14.26

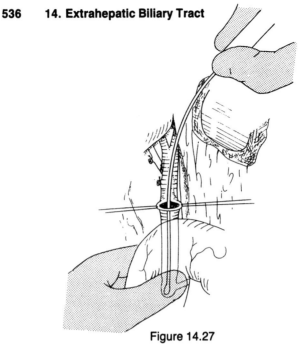

Figure 14.27

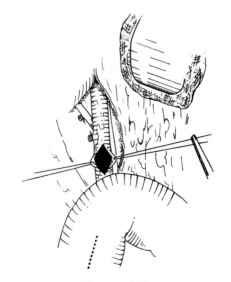

Figure 14.28

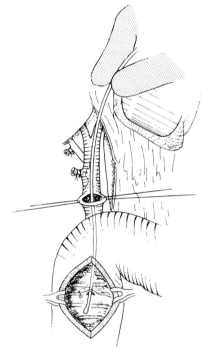

Figure 14.29. Perform the duodenotomy only if it is necessary.

Step 8. Close abdominal wall. Secure T-tube to the skin with 0 silk.

Remember these indications for exploration of the common bile duct:

✓ Presence of a palpable stone

✓ Roentgenographic visualization of a stone

✓ Recent or present jaundice

✓ Dilatation of the common bile duct (we suggest a diameter over 10 mm be considered "dilated")

✓ Multiple stones in the gallbladder together with a large cystic duct

✓ Aspiration of murky bile

✓ When in doubt, explore! Exposure and mobilization of 2–5 cm in length may be obtained by mobilizing the distal common bile duct from the undersurface of the pancreas. Because the duct may be intrapancreatic (Fig. 14.6C), the pancreas and duodenum should be mobilized (Figs. 14.6B, D, E).

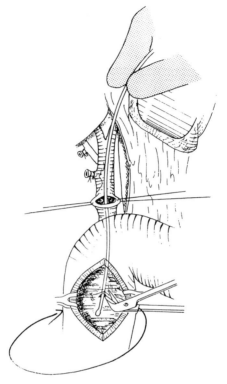

Figure 14.30

■ SPHINCTEROPLASTY

Procedure:

Step 1. Perform cholecystectomy and operating room cholangiogram.

Step 2. Carry out duodenal kocherization (Fig. 14.33) and choledo-chotomy. Insert balloon catheter all the way down through the ampulla. Place stay sutures of 4–0 silk at the duodenal wall in the area of the palpable balloon. Perform duodenotomy using electrocautery (Fig. 14.34).

Step 3. Localize the ampulla.

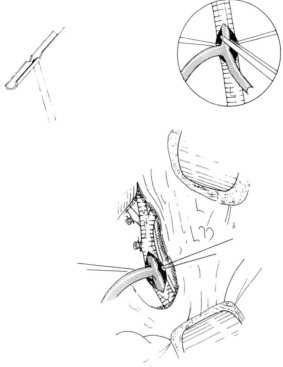

Figure 14.31

Step 4. At the 3 and 9 o'clock positions in the periampullary area, place 5-0 silk stay sutures (Fig. 14.35).

Step 5. Perform a sphincterotomy between the 10 and 11 o'clock positions to a depth of 2–3 mm using electrocautery (Fig. 14.36).

Step 6. Approximate the ductal and duodenal mucosa with interrupted 5-0 synthetic absorbable sutures (Figs. 14.36 and 14.37).

Step 7. Localize the pancreatic duct opening, insert a probe, and carefully perform a septotomy to a depth of 2–4 mm by knife or Pott's scissors. Note: Wirsung's ductoplasty by interrupted sutures, as in step 6, is optional. If the ductal orifice is not found, secretin injection will be very helpful: one unit per kilogram of body weight.

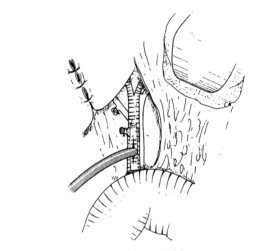

Figure 14.32

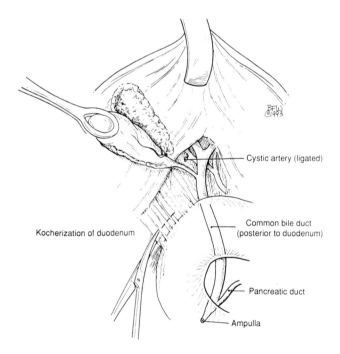

Cystic artery (ligated)

Common bile duct
(posterior to duodenum)

Kocherization of duodenum

Pancreatic duct

Ampulla

Figure 14.33

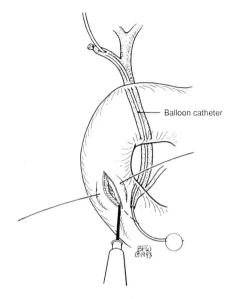

Balloon catheter

Figure 14.34

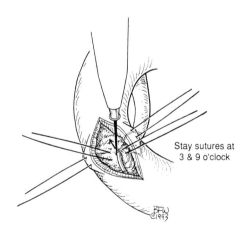

Stay sutures at
3 & 9 o'clock

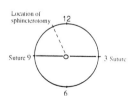

Figure 14.35

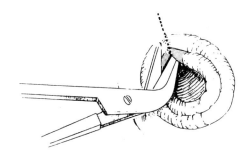

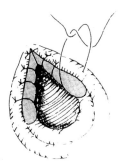

Figure 14.36

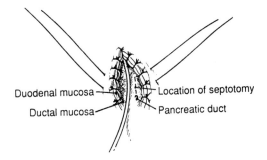

Duodenal mucosa ——
Ductal mucosa ——

Location of septotomy
Pancreatic duct

Figure 14.37

Step 8. Execute duodenorrhaphy in two layers. Place a T-tube into the common bile duct and insert a Jackson-Pratt drain (Fig. 14.38).

■ CHOLEDOCHODUODENOSTOMY

Procedure:

Step 1. Establish good mobilization of the common bile duct and duodenum to avoid anastomotic tension. Anchor the duodenum to the common bile duct by placing a row of 4–0 Vicryl sutures posteriorly (Fig. 14.39).

Step 2. Make a 1.5- to 2-cm transverse incision of the duodenum just below the suture line and a vertical or transverse incision of the common bile duct just above the suture line (Fig. 14.40).

Step 3. Perform the anastomosis in a single layer using interrupted 4–0 Vicryl sutures, full thickness, to the common bile duct and duodenum (Figs. 14.40–14.42).

Note: Alternatively, a side-to-side anastomosis may be performed.

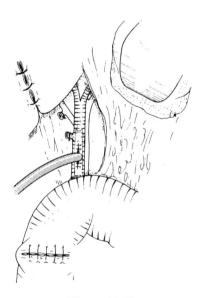

Figure 14.38

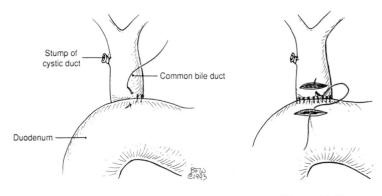

Figure 14.39   Figure 14.40

■ CHOLEDOCHAL CYSTECTOMY

Procedure:

Step 1. Evaluate the extent of the cyst (Fig. 14.43).

Step 2. Execute lysis of pericystic adhesions (Fig. 14.43).

Step 3. Perform cholecystectomy and choledochocystectomy (Fig. 14.44).

Step 4. Perform internal drainage by a 60-cm Roux-en-Y jejunal loop.

    a. Jejunal interrruption at approximately 60 cm

    b. Small opening in transverse mesocolon

    c. Distal jejunal loop, closed with GIA stapler

    d. Distal jejunal Roux-en-Y loop up through the transverse mesocolon opening

    e. End-to-side hepaticojejunal anastomosis in one layer with interrupted 4–0 absorbable sutures (Fig. 14.45)

    f. Secure the jejunum to the transverse mesocolon opening

    g. End-to-side jejunojejunal anastomosis in two layers (Figs. 14.46 and 14.47)

    h. Be sure to secure the Roux-en-Y loop to the vicinity of the gallbladder fossa with two or three interrupted 3–0 silk sutures to avoid possible herniation as well as weight tension.

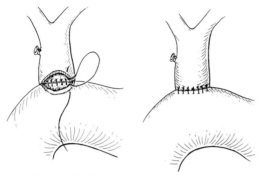

Figure 14.41

Figure 14.42

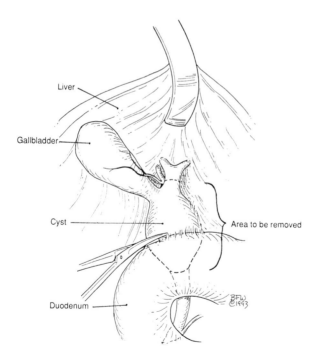

Figure 14.43

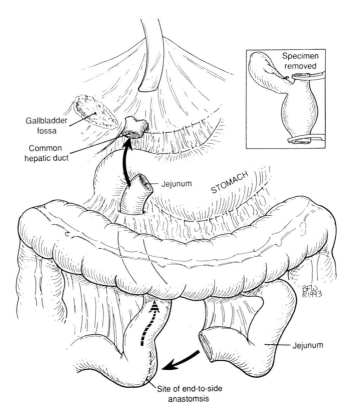

Figure 14.44

i. If there is room, it is advisable to insert a T-tube into the common hepatic duct (Fig. 14.48).

Step 5. Insert Jackson–Pratt drain and close abdominal wall.

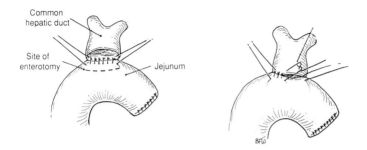

Figure 14.45

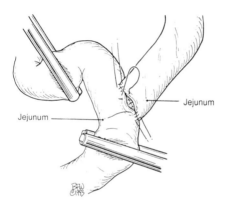

Figure 14.46

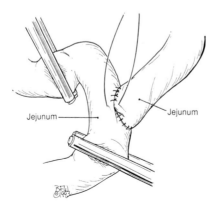

Figure 14.47

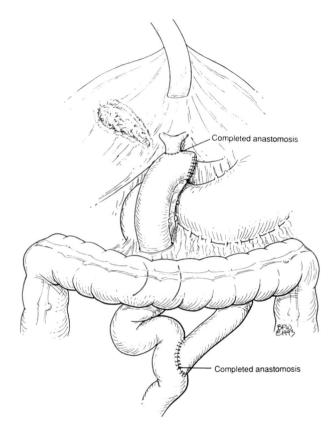

Figure 14.48

15

Spleen

ANATOMY

■ GENERAL DESCRIPTION OF THE SPLEEN

The spleen is concealed at the left hypochondrium and is not palpable under normal conditions. It is associated with the posterior portions of the left 9th, 10th, and 11th ribs, being separated from them by the diaphragm and the costodiaphragmatic recess (Fig. 15.1).

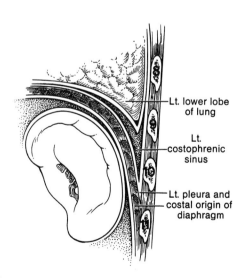

Lt. lower lobe of lung

Lt. costophrenic sinus

Lt. pleura and costal origin of diaphragm

Figure 15.1. Location of the spleen. (By permission of JE Skandalakis, GL Colborn, LB Pemberton, et al., *Prob Gen Surg* 7(1):1–17, 1990.)

If one divides the spleen into three parts, the upper third is related to the lower lobe of the left lung, the middle third to the left costophrenic sinus, and the lower third to the left pleura and costal origin of the diaphragm.

For all practical purposes, the spleen has two surfaces: parietal and visceral (Fig. 15.2). The convex parietal surface is related to the diaphragm, and the concave visceral surface is related to the stomach, the kidney, the colon, and the tail of the pancreas (gastric, renal, colonic, and pancreatic).

The peritoneum covers the entire spleen in a double layer, except for the hilum (Fig. 15.3).

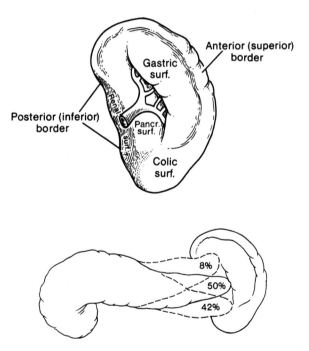

Figure 15.2. Splenic borders. (Top) Anterior and posterior border. (Bottom) Relations of the tail of the pancreas to the spleen. (By permission of JE Skandalakis, GL Colborn, LB Pemberton, et al., *Prob Gen Surg* 7(1):1–17, 1990.)

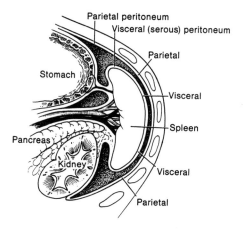

Figure 15.3. Sagittal view of peritoneum covering the spleen. (By permission of JE Skandalakis, GL Colborn, LB Pemberton, et al., *Prob Gen Surg* 7(1):1–17, 1990.)

■ CHIEF SPLENIC LIGAMENTS

At the hilum, the visceral peritoneum joins the right layer of the greater omentum and forms the gastrosplenic and the splenorenal ligaments. These two ligaments form the splenic pedicle. The capsule is formed by the visceral peritoneum, which is as friable as the spleen itself and as easily injured (Fig. 15.4).

The two chief ligaments of the spleen are the gastrosplenic and the splenorenal. The spleen has several minor ligaments, and, except for the presplenic fold, their names indicate their connections (Fig. 15.5): the splenophrenic, splenocolic, pancreatosplenic, phrenicocolic, and pancreatocolic ligaments.

The superior pole of the spleen lies close to the stomach and may be fixed to it. The inferior pole lies 5 to 7 cm from the stomach. The gastrosplenic ligament contains the short gastric arteries above and the left gastroepiploic vessels below; it should be incised only between clamps or preferably after the vessels are ligated one by one. Transfixion sutures may be used.

The splenorenal ligament envelops the splenic vessels and the tail of the pancreas. The outer layer of the splenorenal ligament forms the posterior layer of the gastrosplenic ligament. Careless division of the

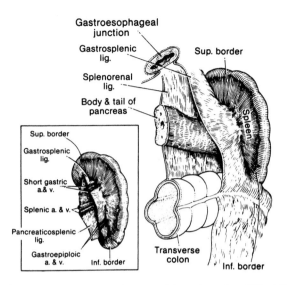

Figure 15.4. The peritoneal attachments of the spleen. (Inset) The hilus of the spleen showing the short gastric and gastroepiploic vessels in the gastrosplenic ligament. (By permission of JE Skandalakis, SW Gray, and JR Rowe, *Anatomical Complications in General Surgery*, New York: McGraw-Hill, 1983.)

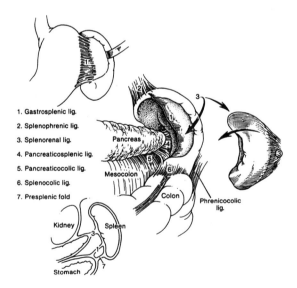

Figure 15.5. Minor splenic ligaments. (By permission of JE Skandalakis, GL Colborn, LB Pemberton, et al., *Prob Gen Surg* 7(1):1–17, 1990.)

former may injure the short gastric vessels. Bleeding from these vessels may be the result of too-enthusiastic deep posterior excavation by the index and middle fingers of an operator seeking to mobilize and retract the spleen to the right. The splenorenal ligament itself is nearly avascular and may be incised, but the fingers should stop at the pedicle (Fig. 15.6).

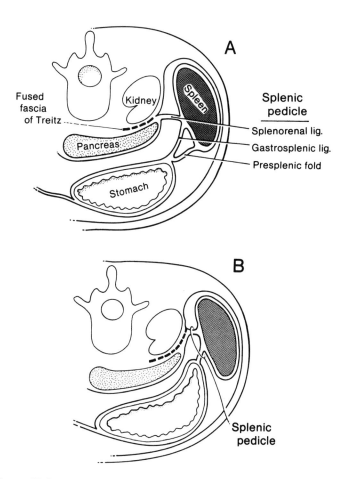

Figure 15.6. The splenic pedicle. (A) Long pedicle with a presplenic fold. (B) Short pedicle. (By permission of JE Skandalakis, SW Gray, and JR Rowe, *Anatomical Complications in General Surgery*, New York: McGraw-Hill, 1983.)

Minor Splenic Ligaments

The splenophrenic ligament (Fig. 15.5) is the reflection of the leaves of the mesentery to the posterior body wall and to the inferior surface of the diaphragm at the area of the upper pole of the spleen close to the stomach. It is usually avascular, but it should be inspected for possible bleeding after section.

Tortuous or aberrant inferior polar vessels or a left gastroepiploic artery may lie close enough to the splenocolic ligament to be injured by careless incision of the ligament, with resulting massive bleeding. The ligament should be incised between clamps.

The pancreatosplenic ligament (Fig. 15.5) exists when the tail of the pancreas does not touch the spleen.

The presplenic fold is a peritoneal fold anterior to the gastrosplenic ligament (Fig. 15.5), often containing the left gastroepiploic vessels. Excessive traction on this fold during upper abdominal operations can result in a tear in the splenic capsule.

The pancreatocolic ligament (Fig. 15.5) is a bridge of the tail or body of the pancreas to the splenic flexure (Fig. 15.7).

The "phrenicocolic ligament" is not a splenic ligament, but the spleen rests upon it. It extends between the splenic flexure and the diaphragm, and constitutes the "splenic floor." It is not connected to the spleen (Fig. 15.5).

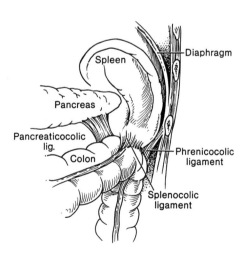

Figure 15.7. Relation of the pancreatocolic, phrenicocolic, and splenocolic ligaments to the transverse mesocolon. (By permission of JE Skandalakis, GL Colborn, LB Pemberton, et al., *Prob Gen Surg* 7(1):1–17, 1990.)

■ SPLENIC VASCULAR SYSTEM

Splenic Artery and Its Branches

The splenic artery, in most people, is a branch of the celiac trunk together with the hepatic and left gastric arteries. The artery varies in length from 8 to 32 cm and in diameter from 0.5 to 1.2 cm. The normal course of the splenic artery crosses the left side of the aorta, passes along the upper border of the pancreas reaching the tail in front, then crosses the upper pole of the left kidney.

The left gastroepiploic artery arises most often from the splenic trunk. Less often it arises from the inferior terminal or its branches, and, rarely, it arises from the middle splenic trunk or the superior terminal branch.

Because the origins of the splenic branches are unpredictable, use of a preoperative arteriogram is paramount in determining the point of ligation of the splenic artery. There is no question that the spleen can tolerate ligation of the splenic artery because of the available collateral circulation. Therefore, the spleen can be saved if necessary. Surgeons should remember that ligation of the splenic artery near its origin can result in hyperamylasemia resulting from deterioration of the pancreatic blood supply. Preoperative splenic arterial occlusion as an adjunct to high-risk splenectomy has been advised.

Splenic Vein and Its Branches

The splenic vein travels with the splenic artery (Fig. 15.8), sometimes crossing over or under it. The anatomy of the splenic vein is summarized in Fig. 15.9. The patterns are highly variable, and, as in the arteries, no one vein resembles the next. The single characteristic of most of the short gastric veins is that they communicate directly with the spleen, entering at its upper part, rather than through the extrasplenic venous vessels. The left gastroepiploic venous drainage is into the splenic veins.

Lymphatic Drainage

The splenic lymphatic chain (Fig. 15.10) is reported to be formed by suprapancreatic nodes, infrapancreatic nodes, and afferent and efferent lymph vessels.

■ SEGMENTAL ANATOMY

Studies indicate that 84 percent of the population has two splenic segments—superior and inferior—and 16 percent has three segments—supe-

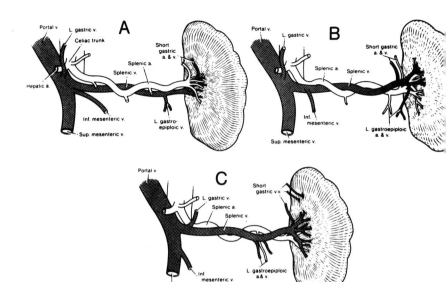

Figure 15.8. Relation of splenic artery and splenic vein. (A) Artery anterior to vein (this is the usual pattern). (B) Artery both anterior and posterior to vein. (C) Artery posterior to vein (this is the least common configuration). (By permission of JE Skandalakis, SW Gray, and JR Rowe, *Anatomical Complications in General Surgery*, New York: McGraw-Hill, 1983.)

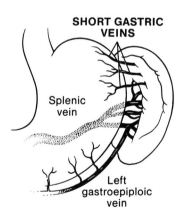

Figure 15.9. Anatomy of the splenic vein. (By permission of JE Skandalakis, GL Colborn, LB Pemberton, et al., *Prob Gen Surg* 7(1):1–17, 1990.)

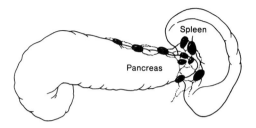

Figure 15.10. Lymphatic drainage of the spleen. (By permission of JE Skandalakis, GL Colborn, LB Pemberton, et al., *Prob Gen Surg* 7(1):1–17, 1990.)

rior, middle, and inferior. More than three segments have been reported. The arterial segments are separated by avascular planes.

■ ACCESSORY SPLEENS

The reported incidence of accessory spleens varies from approximately 10 percent to 30 percent. In most affected patients (approximately 60 percent), only one accessory spleen is present. In 20 percent, two such spleens are present, and in 17 percent, there are three or more splenic structures. Two-thirds to ¾ of accessory spleens are located at or near the hilum of the normal organ, and about 20 percent are embedded in the tail of the pancreas. The remainder are distributed along the splenic artery, in the omentum, in the mesentery, or beneath the peritoneum (Fig. 15.11). They range from 0.2 to 10 cm in size, resembling lymph nodes or miniature spleens.

Notes:

✔ Patients with fractures of the left 9th–11th ribs should be observed closely; they are candidates for an underlying splenic rupture.

✔ In splenomegaly, the spleen is always located in front of the splenic flexure. Adhesions are almost always present and sometimes vascular. Often an enlarged spleen is fixed heavily with the colon.

✔ In elective splenectomies, if splenomegaly is present, intestinal preparation is essential.

✔ After radiologic evaluation of the topography of both the upper splenic pole and the left costophrenic sinus, a left thoracotomy tube should be introduced above the upper pole of the spleen.

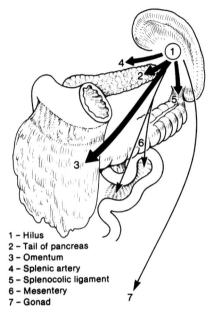

1 – Hilus
2 – Tail of pancreas
3 – Omentum
4 – Splenic artery
5 – Splenocolic ligament
6 – Mesentery
7 – Gonad

Figure 15.11. Sites of accessory spleens in order of frequence: (1) near the splenic hilus; (2) tail of the pancreas (these contain 86 to 95 percent of all accessory spleens); (3) omentum; (4) along the splenic artery; (5) splenocolic ligament; (6) mesentery; and (7) testis or ovary (3 through 7 are unusual locations). (By permission of JE Skandalakis, SW Gray, and JR Rowe, *Anatomical Complications in General Surgery*, New York: McGraw-Hill, 1983.)

TECHNIQUE

■ SPLENECTOMY

A splenectomy is usually performed for one of the four following reasons: hemorrhage, hypersplenism, Hodgkin's disease staging (diagnostic laparotomy), or a problem such as an abscess, cyst, or tumor.

Splenectomy Due to Hemorrhage Secondary to Trauma

Procedure:

Step 1. Make an incision.

Step 2. Mobilize the spleen.

Step 3. Ligate the vessels.

Step 4. Divide the hilum.

Step 5. Obtain hemostasis.

Step 6. Provide drainage.

Step 7. Close the wound.

Splenectomy Due to Hematologic Disorders (Hypersplenism)

Procedure:

Step 1. Make an incision.

Step 2. Ligate the arteries.

Step 3. Mobilize the spleen.

Step 4. Divide the hilum.

Step 5. Obtain hemostasis.

Step 6. Search for accessory spleens.

Step 7. Provide drainage.

Step 8. Close the wound.

Ligation of the Splenic Pedicle

Anterior Approach

Procedure:

Step 1. Incision (Fig. 15.12).

Step 2. Clamp, incise, and ligate the left part of the gastrocolic ligament and the gastroepiploic artery and vein. This will provide access to the lesser sac (Fig. 15.12).

Step 3. Locate the splenic artery at the superior border of the body of the pancreas. Carefully ligate the artery in continuity and doubly, with ligatures being placed as distally as possible (Fig. 15.13).

Step 4. Clamp, divide, and ligate the short gastric arteries and veins, one at a time (Fig. 15.13).

Step 5. Mobilize the spleen by dividing the several ligaments with scissors. Insert the index finger deeply to separate the spleen from

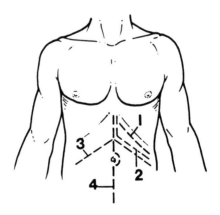

Figure 15.12. Incision for total splenectomy by the anterior approach and access to the lesser sac. 1 = Subcostal; 2 = Kehr subcostal; 3 = Bilateral subcostal; 4 = Midline. (By permission of LB Pemberton and LJ Skandalakis, *Prob Gen Surg* 7(1):85–102, 1990.)

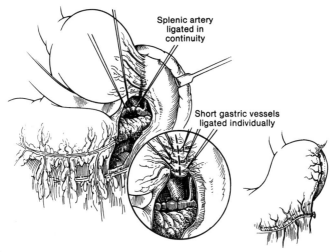

Splenic artery
ligated in
continuity

Short gastric vessels
ligated individually

Figure 15.13. Ligation of the splenic artery and the short gastric arteries and vein. (By permission of LB Pemberton and LJ Skandalakis, *Prob Gen Surg* 7(1): 85–102, 1990.)

the renal covering, with the use of sharp and blunt dissection. Clamp, divide, and ligate the splenocolic and splenophrenic ligaments (Fig. 15.14).

Step 6. Elevate the spleen, tail, and part of the body of the pancreas, being particularly careful with the tail of the pancreas. The spleen is now outside the peritoneal cavity and is attached only by one of the branches of the splenic arteries and veins.

Step 7. Close to the hilum, clamp, divide, and ligate all branches of the splenic artery. The splenic vein and its branches are easily torn and should not be clamped. Ligate and divide the splenic vein and branches in continuity with 2-0 silk. The spleen is now free and should be removed (Fig. 15.15).

Step 8. Inspect the site for bleeding, beginning with the diaphragm and continuing to the greater curvature of the stomach, pancreatic tail, gastrosplenic ligament, splenorenal ligament, splenocolic ligament, and splenic bed and other ligaments.

Remember:

✔ Complete hemostasis is essential. Invert the greater curvature with interrupted 00 suture to prevent postoperative bleeding and possible necrosis. After complete in-

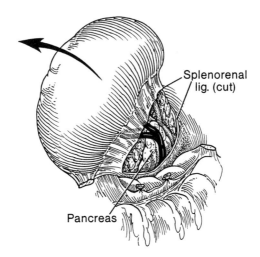

Figure 15.14. Division of the ligaments and delivery of the spleen to the outside of the peritoneal cavity. (By permission of LB Pemberton and LJ Skandalakis, *Prob Gen Surg* 7(1):85–102, 1990.)

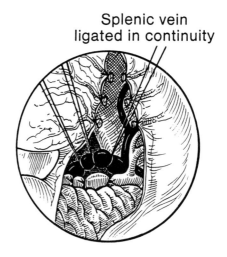

Figure 15.15. Ligation of the splenic vein. (By permission of LB Pemberton and LJ Skandalakis, *Prob Gen Surg* 7(1):85–102, 1990.)

spection for bleeding, search for accessory spleens (Fig. 15.16).

Posterior Approach

Procedure:

Step 1. Hold the spleen medially (Fig. 15.17).

Step 2. Divide the splenorenal, splenophrenic, and splenocolic ligaments (Fig. 15.17).

Step 3. Lift the spleen outside the peritoneal cavity, being particularly careful with the tail of the pancreas.

Step 4. Dissect rapidly and mobilize the bleeding spleen immediately. Bleeding can be controlled by manually compressing the splenic artery and vein and the tail of the pancreas between the thumb and index finger or with a noncrushing clamp (Fig. 15.18).

Step 5. Ligate the arterial and venous branches close to the hilum using 00 and 000 ligatures. Doubly ligate the splenic artery (Fig. 15.19).

Step 6. Ligate the short gastric vessels and invert the area of the greater curvature where the short gastric vessels were ligated (Fig. 15.16).

Step 7. Remove the spleen and secure any bleeding points.

Step 8. Close the abdominal wall.

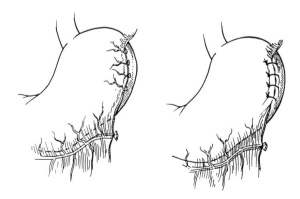

Figure 15.16. Inversion of the greater curvature. (By permission of LB Pemberton and LJ Skandalakis, *Prob Gen Surg* 7(1):85–102, 1990.)

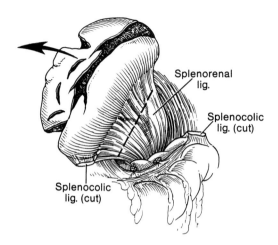

Figure 15.17. Medial position of the spleen during the posterior approach to splenectomy, showing division of the splenocolic ligaments. (By permission of LB Pemberton and LJ Skandalakis, *Prob Gen Surg* 7(1):85–102, 1990.)

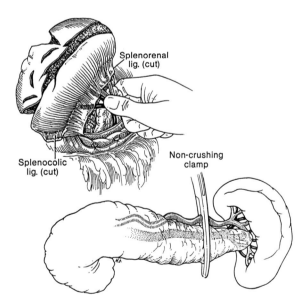

Figure 15.18. Compression of the splenic artery and vein. (By permission of LB Pemberton and LJ Skandalakis, *Prob Gen Surg* 7(1):85–102, 1990.)

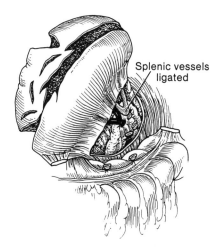

Splenic vessels
ligated

Figure 15.19. Ligation of the splenic artery. (By permission of LB Pemberton and LJ Skandalakis, *Prob Gen Surg* 7(1):85–102, 1990.)

Partial Splenectomy

The major indication for partial splenectomy is trauma to the spleen; it is sometimes performed for nonparasitic splenic cysts, in Gaucher's disease, etc. An effort to save the spleen is paramount. However, it is our opinion that, if there is any doubt, the spleen should be removed and the patient transfused later. Detailed evaluation of the trauma must be done. Decisions must be made about the procedure of choice:

1. Splenorrhaphy
2. Splenorrhaphy with omental fixation (Fig. 15.20)
3. Debridement, perhaps with partial splenectomy and omental fixation
4. Splenic mesh wrap (Fig. 15.21)
5. Autotransplantation (Fig. 15.22)

Technique of Intrasplenic Dissection

With scalpel (not cautery), make a superficial anterior incision (not circumferential) of the splenic capsule on the viable side of the line of demarcation.

Using the scalpel handle, gradually deepen the incision until the entire spleen has been divided.

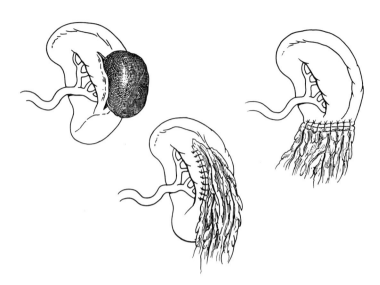

Figure 15.20. (A) Splenic rupture with hematoma; (B) splenorrhaphy with omental fixation; (C) partial splenectomy with omental fixation. (By permission of LB Pemberton and LJ Skandalakis, *Prob Gen Surg* 7(1):85–102, 1990.)

Ligate all vessels with hemoclips or with figure-of-eight 4-0 silk. If oozing occurs, apply a hemostatic substance.

An alternative technique for treating the raw splenic remnant is placement of interlocking mattress sutures of 2-0 chromic catgut, 0.5-1 cm from the divided edge, compressing the splenic parenchyma for hemostasis. Tie these over pledgets of Gelfoam (absorbable gelatin sponge) or Surgicel (oxidized regenerated cellulose). With the proper degree of tension on sutures, we have found pledgets of any kind unnecessary to support the sutures. If the exposed splenic raw area is thin, a running suture of 2-0 chromic catgut will suffice.

Application of a topical hemostatic agent for capsular avulsions or very superficial lacerations may arrest hemorrhage. Partial splenectomy may be handled successfully with stapling devices.

Both an ultrasonic surgical aspirator (Cavitron) and a laser (which produces heat coagulation of blood vessels) have been used for identification and control of the intrasplenic vessels.

Use absorbable mesh in partial splenectomy or a deeply lacerated spleen. Replace and observe the splenic remnant for 10 minutes to ascertain the completeness of hemostasis.

The surgeon should determine whether drainage is required.

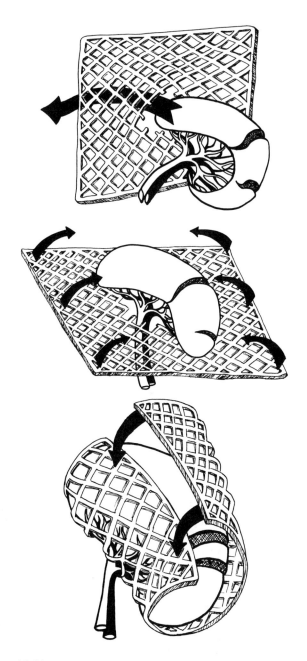

Figure 15.21. Splenic mesh wrap. (Top) Passage of injured spleen through hole in center of mesh; (middle) wrapping spleen in mesh; (bottom) sewing opposite edges of mesh to each other to create tamponade. (By permission of DA Lange, P Zaret, GL Merlotti, et al., *J Trauma* 28(3):269–275, 1988.)

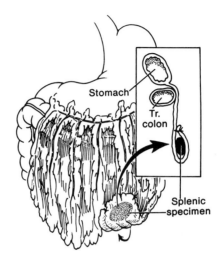

Figure 15.22. Autotransplantation. (By permission of LB Pemberton and LJ Skandalakis, *Prob Gen Surg* 7(1):85–102, 1990.)

■ OCCLUSION OF THE SPLENIC ARTERY

Procedure:

Step 1. Perform temporary occlusion of the main splenic artery.

Step 2. Isolate the segmental branches. Remember, the splenic vasculature is segmental and highly variable. The superior polar artery is, however, quite constant, generally being given off approximately 1–3 cm from the splenic hilum. At or near the splenic hilum, the splenic artery branches further into three to five major branches and into several large and small branches. The splenic veins follow the pattern of the arterial distribution more consistently in the smaller branches than in the larger ones.

Once the segment chosen for preservation is delineated, begin a systematic, stepwise ligation and division of the branches to the segment to be removed. As the ligation proceeds, evidence of the devascularization of the spleen will become increasingly obvious as segment after segment undergoes a color change ranging from dark bluish-purple to bluish-black.

Remove the devascularized splenic parenchyma. The remnant

should be of normal color, size, and consistency, indicating adequate arterial inflow and venous outflow.

■ STAGING PROCEDURE FOR HODGKIN'S DISEASE AND LIMITED NON-HODGKIN'S LYMPHOMA

Procedure:

Step 1. Perform a detailed exploratory laparotomy.

Step 2. Examine the nodes and perform wedge and needle biopsies on both lobes of the liver.

Step 3. Perform total splenectomy with splenic lymph node biopsy.

Step 4. Conduct retroperitoneal exploration (for lymph node biopsies) of: celiac axis, hepatoduodenopancreatic lymph nodes, periaortic lymph nodes, inferior vena caval lymph nodes, iliac lymph nodes, and mesenteric lymph nodes of the small and large intestines.

Step 5. Biopsy iliac crest marrow.

Step 6. Search for accessory spleens.

Step 7. Perform oophoropexy in young women.

Step 8. Place metal clips at the splenic pedicle, the areas where biopsies were performed on lymph nodes, the areas of lymph nodes where biopsies were not performed, and the site of ovarian translocation.

Note: A pathologist should be in the operating room to ensure proper handling of the fresh specimens and to decide if any tissues should be prepared for examination. Touch preparations of the spleen and lymph nodes should be made. Tissues should be placed in a special solution for examination by electron microscope. Slides of bone marrow specimens should be prepared.

Drainage is controversial. It should be done at the surgeon's discretion.

Remember:

✓ The splenorenal ligament is almost avascular, but small veins can cause problems.

✓ The perisplenic adhesions are vascular.

✓ The terminal splenic vessels are fragile and easily torn.

✓ The splenic capsule also is friable.

✓ Dissection of the splenic artery close to the celiac artery through the gastrocolic omentum can be done if moderate splenomegaly and adhesions are present. However, to avoid sudden, large loss of blood, one must be aware of the superfragile splenic vein, which can coil around the artery.

✓ With huge spleens with multiple vascular adhesions, the artery can be ligated along the upper pancreatic border after the gastrocolic ligament is opened.

✓ A healthy ruptured spleen can be delivered easily from the abdomen.

✓ A large, diseased spleen requires careful dissection of the prehilar area and ligation of the vessels.

✓ In thrombocytopenic purpura, the abdomen should be explored after the spleen is removed, to avoid unnecessary bleeding.

✓ In idiopathic thrombocytopenic purpura, the splenic artery should be ligated as soon as possible.

✓ In the presence of hemolytic anemia, transfusions should not be given before the operation. Platelets should be transfused after splenic artery ligation.

✓ Short gastric arteries and veins should be transfixed, and the greater curvature of the stomach should be inverted to avoid bleeding and gastric necrosis.

✓ If the splenic artery is ligated proximally, it should also be ligated distally close to the hilum. This is the most unpredictable artery of the human body.

✓ The pancreatic tail should be handled gently at the hilum, especially when it is located posterior to the pedicle.

✓ Handle the renocolosplenic area gently to avoid bleeding and/or injury to the spleen, kidney or colon.

✓ If the splenic pedicle is ligated en masse the hilar vessels should be religated. The pedicle should be ligated twice with heavy silk.

✓ An autologous splenic capsule should be used over the raw splenic surface; the graft should be secured with fine catgut sutures. Since the authors have had no experience with this, no further details can be provided.

✓ The pancreas should be separated from the spleen by division of the splenic artery and vein distal to the tip of the pancreas. The spleen survives on the short gastric vessels, if carefully preserved.

✓ When there is splenomegaly, heavy adhesions are present between the spleen and the diaphragm above and laterally, the stomach medially, and the splenic flexure below. These adhesions may contain large neoplastic vessels, which can produce tremendous bleeding if not ligated and secured before their division.

✓ If a patient has a hemorrhagic disorder, a nasogastric tube should be inserted in the operating room, not in the patient's room, by an anesthesiologist.

✓ In elective splenectomy with a large spleen, intravenous preoperative antibiotics and occlusion of the splenic artery are advisable. Preoperative splenic embolization should be considered. With such a procedure, the surgeon is committing to a total splenectomy.

✓ If a blood transfusion becomes necessary for a successful splenorrhaphy, splenectomy without transfusion is the safer treatment.

■ POSTOPERATIVE CARE

1. Monitor the patient closely for 24 hours.
2. Perform repeated hematocrit readings.

Avoid chest physiotherapy. Avoid sports for 3 months. A radionuclide scan may be done 3-4 months after surgery to assess the function, size, and location of the splenic remnant.

16

Adrenal Glands

ANATOMY

■ GENERAL DESCRIPTION OF THE ADRENAL GLANDS

Each adrenal gland, together with the associated kidney, is enclosed in the renal fascia (of Gerota) and surrounded by fat.

The glands are firmly attached to the fascia, which is in turn attached firmly to the abdominal wall and to the diaphragm. A layer of loose connective tissue separates the capsule of the adrenal gland from that of the kidney. Because the kidney and the adrenal gland are thus separated, the kidney may be ectopic or ptotic without a corresponding displacement of the gland. Fusion of the kidneys, however, is often accompanied by fusion of the adrenal glands.

Occasionally the fusion of the adrenal gland and the kidney is so extensive that separation is almost impossible. If individuals with such a fusion needed a partial or total nephrectomy, they would also require a coincidental adrenalectomy.

For all practical purposes, each adrenal gland has only an anterior and a posterior surface. Relationships to other structures are as follows: (Fig. 16.1)

I. Right adrenal gland:
   A. Anterior surface:
      1. Superior: "bare area" of liver
      2. Medial: inferior vena cava
      3. Lateral: "bare area" of liver
      4. Inferior: peritoneum and occasionally the first part of the duodenum
   B. Posterior surface:
      1. Superior: diaphragm
      2. Inferior: anteromedial aspect of right kidney

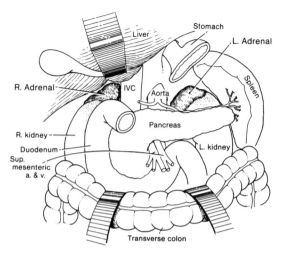

Figure 16.1. The relations of the adrenal glands from the anterior approach. (By permission of JE Skandalakis, SW Gray, and JR Rowe, *Anatomical Complications in General Surgery*, New York: McGraw-Hill, 1983.)

II. Left adrenal gland:
   A. Anterior surface:
      1. Superior: peritoneum (posterior wall of omental bursa) and stomach
      2. Inferior: body of the pancreas
   B. Posterior surface:
      1. Medial: left crus of diaphragm
      2. Lateral: medial aspect of left kidney

The medial borders of the right and left adrenal glands are about 4.5 cm apart. In this space, from right to left, are the inferior vena cava, the right crus of the diaphragm, part of the celiac ganglion, the celiac trunk, the superior mesenteric artery, part of the celiac ganglion, and the left crus of the diaphragm.

■ VASCULAR SYSTEM

Arterial Supply

The arterial supply to the adrenal glands is from three sources: (Fig. 16.2)

   1. A group of six to eight arteries arises separately from the inferior phrenic arteries.

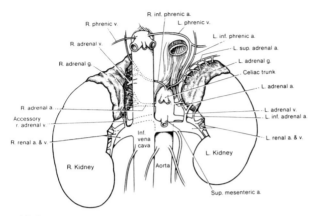

Figure 16.2. The arterial supply and venous drainage of the adrenal glands. As many as 60 arterial twigs may enter the adrenal gland. One or, occasionally, two veins drain the adrenal gland. (By permission of JE Skandalakis, SW Gray, and JR Rowe, *Anatomical Complications in General Surgery*, New York: Mc-Graw-Hill, 1983.)

2. A middle adrenal artery arises from the aorta at or near the level of the origin of the superior mesenteric artery. It may be single, multiple, or absent. It may supply the perirenal fat only.

3. One or more inferior adrenal arteries arise from the renal artery, an accessory renal artery, or a superior polar artery. Small twigs may arise from the upper ureteric artery.

All these arteries branch freely before entering the adrenal gland, so from 50 to 60 arteries penetrate the capsule over the entire surface.

Venous Drainage

The adrenal venous drainage does not accompany the arterial supply and is much simpler (Fig. 16.2). A single vein drains the adrenal gland, emerging at the hilum. The left vein passes downward over the anterior surface of the gland and is joined by the left inferior phrenic vein before entering the left renal vein. The right vein passes obliquely to open into the inferior vena cava posteriorly.

Occasionally there are two veins, one having a normal course and the other being an accessory vein that enters the inferior phrenic vein.

When the posterior approach to the adrenal gland is used, the left adrenal vein is found on the anterior surface of the gland. The right adrenal vein is found between the inferior vena cava and the gland. Careful mobilization of the gland is necessary for good ligation of the vein.

Remember:

✓ The adrenal glands vie with the thyroid gland for having the greatest blood supply per gram of tissue.

Lymphatic Drainage

The lymphatics of the adrenal gland consist of a subcapsular plexus that drains with the arteries and a medullary plexus that drains with the adrenal veins. Drainage is to renal hilar nodes, preaortic nodes, and by way of the diaphragmatic orifices for the splanchnic nerves to nodes of the posterior mediastinum above the diaphragm (Fig. 16.3). Lymphatics from the upper pole of the right adrenal gland may enter the liver.

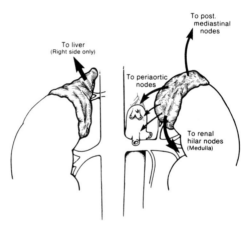

Figure 16.3. The lymphatics of the adrenal glands. (By permission of JE Skandalakis, SW Gray, and JR Rowe, *Anatomical Complications in General Surgery*, New York: McGraw-Hill, 1983.)

TECHNIQUE

■ ADRENALECTOMIES

Anterior Approach

The anterior approach is preferred when (1) the adrenal disease is bilateral (10 percent), (2) the tumor is over 10 cm in size, or (3) the tumor has invaded surrounding structures. Using this approach, both glands can be inspected, palpated, or biopsied. But in spite of these advantages, the use of the posterior approach has increased because of improvements in preoperative diagnosis, such as CT and selective adrenal angiography.

The incision may be vertical, midline or paramedian, transverse, or chevron (Fig. 16.4).

Notes: Exposure and Mobilization of Left Adrenal Gland
Exposure of the left adrenal gland begins with the incision of the posterior parietal peritoneum lateral to the left colon. The incision is carried

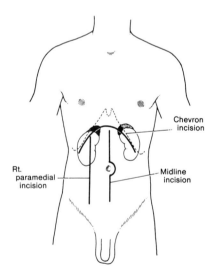

Figure 16.4. Incisions for anterior exposure of the adrenal glands. The chevron transabdominal incision provides bilateral exposure. (By permission of JE Skandalakis, SW Gray, and JR Rowe, *Anatomical Complications in General Surgery*, New York: McGraw-Hill, 1983.)

upward, dividing the splenorenal ligament (Fig. 16.5). Avoid injury to the spleen, the splenic capsule, the splenic vessels, and the tail of the pancreas, which are enveloped by the splenorenal ligament.

Opening the lesser sac through the gastrocolic omentum is another approach to the left adrenal. The incision should be longitudinal outside the gastroepiploic arcade (Fig. 16.6). Care must be taken to avoid traction on the spleen or on the splenocolic ligament. The ligament may contain tortuous or aberrant inferior polar renal vessels or a left gastroepiploic artery.

In both approaches, the peritoneum under the lower border of the pancreas should be incised halfway along the tail and the incision extended laterally for about 10 cm. By retracting the pancreas upward gently, the left adrenal gland on the superior pole of the left kidney will be exposed. Both the kidney and the gland are covered with renal fascia (of Gerota). The gland will be lateral to the aorta, about 2 cm cranial to the left renal vein. By incising the renal fascia, the adrenal gland is completely exposed and the adrenal vein is accessible.

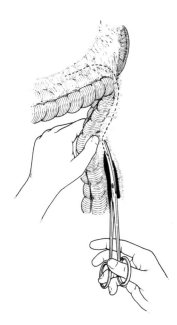

Figure 16.5. Incision of the parietal peritoneum lateral to the left colon. The incision divides the splenorenal ligament. (By permission of JE Skandalakis, SW Gray, and JR Rowe, *Anatomical Complications in General Surgery*, New York: McGraw-Hill, 1983.)

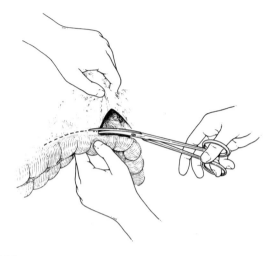

Figure 16.6. Approach to the left adrenal through the gastrocolic omentum opening the lesser sac. (By permission of JE Skandalakis, SW Gray, and JR Rowe, *Anatomical Complications in General Surgery*, New York: McGraw-Hill, 1983.)

If the operation is for pheochromocytoma, the adrenal vein should be ligated at once to prevent the release of catecholamines into the circulation during subsequent manipulation of the gland. If it is impossible to refrain from using retractors in this area, place them gently to avoid tearing the inferior mesenteric vein from the splenic vein.

In patients whose left adrenal lesion is anterior, a third approach is useful. The gland is exposed by an oblique incision of the left mesocolon (Fig. 16.7). The arcuate vessels may be divided, but the major branches of the middle and left colic arteries must be preserved. Injury to the wall of the left colon can be avoided by minimizing retraction.

In some lesions, such as primary aldosteronism, meticulous attention to hemostasis is essential because the adrenal gland is hypervascular and friable. Hematomas from operative trauma may disguise or mimic adenoma. The surgeon may handle the gland with part of the adjacent periadrenal fascia, and manipulation should be with fine forceps only. The numerous arteries can be clipped or electrocoagulated to maintain hemostasis.

The dissection starts at the inferolateral aspect of the left adrenal gland and proceeds superiorly (Fig. 16.8). Remaining alert to the possible presence of a superior renal polar artery, the surgeon should retract the gland

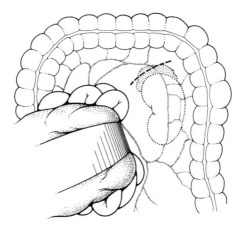

Figure 16.7. Approach to the left adrenal by incision of the left mesocolon near the splenic flexure. The major branches of the middle and left colic arteries must be spared, but the marginal artery may be sectioned. (By permission of JE Skandalakis, SW Gray, and JR Rowe, *Anatomical Complications in General Surgery*, New York: McGraw-Hill, 1983.)

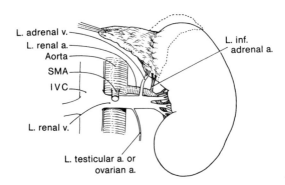

Figure 16.8. Direction of dissection of the left adrenal gland. Note the position of the left adrenal vein. (By permission of JE Skandalakis, SW Gray, and JR Rowe, *Anatomical Complications in General Surgery*, New York: McGraw-Hill, 1983.)

superiorly. Remember that the left adrenal gland extends downward, close to the left renal artery and vein.

After the adrenal gland has been removed, inspect its bed for bleeding points. Check surrounding organs, especially the spleen, for injury. If injuries exist, they may be repaired with sutures over a piece of retroperitoneal fat, Gelfoam, or Avitene. More severe injuries may require partial or even total splenectomy.

Right Adrenalectomy

Notes: Exposure and Mobilization of Right Adrenal Gland
The anterior approach to the right adrenal gland begins with the mobilization of the hepatic flexure of the colon. Posterior adhesions of the liver to the peritoneum are divided by sharp dissection. Keep in mind that medial attachments may contain hepatic veins.

The duodenum is exposed by mobilizing the colon. The duodenum's second portion is freed by incision of its lateral, avascular peritoneal reflection. After separating it from retroperitoneal structures, reflect it forward and to the left (Kocher maneuver) (Fig. 16.9). The vena cava, right adrenal gland, and upper pole of the right kidney are now exposed (Fig. 16.10). The surgeon must remember that the common bile duct and the gastroduodenal artery are in this area.

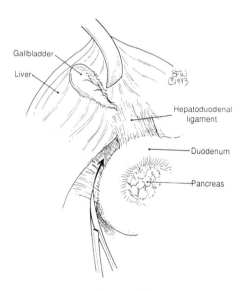

Figure 16.9

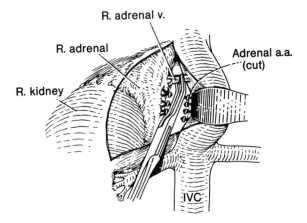

Figure 16.10. (By permission of JE Skandalakis, SW Gray and JR Rowe, *Anatomical Complications in General Surgery*, New York: McGraw-Hill, 1983.)

The right adrenal gland rarely extends downward to the renal pedicle, unlike the left adrenal gland. Usually the right adrenal vein leaves the gland on its anterior surface close to the cranial margin and enters the vena cava on its posterior surface (Fig. 16.10). Place hemostatic clips as soon as both borders of the vein are visible to prevent release of catecholamines and to avoid stretching the vein. Hemorrhage from the vena cava may follow if the vein is stretched.

Unilateral or Bilateral Adrenalectomy

Right Anterior
Procedure:

Step 1. Patient should be in supine position.

Step 2. Make a long midline incision from the xiphoid process to the lower midline or bilateral subcostal. If exploring for pheochromocytoma, use a longer midline (Fig. 16.4).

Step 3. Lysis of the hepatocolic, hepatoduodenal, and gastrohepatic ligaments with downward and left mobilization of the hepatic flexure and upward retraction of the right lobe of the liver.

Step 4. Kocherize the duodenum, which is retracted medially (Fig. 16.9).

Step 5. Visualize the adrenal gland, kidney, and inferior vena cava (Fig. 16.10).

Step 6. Gently and carefully dissect the adrenal gland downward with the finger. Maintain good hemostasis, and apply downward retraction to the kidney (Fig. 16.11).

Step 7. Remember:

✓ The adrenal vein empties into the lateral surface of the inferior vena cava and should be clipped or ligated carefully.

✓ The arterial supply, by branches of the inferior phrenic artery superiorly, the renal artery inferiorly, and the aorta medially, is very rich. Perform careful ligation and lysis of any adhesions (Fig. 16.10).

Step 8. The surgeon decides whether a Jackson-Pratt drain is required. Close in layers.

Left Anterior

Study the previous notes on left anterior adrenal mobilization, then proceed. If the left adrenal tumor involves the pancreatic tail as well as the splenic portae, or the splenic flexure of the colon, en bloc resection is advised. On large adrenal tumors, bowel preparation is a wise step prior to surgery.

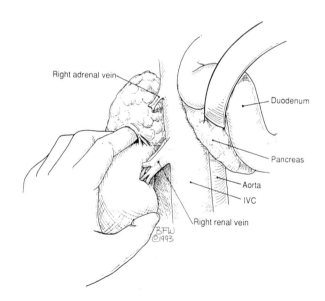

Figure 16.11

Posterior Approach

Use the posterior approach for any adrenalectomy except that in which a large or ectopic tumor is a strong possibility. Because peritoneal metastases often make an anterior approach difficult, the posterior approach is the procedure of choice in palliative adrenalectomy for breast carcinoma.

With the patient prone, make a curvilinear incision through the latissimus dorsi muscle to the posterior lamella of the lumbodorsal fascia. The sacrospinalis muscle is exposed and the lumbar cutaneous vessels must be ligated or cauterized. Because dissection of the pleural fold at the 11th rib may result in pneumothorax, the surgeon must be sure to be over the 12th, not the 11th, rib. However, some surgeons prefer to remove the 11th rib on the right.

By detaching the sacrospinalis muscle attachments to the dorsal aspect of the 12th rib, the rib is exposed. It must be removed subperiosteally to avoid damaging the underlying pleura. Periosteum should be stripped on the superior surface from medial to lateral and on the inferior surface from lateral to medial. Be careful not to injure the 12th intercostal nerve bundle at the inferior angle of the rib. The nerve is separate from, but parallel to, the blood vessels, which may, if necessary, be ligated.

Separate the pleura from the upper surface of the diaphragm, and incise the diaphragm from lateral to medial. Open the fascia, and identify the upper pole of the kidney. The adrenal gland can usually be brought into the field with interior retraction of the kidney. Avoid tearing the renal capsule or stretching any artery that might be the superior polar artery.

Left Adrenalectomy

Begin dissection of the left adrenal gland on the medial aspect, clipping the arteries encountered. Remember that the pancreas lies just beneath the gland and is easily injured. Identify the left adrenal vein, which usually emerges from the medial aspect of the gland and courses obliquely downward to enter the left renal vein. Avoid undue traction on the gland, so the renal vein will not be torn.

Right Adrenalectomy

Approach the right adrenal gland by retracting the superior pole of the right kidney inferiorly; the posterior surface of the adrenal gland can then be dissected free from fatty tissue. When the apex of the gland is reached, retract the liver upward. After freeing the lateral borders, the only attachments are the medial margins.

Retract the right adrenal gland laterally, and ligate the arterial branches from the aorta and the right renal artery to the gland. Also ligate the right adrenal vein. Because of the possibility of hemorrhage from the vena cava or the adrenal vein, we recommend freeing up the vena cava far enough to ensure room for an angle clamp. After removing the gland and inspecting for air leaks and bleeding, the incision is closed.

Unilateral or Bilateral Adrenalectomy

Right Posterior
  Procedure:

> **Step 1.** Place patient in prone position with flexion of hips and shoulders and rolls under them.

> **Step 2.** Incise skin and subcutaneous fat along the length of the 11th rib, using knife or electrocautery (Fig. 16.12).

> **Step 3.** Divide the latissimus dorsi and serratus posterior muscles with electrocautery (Fig. 16.13).

> **Step 4.** Subperiosteal resection of the 11th rib (Fig. 16.14).

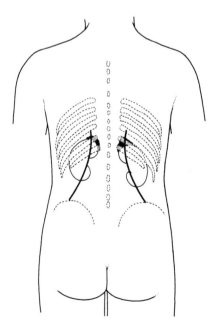

Figure 16.12. Incisions for a posterior approach to the adrenal glands. (By permission of JE Skandalakis, SW Gray, and JR Rowe, *Anatomical Complications in General Surgery*, New York: McGraw-Hill, 1983.)

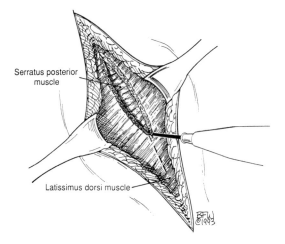

Serratus posterior
muscle

Latissimus dorsi muscle

Figure 16.13

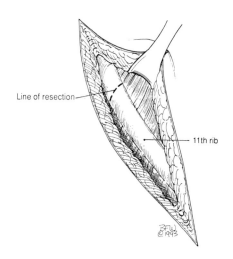

Line of resection

11th rib

Figure 16.14

Step 5. Carefully push the plura upward, or, if necessary, incise the pleura and the diaphragm.

Step 6. Incise Gerota's fascia and push the kidney downward carefully (Fig. 16.15).

Step 7. Perform very careful finger dissection of the adrenal gland. Any palpated cordlike formation should be clipped (Fig. 16.16).

Step 8. After good mobilization, divide the adrenal vein between clips (Fig. 16.17).

Remember:

✔ The adrenal vein on the right is very short and, in most cases, drains into the inferior vena cava; but on the left side the adrenal vein is, in most cases, long and drains into the left renal vein.

Step 9. If pleura and diaphragm are incised, close diaphragm with interrupted nonabsorbable sutures. Use a thoracotomy tube through a stab wound and close the wound in layers. The surgeon determines whether a Jackson–Pratt drain is required.

Note: The left posterior approach will not be presented.

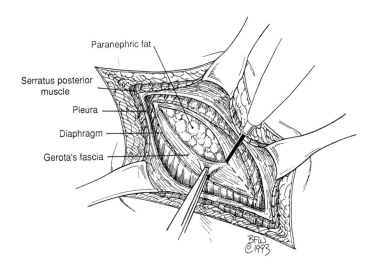

Paranephric fat

Serratus posterior muscle

Pleura

Diaphragm

Gerota's fascia

BFW
© 1993

Figure 16.15

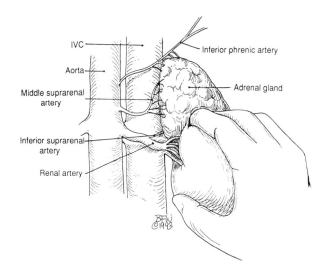

Figure 16.16

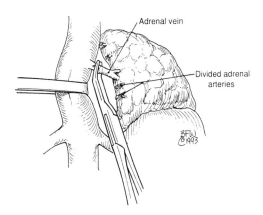

Figure 16.17

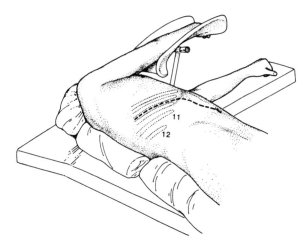

Figure 16.18. Incision for a thoracolumbar approach to the adrenal gland. (By permission of JE Skandalakis, SW Gray, and JR Rowe, *Anatomical Complications in General Surgery*, New York: McGraw-Hill, 1983.)

Thoracoabdominal Approach

Better exposure for large tumors of a single adrenal gland is achieved through the thoracoabdominal approach. It facilitates removal of the spleen and distal pancreas should they be involved with the adrenal tumor. Splenectomy is to be avoided whenever possible.

Start the incision at the angle of the 8th to the 10th ribs and extend it across the midline to the midpoint of the contralateral rectus muscle just above the umbilicus (Fig. 16.18). Remove the 10th rib, open the pleura, and incise the diaphragm from above. Follow the anterior approach procedure to complete the surgery.

17

Carpal Tunnel

ANATOMY

This is a pictorial presentation of the surgical anatomy and anatomical entities related to the carpal tunnel syndrome (Figs. 17.1–17.8; Tables 17.1–17.3).

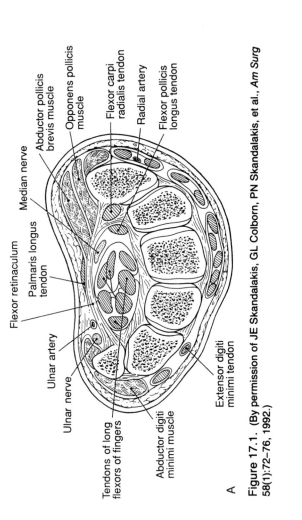

Flexor retinaculum

Palmaris longus tendon

Median nerve

Abductor pollicis brevis muscle

Opponens pollicis muscle

Flexor carpi radialis tendon

Radial artery

Flexor pollicis longus tendon

Ulnar artery

Ulnar nerve

Tendons of long flexors of fingers

Abductor digiti minimi muscle

Extensor digiti minimi tendon

A

Figure 17.1. (By permission of JE Skandalakis, GL Colborn, PN Skandalakis, et al., *Am Surg* 58(1):72–76, 1992.)

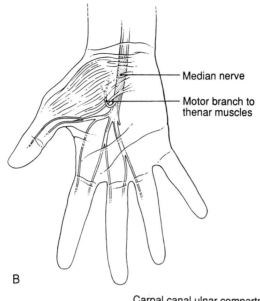

Median nerve

Motor branch to
thenar muscles

B

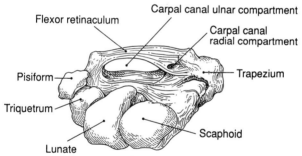

Flexor retinaculum

Carpal canal ulnar compartment

Carpal canal
radial compartment

Pisiform

Trapezium

Triquetrum

Lunate

Scaphoid

C   **Carpal canal (proximal view)**

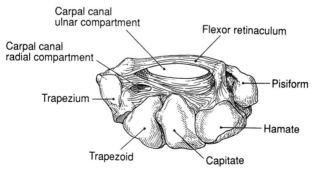

Carpal canal
ulnar compartment

Flexor retinaculum

Carpal canal
radial compartment

Trapezium

Pisiform

Hamate

Trapezoid

Capitate

D   **Carpal canal (distal view)**

Figure 17.1. Continued.

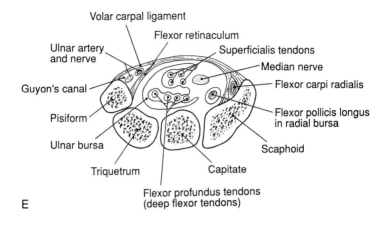

Volar carpal ligament

Flexor retinaculum

Ulnar artery and nerve

Superficialis tendons

Median nerve

Guyon's canal

Flexor carpi radialis

Pisiform

Flexor pollicis longus in radial bursa

Ulnar bursa

Scaphoid

Triquetrum

Capitate

Flexor profundus tendons (deep flexor tendons)

E

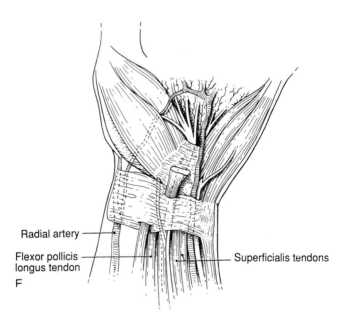

Radial artery

Flexor pollicis longus tendon

Superficialis tendons

F

Figure 17.1. Continued.

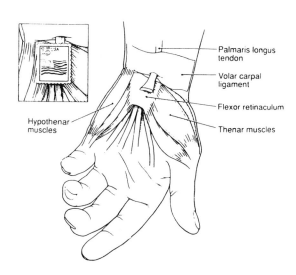

Superficial palmar arterial arch

Deep palmar arterial arch

Motor branch of median nerve

Median nerve

Figure 17.2. The superficial and deep palmar arches and the topography of the motor branches of the median nerve. (By permission of JE Skandalakis, GL Colborn, PN Skandalakis, et al., *Am Surg* 58(1):72–76, 1992.)

Palmaris longus tendon

Volar carpal ligament

Flexor retinaculum

Thenar muscles

Hypothenar muscles

Figure 17.3. The "postage stamp" size of the flexor retinaculum. (By permission of JE Skandalakis, GL Colborn, PN Skandalakis, et al., *Am Surg* 58(2):77–81, 1992.)

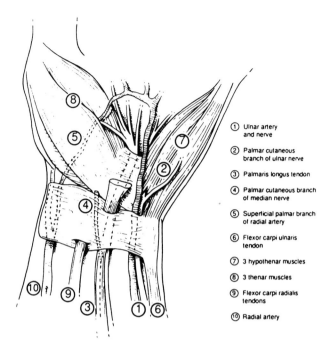

① Ulnar artery
  and nerve

② Palmar cutaneous
  branch of ulnar nerve

③ Palmaris longus tendon

④ Palmar cutaneous branch
  of median nerve

⑤ Superficial palmar branch
  of radial artery

⑥ Flexor carpi ulnaris
  tendon

⑦ 3 hypothenar muscles

⑧ 3 thenar muscles

⑨ Flexor carpi radialis
  tendons

⑩ Radial artery

Figure 17.4. Superficial relations of the flexor retinaculum. (By permission of JE Skandalakis, GL Colborn, PN Skandalakis, et al.,*Am Surg* 58(2):77–81, 1992.)

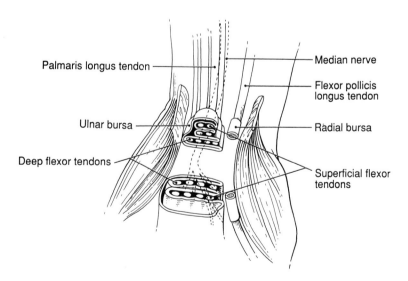

Palmaris longus tendon — Median nerve

— Flexor pollicis longus tendon

Ulnar bursa — Radial bursa

Deep flexor tendons — Superficial flexor tendons

Figure 17.5. The canals within the carpal tunnel (the middle surgical zone). (By permission of JE Skandalakis, GL Colborn, PN Skandalakis, et al.,*Am Surg* 58(2): 77–81, 1992.)

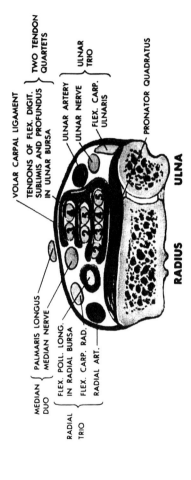

PALMARIS LONGUS

MEDIAN NERVE

FLEX. POLL. LONG.
IN RADIAL BURSA

FLEX. CARP. RAD.

RADIAL ART.

MEDIAN DUO

RADIAL TRIO

VOLAR CARPAL LIGAMENT

TENDONS OF FLEX. DIGIT.
SUBLIMIS AND PROFUNDUS
IN ULNAR BURSA

TWO TENDON QUARTETS

ULNAR ARTERY

ULNAR NERVE

FLEX. CARP. ULNARIS

ULNAR TRIO

PRONATOR QUADRATUS

RADIUS

ULNA

Figure 17.6. The proximal surgical zone. (From EW Lampe *Clin Symp* 21(3):66–109, 1969. Copyright by Ciba-Geigy.)

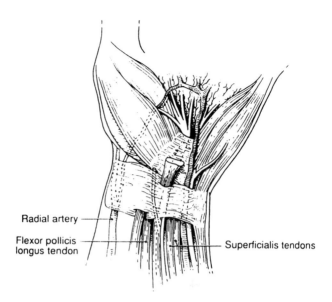

Radial artery

Flexor pollicis
longus tendon

Superficialis tendons

Figure 17.7. The distal surgical zone. (By permission of JE Skandalakis, GL Colborn, PN Skandalakis, et al., *Am Surg* 58(3):158–166, 1992.)

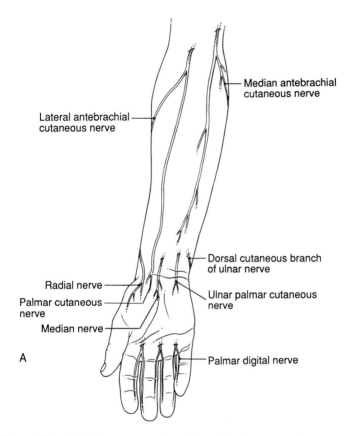

Median antebrachial
cutaneous nerve

Lateral antebrachial
cutaneous nerve

Dorsal cutaneous branch
of ulnar nerve

Radial nerve

Ulnar palmar cutaneous
nerve

Palmar cutaneous
nerve

Median nerve

A

Palmar digital nerve

Figure 17.8. (A) Palmar cutaneous branches of the ulnar, musculocutaneous, radial, and median nerves; (B) palmar cutaneous branch of the median nerve. (By permission of JE Skandalakis, GL Colborn, PN Skandalakis, et al., *Am Surg* 58(3):158–166, 1992.)

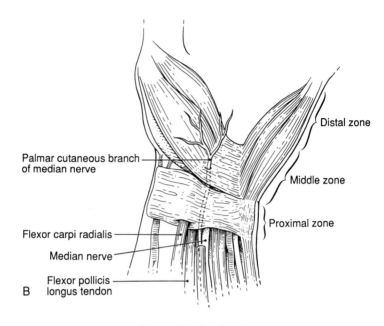

Figure 17.8 Continued.

Table 17.1 Upper Proximal Zone Divisions

Ulnar side
   Ulnar trio: flexor carpi ulnaris
                 ulnar nerve
                 ulnar artery
Central (median) area
   Ulnar bursae with flexor digitorum superficialis and profundus tendons
   Median duo: palmaris longus
                    median nerve
Radial side
   Radial trio: radial artery
                 flexor carpi radialis
                 flexor pollicis longus within the radial bursa

(By permission of JE Skandalakis, GL Colborn, PN Skandalakis et al., *Am Surg* 58(2):77–81, 1992.)

Table 17.2 Central Zone (Carpal Tunnel) Divisions

Ulnar side
  Ulnar bursa: eight tendons (sublimis and profundus)
Central area
  Median nerve and its branches (with possible variations)
Radial side
  Radial bursa and flexor pollicis

(By permission of JE Skandalakis, GL Colborn, PN Skandalakis et al., *Am Surg* 58(2):77–81, 1992.)

Table 17.3 Distal Zone Divisions

Ulnar side
  Ulnar nerve branches
  Ulnar artery and superficial arch
  Ulnar bursa: four profundus tendons
                 four superficialis tendons
Central (median) side
  Median nerve branches
    Recurrent branch thenar muscles
    One or two digital nerves for thumb
    Four or five digital nerves for index, middle, and radial side of ring finger
Radial side
  Flexor pollicis longus with radial bursa
  Median nerve palmar cutaneous branch

(By permission of JE Skandalakis, GL Colborn, PN Skandalakis et al., *Am Surg* 58(2):77–81, 1992.)

TECHNIQUE

■ SURGICAL TREATMENT OF CARPAL TUNNEL SYNDROME (Fig. 17.9)

When the surgeon is satisfied that the patient has all the signs and symptoms and, therefore, all the indications for division of the flexor retinaculum, surgical intervention is the procedure of choice.

Procedure:

Step 1. Apply an upper arm tourniquet. Elevate the upper extremity. Use elastic bandages for exsanguination. Inflate the tourniquet.

Step 2. Make a curved skin incision at the ulnar side of the palm across the thenar crease and along the long axis of the ring finger, from the lower border of the flexor retinaculum to the proximal wrist crease (Fig. 17.10).

Step 3. Carefully separate the subcutaneous fat. Find and protect the palmar cutaneous branch of the median nerve. It is located close to the palmaris longus, flexor carpi radialis, and flexor

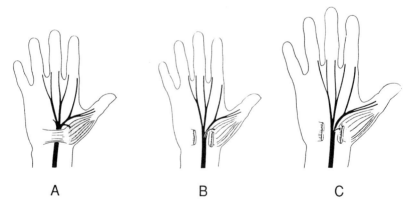

A   B   C

Figure 17.9. Anatomical variations of the median nerve in the carpal tunnel. (A) Regular branching of the median nerve, 55 percent; (B) thenar branch leaving the median nerve within the carpal tunnel (subligamentous), 31 percent; (C) transligamentous course of the thenar branch, 14 percent. (By permission of JE Skandalakis, GL Colborn, PN Skandalakis, et al., *Am Surg* 58(3):158–166, 1992.)

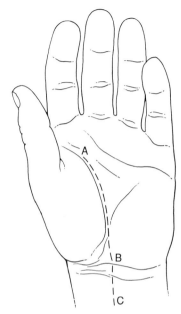

Figure 17.10. Skin incision. This incision follows the natural crease and not the axis of the fourth finger. (By permission of JE Skandalakis, GL Colborn, PN Skandalakis, et al., *Am Surg* 58(3):158–166, 1992.)

pollicis longus at the thenar side of the median nerve (Figs. 17.11A and B). Incise the palmar fascia in a longitudinal fashion, starting at the proximal part of the incision.

Step 4. Open the superficial transverse carpal ligament (antebrachial fascia) in a similar fashion and identify the median nerve (Fig. 17.12). Dissect, observe, and isolate the median nerve and the recurrent branch. Use magnification glasses, if necessary. Incise the epineurium longitudinally. Take care to open (divide) only the volar carpal ligament.

Step 5. Divide the flexor retinaculum at the ulnar side close to the hamate bone. Locate and protect the motor branch of the recurrent nerve (Fig. 17.13).

Step 6. Evaluate the canal and anatomical entities for any other pathology, congenital or acquired.

Step 7. Close the wound, skin only, with interrupted 4-0 or 5-0 silk or nylon. A volar plaster splint is applied for 2 weeks.

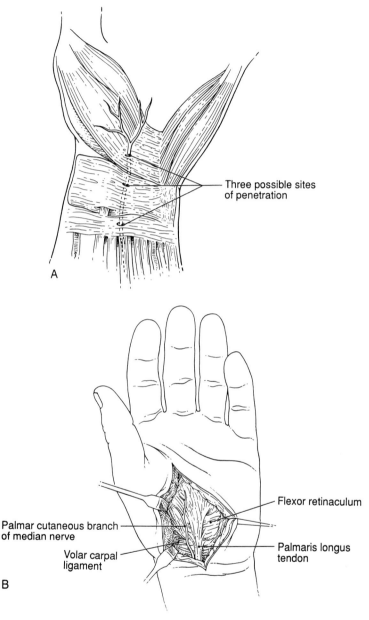

Figure 17.11. (A) Three possible sites of penetration of the palmar cutaneous nerve. (B) Note the palmar cutaneous branch of the median nerve that parallels the palmaris longus tendon. (By permission of JE Skandalakis, GL Colborn, PN Skandalakis, et al., *Am Surg* 58(3):158–166, 1992.)

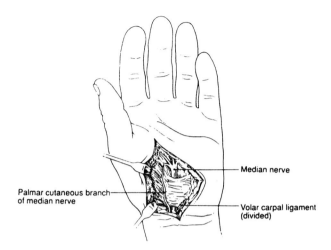

Figure 17.12. Division of the volar carpal ligament. (By permission of JE Skandalakis, GL Colborn, PN Skandalakis, et al., *Am Surg* 58(3):158–166, 1992.)

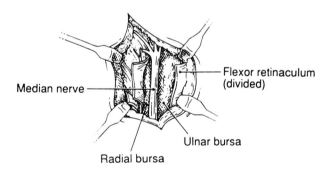

Figure 17.13. Division of the flexor retinaculum. (By permission of JE Skandalakis, GL Colborn, PN Skandalakis, et al., *Am Surg* 58(3):158–166, 1992.)

18

Varicosities of the Lower Extremity

ANATOMY

■ VEINS OF THE LOWER EXTREMITY

The veins of the lower extremity may be divided into three groups: superficial, perforating, and deep (Fig. 18.1). Here, we will describe the deep veins only briefly, and concentrate on the superficial and perforating vessels.

Deep Veins

The deep veins of the lower extremity lie beneath the deep fascia and accompany the arteries bearing the same names. They originate from venous plexuses on the plantar surface of the toes (plantar digital veins) and form four plantar metatarsal veins which, in turn, unite to form the deep plantar arch. From the arch, medial and lateral plantar veins pass backward to form the posterior tibial vein behind the medial malleolus of the tibia.

The anterior tibial vein arises from the dorsum of the foot. It passes between the tibia and the fibula through the interosseous membrane and joins the posterior tibial vein to form the popliteal vein.

The popliteal vein passes through the aperture in the adductor magnus muscle and continues upward as the femoral vein. It enters the middle compartment of the femoral sheath and, at the level of the inguinal ligament, continues as the external iliac vein.

The deep veins communicate with each other and with the superficial veins by way of the perforating veins. The deep veins also receive a

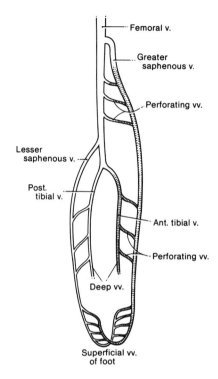

Figure 18.1. Diagram of the relation of the deep and superficial veins of the lower extremity. Only the direct perforating vessels are shown. (By permission of JE Skandalakis, SW Gray, and JR Rowe, *Anatomical Complications in General Surgery*, New York: McGraw-Hill, 1983.)

number of tributaries, the largest being the deep femoral vein (profunda femoris).

Superficial Veins

The superficial veins of the lower extremity are the great and short saphenous veins and their many tributaries, both named and unnamed. They lie between the skin and the deep fascia.

The great saphenous vein originates from the dorsal digital and dorsal metatarsal veins by way of the dorsal venous arch and the medial marginal vein, and begins 2.54 cm in front of the medial malleolus of the tibia as a continuation of the medial marginal vein. It ascends the leg in front of the medial malleolus, behind the saphenous nerve, and along the medial border of the tibia and the posteromedial aspect of the knee. It enters the saphenous opening to end in the femoral vein at or about 1 cm below and 4 cm lateral to the pubic tubercle and 2.5 cm below the inguinal ligament (Fig. 18.2).

The named tributaries of the great saphenous vein fall into three natural groups: those below the knee, those above the knee, and those in the inguinal area (upper part of the femoral triangle). Below the knee are the anterior arch vein of the leg and the posterior arch vein. Above the knee are the anterior lateral vein, the posterior medial vein, and the accessory saphenous vein. The superficial circumflex iliac, the superficial epigas-

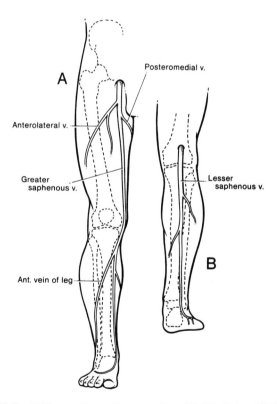

Figure 18.2.   (A) The greater saphenous vein and its tributaries. (B) The lesser saphenous vein and its tributaries. (By permission of JE Skandalakis, SW Gray, and JR Rowe, *Anatomical Complications in General Surgery*, New York: McGraw-Hill, 1983.)

tric, and the deep and superficial external pudendal veins are in the inguinal area (Fig. 18.3). The external and internal pudendal veins and the veins of the round ligaments are responsible for vulval varicosities in pregnancy.

The great saphenous vein may lie anterior or posterior to the superficial external pudendal artery, or the artery may cross the common femoral vein above the junction with the great saphenous vein.

The short saphenous vein, also called the small or internal saphenous vein, originates from the junction of the lateral marginal vein of the foot with small veins from the lateral side of the heel behind the lateral malleolus. It passes between the Achilles tendon and the posterior border of the lateral malleolus to ascend in the center of the calf up to the popliteal fossa about 1.25 cm below the posterior transverse skin crease

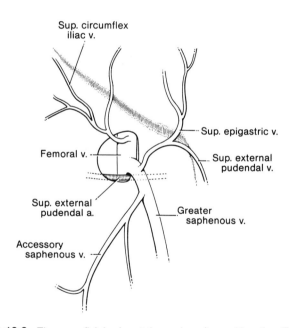

Figure 18.3. The superficial veins at the saphenofemoral junction. There are many variations of this pattern. The accessory saphenous vein may be medial, lateral, or absent. The superficial pudendal artery usually passes over the femoral vein and behind the greater saphenous vein. It may cross the femoral vein above the saphenofemoral junction. (By permission of JE Skandalakis, SW Gray, and JR Rowe, *Anatomical Complications in General Surgery*, New York: McGraw-Hill, 1983.)

of the knee. From this level to about 10 cm above the crease, the lesser saphenous vein joins the popliteal vein (Fig. 18.2B).

There is considerable variation in the level of this termination. In about 13 percent of subjects, the vein ends in midthigh and joins the great saphenous rather than the popliteal vein. In 15 percent of subjects, the short saphenous vein divides in the popliteal space, with one branch entering the popliteal vein and the other branch continuing upward in the superficial fascia to join the great saphenous vein. At the other extreme, the short saphenous vein may join the great saphenous vein at the level of the knee.

Perforating Veins

Perforating veins provide communications between the deep and superficial systems of veins with valves arranged to facilitate this flow. Failure of these valves or the absence of them permits blood to pass to the superficial veins during contraction of the calf muscles. This results in superficial venous hypertension and the eventual formation of varicosities.

Perforating veins may be indirect or direct (Figs. 18.4 and 18.5). Indirect perforating veins are small, superficial vessels that pierce the deep fascia and join small intermuscular veins which in turn join tributaries of the deep veins.

The obvious direct perforating veins are the great and short saphenous veins themselves. In addition, there is a series of smaller direct perforating veins in the extremity associated with the great and short saphenous veins (Fig. 18.3).

There are five perforating veins of the leg:

1. A vein, just distal to the knee, arises from the great saphenous or posterior arch vein and opens into the posterior tibial vein.

2. The external or lateral perforating vein is on the outer side of the leg at the junction of the middle and lower thirds of the leg. In the lower half of the leg are three internal-valved perforating veins called, for lack of a better name, "ankle" perforating veins.

3. The upper ankle perforating vein is located about halfway up the leg at the posterior tibial margin. It connects the great saphenous or a tributary vein with the posterior tibial vein.

4. The middle ankle perforating vein is 7.5–10 cm above the medial malleolus.

5. The lowest ankle perforating vein arises behind and below the medial malleolus.

6. Other smaller and inconstant perforating veins have been described.

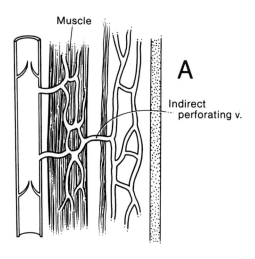

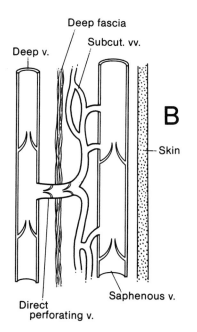

Figure 18.4. Perforating veins. (A) Indirect perforating veins. (B) Direct perforating veins. The sites of direct perforators are shown in Fig. 18.5. (By permission of JE Skandalakis, SW Gray, and JR Rowe, *Anatomical Complications in General Surgery*, New York: McGraw-Hill, 1983.)

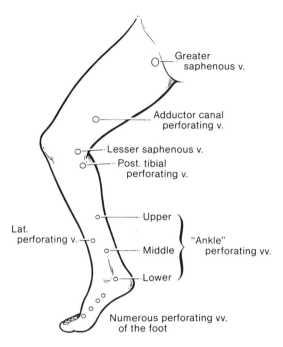

Figure 18.5. The sites of direct perforating veins of the lower extremity. Some are more constant than others. (By permission of JE Skandalakis, SW Gray, and JR Rowe, *Anatomical Complications in General Surgery*, New York: McGraw-Hill, 1983.)

A detailed description of the perforating veins is found in *The Pathology and Surgery of the Veins of the Lower Limb*, 2nd ed. by H. Dodd and F. B. Cockett. Edinburgh: Churchill Livingstone, 1976. Their book is indispensable to anyone wishing to understand the circulation of the lower extremity.

Variations in Veins

Below are some of the most common variations in veins:

1. The short saphenous vein may empty into the great saphenous vein, into the deep veins below the knee, or into the posteromedian vein.

2. There are many variations of the entrances of deep and superficial pudendal veins, the superficial circumflex iliac vein, and the super-

ficial epigastric vein into the great saphenous vein at the saphenous opening (fossa ovalis).

3. The great saphenous vein may enter the femoral vein as far as 5 cm below the saphenous opening.

4. There may be an accessory saphenous vein at the medial aspect of the inner thigh, not to be confused with a posteromedial vein.

5. The inguinal tributaries may enter the femoral vein rather than the great saphenous vein. Be careful to ligate the great saphenous vein and not the femoral vein.

6. The great saphenous vein may be duplicated below the knee.

7. The superficial external pudendal vein may be duplicated or even triplicated.

Valves

The anterior and posterior tibial veins, the peroneal veins, the femoral vein, and the internal iliac vein have valves about every 2.54 cm or so. All the perforating veins have valves to allow blood to pass only from superficial to deep veins (Fig. 18.4).

TECHNIQUE

■ SAPHENECTOMY

The surgeon should mark all varicosities. The great saphenous vein and all tributaries should be ligated at the saphenous opening. The short saphenous vein should be ligated at the popliteal fossa. All tributaries and perforating veins should be ligated by separate incisions that extend through the deep fascia.

Great Saphenous Vein

Procedure:

Step 1. Make an incision 6–8 cm in length, 3 cm below and parallel to the inguinal ligament from the point of the femoral artery pulsation to the medial border of the adductor magnus (Fig. 18.6).

Step 2. The great saphenous vein is just below the fascia of Scarpa, at the fossa ovalis. Isolate the vein and ligate all tributaries, including tributaries draining into the femoral vein just above and below the saphenofemoral junction. Complete the isolation of the vein, as distally as possible, between clamps. Doubly ligate the saphenous stump with 00 absorbable synthetic suture, applying one ligature by transfixion (Fig. 18.7).

Step 3. Make an incision 1–2 cm over and parallel to the vein at the medial malleolus, at a point superior and lateral. Locate the vein beneath the superficial fascia, elevate it, transect it between two clamps, and ligate it distally. Dissect the saphenous nerve carefully to avoid avulsion (Fig. 18.8).

The saphenous nerve is the largest cutaneous branch of the femoral nerve. In the femoral triangle, it lies lateral to the femoral artery. In the adductor canal, it crosses the artery anteriorly to reach the medial side of the thigh. Below the knee, the saphenous nerve becomes cutaneous between the sartorius and gracilis muscles, passing down the medial border of the tibia together with the great saphenous vein. One branch supplies the skin of the medial side of the foot; another follows the great saphenous artery to supply the posterior medial skin of the leg.

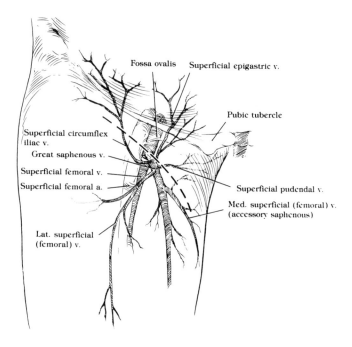

Figure 18.6. (By permission of WV McDermott, *Atlas of Standard Surgical Procedures*, Philadelphia: Lea & Febiger, 1983, pp 176–179.)

Injury to the saphenous nerve may be avoided by careful dissection of the vein in the leg, especially near the medial malleolus. Incision parallel to the vein is best, but if the surgeon prefers a transverse incision, separation of subarterial fat by a curved hemostat will help avoid injury to the nerve with its resulting neuromas and paresthesias of the dorsum of the foot.

Step 4. Insert the smaller tip of the stripper into the proximal opening of the great saphenous vein at the ankle, manipulating it carefully until the tip is palpated in the groin at the ligated part of the great saphenous vein (Fig. 18.9).

Step 5. With 00 chromic catgut, secure the lower opening of the great saphenous vein to the distal end of the stripper. The proximal end comes out the proximal opening of the vein at the fossa ovalis. Provide traction from above and remove the vein. If you are unsuccessful, remove the remaining segment by traction from below, making a small incision at the point where the previous procedure stopped (Fig. 18.10).

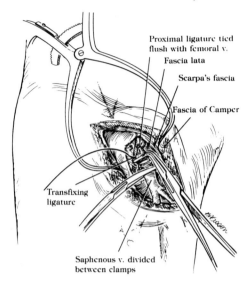

Proximal ligature tied
flush with femoral v.

Fascia lata

Scarpa's fascia

Fascia of Camper

Transfixing
ligature

Saphenous v. divided
between clamps

Figure 18.7. (By permission of WV McDermott, *Atlas of Standard Surgical Procedures*, Philadelphia: Lea & Febiger, 1983, pp 176–179.)

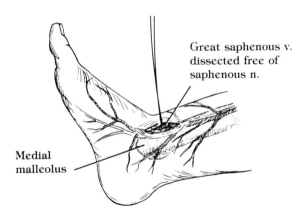

Great saphenous v.
dissected free of
saphenous n.

Medial
malleolus

Figure 18.8. (By permission of WV McDermott, *Atlas of Standard Surgical Procedures*, Philadelphia: Lea & Febiger, 1983, pp 176–179.)

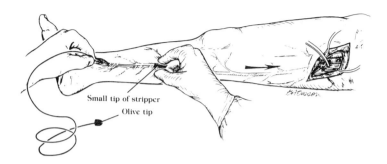

Small tip of stripper

Olive tip

Figure 18.9. (By permission of WV McDermott, *Atlas of Standard Surgical Procedures*, Philadelphia: Lea & Febiger, 1983, pp 176–179.)

Step 6. During the procedure, a sterile towel may be used to provide pressure on the lower extremity along the vein. After all incisions are closed, apply an Ace bandage, starting from the foot.

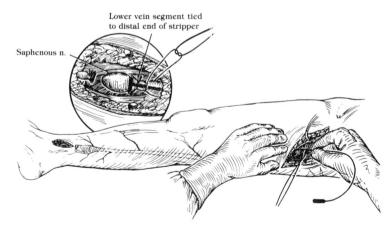

Lower vein segment tied to distal end of stripper

Saphenous n.

Figure 18.10. (By permission of WV McDermott, *Atlas of Standard Surgical Procedures*, Philadelphia: Lea & Febiger, 1983, pp 176–179.)

Short (Small) Saphenous Vein (Fig. 18.11)

Notes:

✓ Do not strip the short saphenous vein; make multiple incisions and ligate.

✓ At the popliteal fossa, ligate the short saphenous vein carefully to prevent injury to the popliteal vein.

✓ Be careful not to injure the sural nerve.

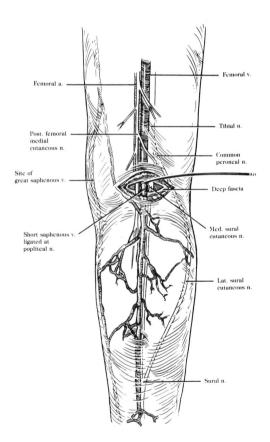

Figure 18.11. (By permission of WV McDermott. *Atlas of Standard Surgical Procedures*. Philadelphia: Lea & Febiger, 1983, pp 176–179.)

Procedure:

Step 1. Make a small incision behind the lateral malleolus, followed by a similar incision at the popliteal fossa, just above the posterior transverse skin crease.

Step 2. Doubly ligate the short saphenous vein just below the popliteal crease, and at the incision behind the lateral malleolus. Divide the proximal and distal ends and proceed accordingly. Pay special attention to the sural nerve, which is a branch of the tibial nerve that lies anterior to the soleus muscle behind the knee. It travels with the short saphenous vein and may be injured during ligation of that vein. The nerve supplies the skin of the dorsolateral leg and the lateral side of the foot.

The posterior cutaneous nerve lies medial or posterior to the sciatic nerve. It accompanies the short saphenous vein through the popliteal fossa as far as the upper part of the calf of the leg and may be injured during dissection of the vein. It supplies the skin of the posterior popliteal area of the thigh and the upper central part of the skin of the calf.

19

Laparoscopic Surgery

ANATOMY

During the past 3–4 years, we have witnessed the genesis of laparoscopic surgery. Laparoscopists are extremely enthusiastic about it and want to perform every abdominal operation laparoscopically. Being a surgical anatomist and a retired general surgeon who has observed laparoscopic surgery but never performed one, I have my doubts about the ability of the laparoscopist to perform *all* abdominal operations through the laparoscope.

Having said this, I am reminded of the story of the firing of Sauerbruch by Mikulicz because a dog's lung collapsed during experimental surgery (Haeger K. *The Illustrated History of Surgery*. London: Harold Starke, 1988; p. 252). My professor at the First Surgical Clinic of the University of Athens (Greece) told us the story in another way. When Mikulicz was out of town, Sauerbruch opened the chest of a patient. Mikulicz came back and fired Sauerbruch. About 3 months later, the patient returned, well, and Mikulicz asked Sauerbruch to come back to the clinic. I have never found a written report about this case, but it sounds very plausible.

I am not against laparoscopic surgery; progress is our most important product. However, we do not yet know laparoscopic anatomy, which must be understood in detail. At the present time, I am trying to learn it myself so I will be able to present it to the surgical profession. We must, by all means, learn laparoscopic anatomy, because it is not topographico-anatomically the same as typical orthodox anatomy from skin to peritoneum as known. An example is the anatomy of the inguinal area from the peritoneum to the skin, which, I repeat, is not the same—at least topographico anatomically—as the anatomy from the skin to the peritoneum.

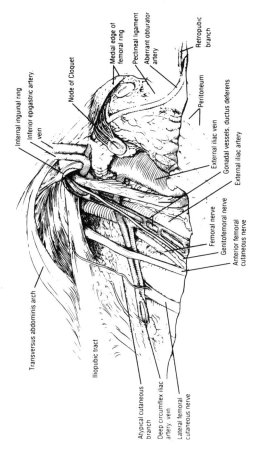

Figure 19.1 (By permission of WK Brick, GL Colborn, TR Gadacz, JE Skandalakis. *Am Surg* 1995;61(2). In press.)

We apologize to our readers that we are not ready yet to present laparoscopic anatomy. Emphatically and categorically, the laparoscopic anatomy that has been presented for the past 3–4 years is not 100 percent correct, and it must be correct to avoid medicolegal problems.

Preliminary drawings (Figs. 19.1 and 19.2) of laparoscopic anatomy in the inguinal area are included in the hope that they will help the surgeon avoid anatomical complications.

One of the co-authors of this book, Lee John Skandalakis, does perform laparoscopic surgery, though, and he has provided the sections on laparoscopic cholecystectomy and laparoscopic appendectomy. The sections on laparoscopic gastrostomy, jejunuostomy, Nissen fundoplication, highly selective vagotomy, and inguinal hernia repair were written by John G. Hunter, MD, FACS, and William S. Laycock, MD. Dr.

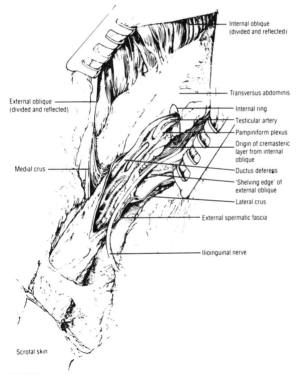

Figure 19.2 (By permission of WK Brick, GL Colborn, TR Gadacz, JE Skandalakis. *Am Surg* 1995:61(2). In press.)

Hunter is associate professor of surgery at Emory University School of Medicine, Atlanta, Georgia, and chief of gastrointestinal surgery at Emory University Hospital. Dr. Laycock is an instructor in surgery at Emory University Hospital.

J.E.S.

TECHNIQUE

■ LAPAROSCOPIC CHOLECYSTECTOMY

At the present time, laparoscopic cholecystectomy is the most sound laparoscopic procedure and, with use of special laparoscopic instruments, can replace the open method in most cases.

The anatomical and technical destiny of each port: (Fig. 19.3).

UMBILICAL: Laparoscopic examination of the peritoneal cavity. Gallbladder localization. Removal of the gallbladder.

UPPER MIDLINE: Surgical dissection of the gallbladder and partially of the hepatic triad at the hilum. Clips may be accommodated through this port.

RIGHT ANTERIOR AXILLARY LINE: Retraction of the gallbladder.

RIGHT MIDCLAVICULAR LINE: Retraction of the gallbladder.

Procedure:

POSITION: Supine on x-ray operating room table

ANESTHESIA: General

OTHER: Place Foley catheter, nasogastric tube, and knee-high pneumatic apparatus.

> **Step 1.** Using a No. 10 scalpel blade, make a longitudinal 10-mm incision in the umbilical area long enough to permit the entrance of a 10 to 11-mm trocar.

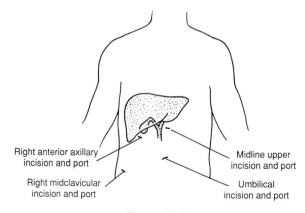

Right anterior axillary incision and port

Right midclavicular incision and port

Midline upper incision and port

Umbilical incision and port

Figure 19.3

Step 2. Insert a Veress needle into the peritoneal cavity at a 45-degree angle toward the pelvic cavity. This may be facilitated with upward traction of the abdominal wall using two towel clamps on each side of the incision. Aspirate with a 10 to 20-cc syringe, and if there is no return with the aspiration, inject normal saline through the syringe. If normal saline is easily injected, then insufflate CO_2.

Step 3. Start to slowly insufflate the peritoneal cavity (pneumoperitoneum) with carbon dioxide.

Remember:

✓ During insufflation, the intraperitoneal pressure should be 0–5 mm, except when the Veress needle is not well placed. With obesity, initial pressure may be a little higher.

Step 4. If abdominal distention is satisfactory, proceed with the following "trocar steps":

a. Insert a 10- or 11-mm trocar at the umbilical area at a 45-degree angle cephalad.

b. Insert the laparoscope with the attached camera.

c. Perform laparoscopic inspection and begin exploration for any gross pathology.

d. Visualize the gallbladder.

e. Under direct vision, insert a 10-mm trocar through the incision at the upper midline or to the right of the midline or a similar incision. The need for narrow or wide coastal margins and the patient's length of trunk should be considered because low placement will clash with the laparoscope, while in high placement the liver will interfere with dissection.

f. Place the remaining two 5–mm trocars, also under direct vision, at the right anterior axillary line and the right midclavicular line.

g. The table should be set in reverse Trendelenburg with rolling to the left.

Step 5. Retract the dome of the gallbladder anteriorly and upward by grasping the fundus with the port of the anterior axillary line. Grasp Hartmann's pouch with the port at the midclavicular line and retract laterally (Fig. 19.4).

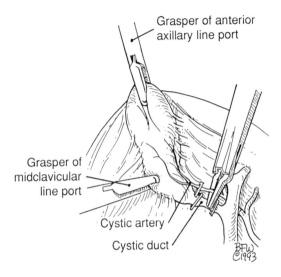

Figure 19.4

Step 6. Dissect and visualize the cystic duct artery and common bile duct. If a cholangiogram is required, it may be done through the cystic duct prior to its ligation.

Step 7. Carefully ligate the cystic artery and cystic duct by proximal and distal clipping. Divide both entities (Figs. 19.4 and 19.5).

Step 8. Dissect the gallbladder from the liver using the "hook" electrocautery (Fig. 19.6).

Step 9. Slowly and carefully separate the gallbladder from its bed. Obtain hemostasis. Perform repeated irrigations (Fig. 19.7).

Step 10. Remove the gallbladder through the umbilical port with the help of a 10- to 11-mm forceps and under direct vision. Occasionally, the umbilical incision should be enlarged to permit the cholecystic exodus.

Step 11. After ascertaining there is no bleeding, remove all trocars under direct vision.

Step 12. Close the umbilical incision by suturing the fascia and the skin. Close the skin of the other ports.

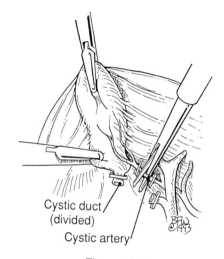

Cystic duct
(divided)

Cystic artery

Figure 19.5

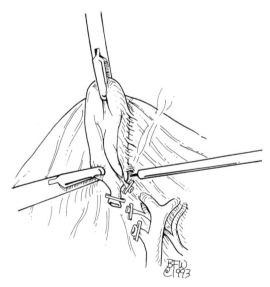

Figure 19.6. (Used with permission of Ross Products Division, Abbott Laboratories, Columbus, OH 43216. Flexiflo Lap G. © 1992 Ross Products Division, Abbott Laboratories.)

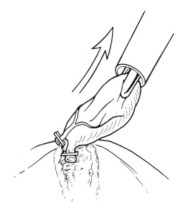

Figure 19.7

■ LAPAROSCOPIC APPENDECTOMY

Procedure:

Step 1. Make an umbilical incision and insufflate the abdominal cavity with a Veress needle, as in a cholecystectomy.

Step 2. Place three 5-mm trocars as follows: the first in the superpubic region, approximately 2–4 cm cephalad to the symphysis pubis; the second in the right upper quadrant below the costal margin at the midclavicular line; the third in the right lower quadrant (Fig. 19.8).

Step 3. Visualize the intraperitoneal contents to ascertain that the patient has appendicitis. After inserting the right upper quadrant trocar, grasp the cecum gently using bowel forceps or laparoscopic Babcock. Apply gentle traction cephalad (Fig. 19.9).

Step 4. Grasp the appendix through the right lower quadrant trocar and apply traction caudally. Visualize the mesoappendix.

Step 5. Insert a 5-mm laparoscope through the superpubic port and place the clip applier through the umbilical port.

Step 6. Clip the mesoappendix and divide it (Fig. 19.10).

Step 7. Insert two endoloops through the right lower quadrant trocar and doubly ligate the base of the appendix. Place a third endoloop more distally, then divide the appendix (Fig. 19.11).

Step 8. Grasp the appendix and remove it via the umbilical trocar. Irrigate as required and close all incisions.

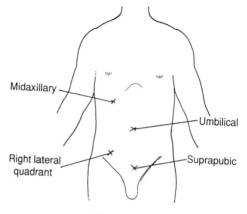

Midaxillary

Umbilical

Right lateral
quadrant

Suprapubic

Figure 19.8

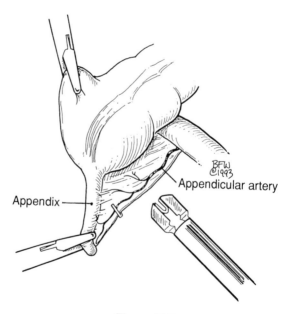

Appendicular artery

Appendix

Figure 19.9

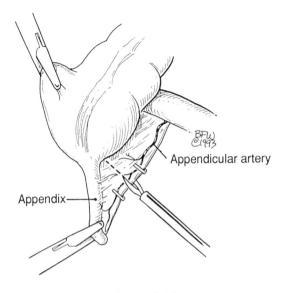

Appendicular artery

Appendix

Figure 19.10

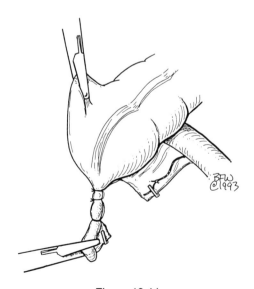

Figure 19.11

■ LAPAROSCOPIC GASTROSTOMY

By John G. Hunter, MD, FACS, and
William S. Laycock, MD

Patient and Room Preparation

Laparoscopic gastrostomy can be performed under general anesthesia or local anesthesia with intravenous sedation. If the latter technique is chosen, peritoneal pressures should be kept low (7–8 mm Hg).

The patient is placed supine on the operating table. The surgeon and the camera operator stand on the patient's right, and the first assistant stands on the patient's left. The desired position for gastrostomy placement is chosen in the left upper quadrant several finger breadths from the costal margin. A pneumoperitoneum is obtained through the umbilicus and a 10 mm, 30-degree telescope is placed through the umbilicus. Two 5-mm trocars are positioned equidistant from the operating telescope. These trocars should be positioned approximately 10 cm from the gastrostomy site, as marked in the skin earlier, with the one on the left slightly lower (Fig. 19.12).

Operative Technique

The surgeon works in a two-handed fashion. The first assistant's job is to introduce the elements of the gastrostomy tube. The surgeon, using two atraumatic Glassman-type bowel clamps, elevates the stomach to the desired position for the gastrostomy tube. A small nick is made in the skin by the assistant and a thin-walled needle and guide wire are introduced through the abdominal wall and into the stomach. The needle is removed, leaving the guide wire in position. A 24 French dilator and peel-away introducer (Cook Surgical, Inc., Bloomington, IN) is then passed into the stomach over the guide wire (Fig. 19.13). The dilator and guide wire are removed. A 22 French Foley catheter is passed through the center of the peel-away sheath, the Foley catheter balloon is then inflated with saline, and the peel-away sheath is slowly separated.

The stomach wall now needs to be fixed to the posterior abdominal wall. This can be done in several fashions. (1) One method involves the placement of three interrupted sutures 120 degrees apart spanning the gap between stomach and posterior abdominal wall. These sutures may be tied with intracorporeal or extracorporeal techniques (Fig. 19.14). Because these skills are beyond those of many surgeons, two alternative techniques have been developed. (2) A Kithe needle may be introduced

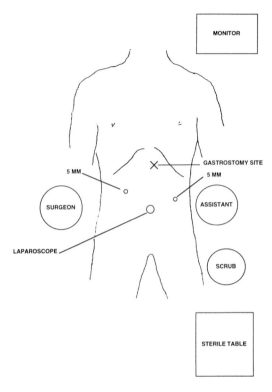

Figure 19.12. Operating room setup and trocar placement for laparoscopic gastrostomy.

through the skin into the peritoneal cavity and then grasped and passed through the gastric wall and back out the anterior abdominal wall. The suture is tied on the outside over a gauze or rubber bolster (Fig. 19.15). Two additional sutures are placed, each 120 degrees apart. (3) Use T-fasteners (Ross Laboratories, Columbus, OH), which are placed through specialized needles into the gastric wall and secured at the skin level over a cotton bolster (Fig. 19.16). T-fasteners or extracorporeal sutures are left in place for 10 days to 2 weeks and then removed. The T-fasteners are merely cut at their nylon attachment and the T bar is allowed to pass with the stool. An intraoperative contrast study can be perfomed using fluoroscopy to check for extravasation. The gastrostomy tube may be used the day following the procedure, although residuals should be checked to make sure a gastric ileus has not occurred. The tube can

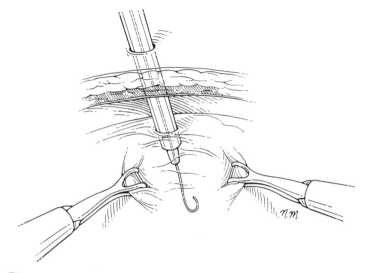

Figure 19.13. Peel-away catheter passed over dilator and guide wire into stomach.

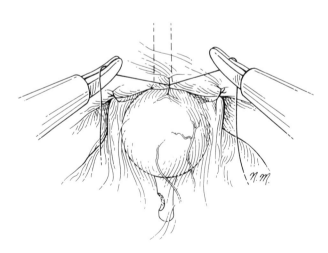

Figure 19.14. Stomach being fixed to posterior abdominal wall using intracorporeal suturing techniques.

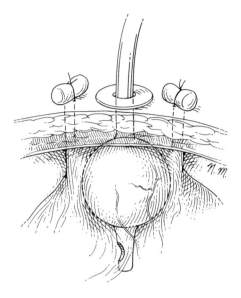

Figure 19.15. Stomach fixed to posterior abdominal wall with suture tied over a cotton bolster at the skin level.

T-Fastener/Needle Device

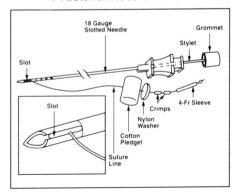

Figure 19.16. Detail of the T-fastener. (Used with permission of Ross Products Division, Abbott Laboratories, Columbus, Ohio 43216. From Flexiflo Lap G.)

otherwise be managed in the fashion of a standard surgical gastrostomy tube.

■ LAPAROSCOPIC JEJUNOSTOMY

By JOHN G. HUNTER, MD, FACS, AND
WILLIAM S. LAYCOCK, MD

Patient Preparation

Patient preparation, position, and anesthesia are identical to that of laparoscopic gastrostomy. A broad-spectrum antibiotic is administered preoperatively.

Operative Technique

A major difference between this procedure and gastrostomy is that the small bowel will be brought up to the abdominal wall in a significantly lower position, about at the level of the umbilicus to the left of the midline. For this reason, it is necessary to put all three ports — camera, left hand, and right hand — lower down and farther to the left (Fig. 19.17). Specifically, the umbilicus is a poor area for camera position. For this reason, after insufflating the abdomen, a 5-mm trocar and 5-mm telescope placed through the umbilicus will allow placement, under direct vision, of a 10-mm trocar in the right lower quadrant. A 5-mm trocar is then placed in the right upper quadrant. Again the surgeon stands on the patient's right with the camera operator. The assistant stands on the left. The patient is placed in the Trendelenburg position. The first assistant, using a Glassman-type grasper through the umbilical trocar, pushes the transverse colon cephalad. Operating with a two-handed technique, the surgeon walks the small bowel back toward the ligament of Treitz. When the ligament is reached, the surgeon comes down the small bowel 20 or 30 cm searching for a convenient long vascular arcade. The chosen loop is brought up to the abdominal wall. The small bowel is oriented in the proper position and the cephalad end of the bowel may be approximated to the abdominal wall with an interrupted suture tied extracorporeally. This first suture is placed before the jejunostomy tube is introduced, as there will be no balloon to help hold the viscus to the abdominal wall with this procedure.

With the small bowel held up to the abdominal wall, the first assistant then places a needle through the abdominal wall and into the jejunum.

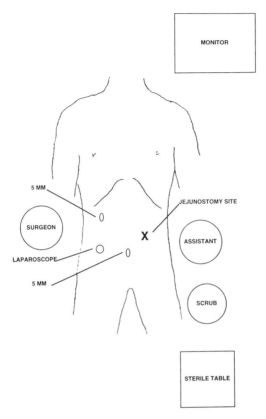

Figure 19.17. Operating room setup and trocar placement for laparoscopic jejunostomy.

Again, a guide wire is passed and slid distally in the jejunum (Fig. 19.18). The needle is removed and, using a Seldiner technique, a 12 French peel-away introducer is placed into the jejunum followed by removal of the dilator and guide wire. A 10 French red rubber catheter is then passed through the center of the peel-away introducer, which is then peeled away. The surgeon must be certain that 8–10 cm of tube are in the jejunum. The tube is then secured at the skin level with a single silk suture so that it will not accidentally become dislodged. The jejunum is then secured to the posterior abdominal wall with interrupted sutures placed totally intra-corporeally, or utilizing T-fasteners as previously mentioned in the technique of laparoscopic gastrostomy, pp. 632–633 (Fig. 19.19). Because these tubes are easier to dislodge than gastrostomy tubes, it is probably

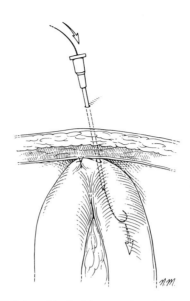

Figure 19.18. Small bowel tacked to posterior abdominal wall with needle and guide wire introduced.

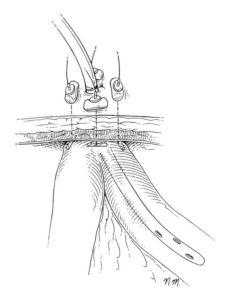

Figure 19.19. Small bowel approximated to posterior abdominal wall using T-fastener. Jejunostomy tube passed distally for 8–10 cm.

wise to perform a Gastrografin tube study before initiating tube feedings. These studies can be performed on the first postoperative day.

■ LAPAROSCOPIC NISSEN FUNDOPLICATION

BY JOHN G. HUNTER, MD, FACS, AND
WILLIAM S. LAYCOCK, MD

Patient Preparation

After thorough preoperative evaluation with a 24-hour pH probe, esophageal motility studies, esophagoscopy, and barium swallow, the patient with a firm diagnosis of symptomatic gastroesophageal reflux is brought to the operating room and placed in a supine position on the operating table. After general anesthesia is obtained, the legs are spread out into a Y position to allow the surgeon to operate from between the patient's legs. An orogastric tube is placed, as well as a Foley catheter. At the beginning of the procedure the surgeon stands on the patient's right and the first assistant on the patient's left. The camera operator starts between the legs. Pneumoperitoneum is obtained through the umbilicus to 15 mm Hg pressure.

The initial trocar, 10 mm, is placed through the left rectus muscle, approximately 15 cm from the xiphoid. This allows the most direct in-line access to the esophageal hiatus. A second trocar, also 10 mm, is placed 10 cm from the xiphoid along the left costal margin. It is critical that this trocar be aimed toward the left shoulder as it is placed through the fascia in order to get the appropriate alignment for easy dissection. Through this subcostal trocar, a blunt rod is used to elevate the round ligament and allow access to the right upper quadrant. A third 10-mm trocar, 15 cm from the xiphoid along the right costal margin, is placed, and the trocar is brought beneath the round ligament. Through this trocar an expandable liver retractor is introduced and opened under the left lobe of the liver. Laceration of the left lobe of the liver can be avoided if this retractor is attached to a mechanical robotic arm. The fourth trocar placed, which is 5 mm, is immediately beneath the left lobe of the liver just to the left of the round ligament. The fifth trocar, 5 mm, is placed along the left costal margin, approximately 20 cm from the xiphoid (Fig. 19.20). Through this port the first assistant will retract the gastroesophageal junction inferiorly.

The surgeon works through the two highest ports, initially with the scissors in the right hand and an atraumatic grasper in the left hand. The

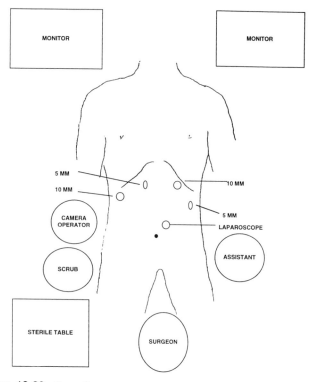

Figure 19.20. Operating room setup and trocar placement for laparoscopic Nissen fundoplication.

dissection starts to the right of the esophagus by opening the gastrohepatic omentum above the hepatic branch of the vagus nerve (Fig. 19.21). This allows immediate access to the caudate lobe of the liver. This incision is taken to the patient's left across the phrenoesophageal ligament above the epiphrenic fat. The gastrophrenic attachments to the left of the left crus are divided and the crus is identified.

Returning to the right side, the right crus of the diaphragm is identified and cleaned of all fat, sweeping fat and the hepatic branch of the vagus inferiorly. When several centimeters of right crus have been laid bare, the dissection proceeds between the esophagus and the right crus using blunt dissection techniques teasing the crus to the left and the esophagus to the right. The posterior vagus is usually readily seen in the posterior mediastinum at this point. Generally, the dissection hugs the esophagus, leaving the posterior vagus back into the crura of the diaphragm.

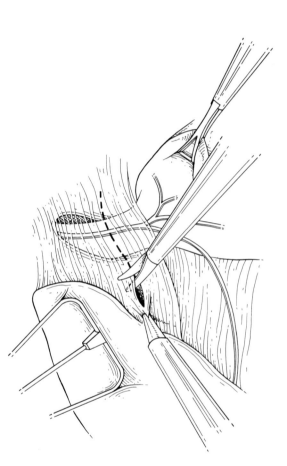

Figure 19.21. Dissection begins by opening the gastrohepatic omentum over the caudate lobe of the liver and cephalad to the hepatic branch of the vagus nerve. The incision is carried across the phrenoesophageal ligament (broken line).

Remaining under direct vision, the dissection proceeds posteriorly until the left crus of the diaphragm is identified. It may be necessary to return to the left side of the esophagus to facilitate this posterior dissection. Generally, the majority of the dissection can be done from the right side of the esophagus.

After identification of the left crus, further posterior dissection will open the remaining retroesophageal tissue and lead back into the peritoneal space. The surgeon will see the gastric fundus, epiphrenic fat, or the spleen through the posterior esophageal hiatus (Fig. 19.22). The grasper is advanced and a Penrose drain is brought into the abdomen and placed in the jaws of the clamp behind the esophagus (Fig. 19.23). The gastroesophageal junction is pulled anteriorly and a single hemoclip approximates both arms of the Penrose drain. The first assistant then moves his point of traction from the gastroesophageal junction to the Penrose drain. Traction inferiorly and to the left will open up the posterior esophgeal window so that a thorough posterior dissection can be performed.

Dissection is complete when the posterior vagus nerve is separate from the esophagus over a distance of approximately 4 cm. A minimum of 4

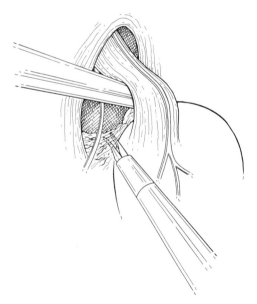

Figure 19.22. A thorough posterior esophageal dissection allows visualization of the gastric fundus, epiphrenic fat, or spleen through the posterior esophageal hiatus.

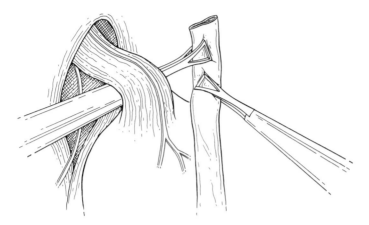

Figure 19.23. A grasping forceps is passed, under direct vision, posterior to the esophagus and a Penrose drain is used to encircle and retract the esophagus.

cm of the esophagus will be brought down into the abdomen. After release of the Penrose drain, the majority of this 4 cm should rest comfortably within the abdomen. If this does not occur, it will be necessary to dissect the esophagus further cephalad. Upon completion of the posterior dissection, the crura are approximated with two or three interrupted sutures of heavy (No. 0) nonabsorbable suture material. These knots may be tied extracorporeally using a knot pusher or totally intracorporeally (Fig. 19.24).

Next, the gastric fundus is mobilized off the diaphragm by dividing all gastrophrenic attachments with an "L" hook from the angle of His to the tip of the spleen. If the fundus is floppy and redundant, it may be possible to perform a loose floppy fundoplication without taking down the short gastric vessels. To determine if the fundus is floppy enough, the surgeon brings the fundus around posterior to the esophagus and then drops it. If the fundus stays to the right of the esophagus without tension or retraction, it will be possible to perform a Rosetti modification (short gastrics not taken down) of the Nissen procedure. If the fundus fails to stay behind the esophagus, it will be necessary to take down the short gastric vessels.

The easiest way to divide short gastric vessels is to start approximately a third of the way down the stomach. The first assistant grasps the gastrosplenic omentum and holds it anteriorly. With the surgeon's left hand, the stomach is held inferiorly. A nick is made in the peritoneum

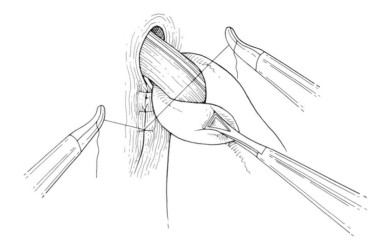

Figure 19.24. The crura are approximated using interrupted sutures tied extracorporeally or intracorporeally.

with a pair of scissors and the lesser sac is entered. Using a right-angle clamp and a clip applier, each short gastric artery is individually identified and divided between clips (Fig. 19.25). As one approaches the superior pole of the spleen, the distance between the stomach and the spleen becomes very short. Great care must be taken in this area to secure these vessels without injuring the spleen tip or the stomach, or starting uncontrollable bleeding. When the fundus of the stomach is free, it can be passed behind the esophagus and will always stay there without a tendency to retract.

At this point, a large dilator, preferably 60 French, is passed through the mouth and down into the esophagus if there is no stricture present. A smaller dilator, equivalent to the size of the last dilation, is used in patients with peptic stricture. A 2-cm wrap is then created using three or four nonabsorbable sutures, either 2-0 or 3-0 in caliber. It is probably best to tie these knots intracorporeally, as extracorporeal knot tying has a tendency to pull the sutures out of the esophagus. It is clearly necessary to get a bite of the esophagus with each stitch. The total length of the wrap should not exceed 2.5 cm (Fig. 19.26). The dilator is then removed. The apex of the wrap is secured to the diaphragm in three places to make sure the wrap will not migrate into the chest (usually two stitches on the right and one on the left). The field is then thoroughly irrigated and all fluid is removed. The liver retractor is removed under direct vision, as are all trocars.

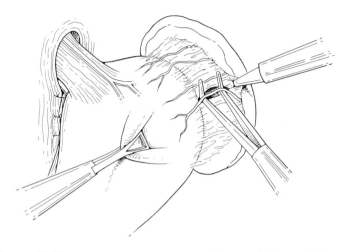

Figure 19.25. The short gastrics are taken down beginning ⅓ of the way down the greater curvature of the stomach and working cephalad.

The patient is returned to the room and started on liquids when awake. It is possible to discharge the patient on a full liquid diet on postoperative day 1 or on a blenderized soft diet on postoperative day 2. A full regular diet is not resumed for 3–4 weeks after surgery to allow the postoperative edema to subside. A postoperative contrast swallow is performed on a selective basis.

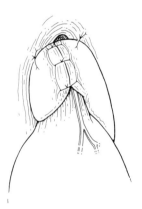

Figure 19.26. The completed Nissen fundoplication should not exceed 2.5 cm in length.

■ LAPAROSCOPIC HIGHLY SELECTIVE VAGOTOMY

By John G. Hunter, MD, FACS, and
William S. Laycock, MD

Patient Preparation

Patient preparation is identical to that used for the laparoscopic Nissen fundoplication previously presented. A five-trocar technique is used and all the trocars are positioned identically to the Nissen procedure (Fig. 19.27).

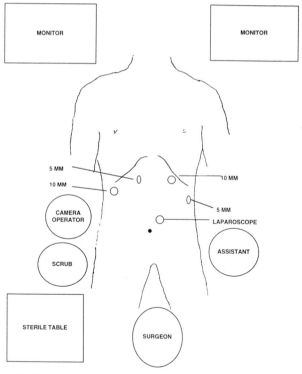

Figure 19.27. Operating room setup and trocar positions for laparoscopic highly selective vagotomy.

Operative Technique

The operation starts in the same manner as did the fundoplication, by taking down the phrenoesophageal ligament and dissecting the esophagus circumferentially. Again a Penrose drain is placed to provide traction on the gastroesophageal junction. The only difference in this case is that the Penrose drain excludes the anterior vagus nerve, which is carefully lifted from the anterior surface of the stomach. Delicately retracting the vagi to the patient's right, all connections to the major vagal trunks are taken off the anterior surface of the esophagus for a distance of 6 cm above the gastroesophageal junction (Fig. 19.28). When this portion of the dissection is complete and the vagi are all separated from the esophagus, attention is turned to the stomach.

The pyloric valve is identified and a point on the lesser curvature 6 cm from the pyloric valve is marked with a small electrocautery coagulation or a stitch (Fig. 19.29). This usually is in the midportion of the crow's foot.

Dissection along the lesser curvature starts by opening the gastrohepatic omentum from the crow's foot to the gastroesophageal junction. A row of small vessels will be encountered next. The smallest of these can be handled with monopolar electrocautery. Bigger vessels will need to be divided between clips (Fig. 19.30). Some of these larger vessels may be managed with bipolar electrocoagulation, effectively mitigating the need

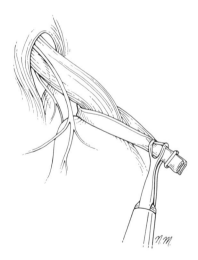

Figure 19.28. With retraction of the esophagus to the left, all connections to the major vagal trunks are divided for a distance of 6 cm above the gastroesophageal junction.

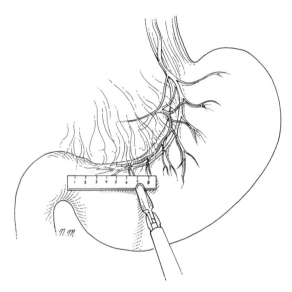

Figure 19.29. A disposable ruler is introduced and a point 6 cm from the pylorus is marked, usually in the midportion of the crow's foot. Dissection will begin here and proceed cephalad to the gastroesophageal junction.

for a large number of clips. Again the dissection in the second layer is carried cephalad to the gastroesophageal junction.

The third layer encountered, staying close to the lesser curvature, is the posterior leaf of the gastrohepatic omentum, including blood vessels and nerve branches of the posterior vagus. This is taken down in an identical fashion with clips or electrocautery. When this is divided, the surgeon enters the lesser sac. Moving up and across the gastroesophageal junction includes the separation of both vagal trunks from the esophagus and stomach (Fig. 19.31). Care must be exercised not to follow the posterior gastroesophageal junction around too far, as it is possible to get all the way around to the greater curvature into the short gastric vessels.

At this point, the procedure can be completed, or the surgeon may elect to close the posterior leaflet of the gastrohepatic ligament to the anterior leaflet, thus closing in the severed branches of the nerve of Latarjet. Not only does this step make the surgical field look neater, but it may prevent vagal nerve fiber regrowth across the gap to the stomach. At this point, it may be wise to perform a Congo red test to assess for completeness of denervation.

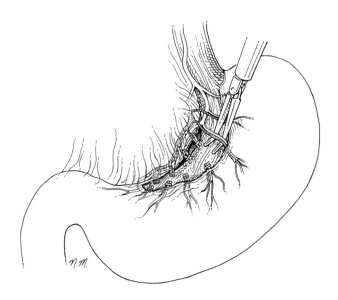

Figure 19.30. Larger vessels along the lesser curvature will be divided between clips.

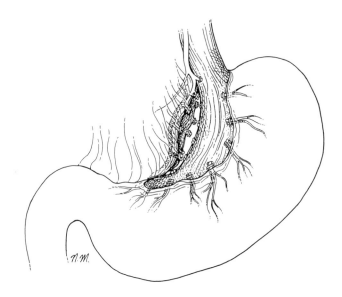

Figure 19.31. Completion of the highly selective vagotomy.

Postoperative Care

Because of the extensive mobilization performed in this operation, a nasogastric tube may be left overnight to prevent gastric dilatation. Liquids may be started on the first postoperative day, and if they are well tolerated, the patient may be discharged on the second postoperative day. If the patient has a gastric outlet obstruction or duodenal stricture, this operation can be combined with a gastrojejunostomy in order to promote gastric drainage.

■ LAPAROSCOPIC INGUINAL HERNIA REPAIR

By John G. Hunter, MD, FACS, and
William S. Laycock, MD

Patient Preparation

The patient is placed in a supine position upon the operating table. For this procedure, the TV monitors are mounted off the foot of the table to allow the surgeon to see the monitor while facing the groin from above. The patient is placed in the Trendelenburg position. A Foley catheter is placed and a first-generation cephalosporin is administered. One of two repairs, either transabdominal preperitoneal hernia repair or extraperitoneal hernia repair, should be employed. Both these procedures will be described.

Extraperitoneal Hernia Repair (Fig. 19.32)

Extraperitoneal hernia repair starts by establishing a pneumopreperitoneum. There are several methods of establishing such an inflated preperitoneal field. One method starts by making an infraumbilical transverse incision and dissecting down with S-shaped metal retractors to the level of the fascia. Long 0-Vicryl sutures are placed in the fascia at the 3 and 9 o'clock positions. A vertical incision is made in the fascia between these two stay sutures, and with gentle spreading of a Kelly clamp the preperitoneal space is identified. The S-retractor is placed in the preperitoneal space and further spreading allows a blunt-tipped (Hasson-type) trocar to be placed in the preperitoneal space. The obturator is removed and an operating telescope with a blunt rod in the channel is passed through the trocar. Pneumoperitoneum is then begun with the insufflator set on 10 mm Hg.

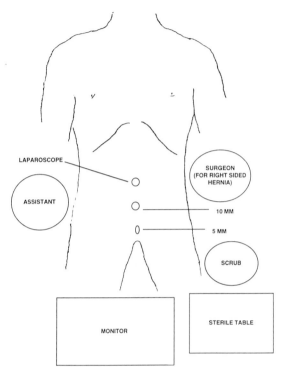

Figure 19.32. Operating room setup and trocar positions for extraperitoneal hernia repair.

Gentle, blunt, teasing dissection opens up the preperitoneal space (Fig. 19.33). The first move is to identify the pubic symphysis by sweeping the rod directly down the midline and contacting the bone. The tunnel is extended laterally toward the hernia side to be repaired. Once an adequate tunnel has been created, the operating telescope is removed and a 45-degree obliquely-angled telescope is placed through the Hasson cannula. A 5-mm trocar is then placed in the suprapubic midline position. A 10-mm trocar is placed half the distance between these two trocars, again in the midline. Great care is taken when placing these trocars to avoid penetration of the peritoneum.

Dissection starts by following the pubic tubercle down along Cooper's ligament to the femoral vein. In the course of this dissection, it is not unusual to encounter an aberrant obturator artery, which occurs in 43 percent of patients. When the femoral vein is reached, dissection proceeds cephalad along the inferior epigastric vessels until the deep inguinal

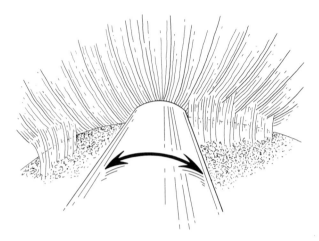

Figure 19.33. Using the operating telescope with a blunt rod in the channel, the preperitoneal space is developed using gentle dissection between the rectus muscle and the peritoneum.

ring is encountered. Defects medial to these vessels represent direct inguinal hernias; defects lateral to these vessels represent indirect inguinal hernias (Fig. 19.34). Upon identifying this anatomy, attention is redirected to the transversalis fascia in Hesselbach's triangle. The iliopubic tract, at the inferior edge of this angle, is identified and the femoral space is also inspected to make sure it is clear of hernias. After inspecting for femoral and direct hernias, attention is directed to the structures traversing the internal inguinal ring. With gentle, teasing dissection using atraumatic graspers in both hands, the cord vessels and vas deferens can be separated away from an indirect inguinal hernia sac.

Occasionally, a cord lipoma will be encountered. This can be reduced off the cord and removed. To make sure that no sac is present, the infundibulum of the peritoneum should be visualized adjacent to the cord structures. If exposure is difficult, it is occasionally helpful to place a vessel loop or a thin Penrose drain around the cord structures to aid in their retraction.

When the sac has been dissected out, a loop ligature is placed around it and tightened down partially. The sac is then carefully opened and the contents carefully inspected to make sure there is no sliding component (Fig. 19.35). Once this has been verified, the suture on the sac can be further tightened to secure the closure of the sac.

In the large scrotal hernia with a long distal sac, no attempt is made to

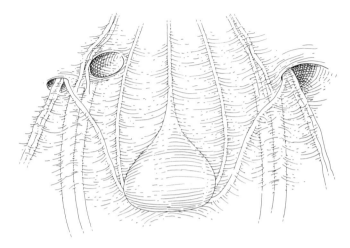

Figure 19.34. Laparoscopic view of the inguinal region. There is an indirect hernia on the right and a direct hernia on the left.

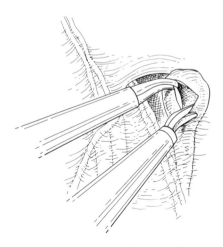

Figure 19.35. The hernia sac has been dissected off the cord structures and is being carefully opened to inspect its contents.

reduce the whole sac; instead, the sac is divided after proximal ligature. The distal sac is allowed to retract back down toward the scrotum.

Mesh Placement

After the hernia has been identified and reduced, repair can be completed by placing prosthetic mesh over the defect. A 7.5 × 13 cm piece of Prolene mesh (Ethicon, Inc., Somerville, NJ) is keyholed 5 cm from the lateral end of the mesh (Fig. 19.36). The mesh is now grasped at the midsection and passed down the 10-mm trocar into its position behind the cord. The suture is then cut, and the two wings of the mesh are allowed to unfold in an anterior and superior direction. Two or three staples are placed medial to the epigastric vessels to hold the two wings of the mesh back together. Two additional staples are placed in the upper outer corner. One or two staples are passed into the posterior transversalis fascia in Hesselbach's triangle, and three additional staples are placed in the pubic tubercle and down Cooper's ligament to the obturator or femoral vein.

It is most important that sutures lateral to the spermatic cord are not placed near or below the iliopubic tract (Fig. 19.37). A safe trick to avoid staple injury to the cutaneous nerves of the thigh is to indent the abdominal wall with a finger at the inguinal ligament and only staple above that level when lateral to the cord.

Once the mesh is in place, the field is irrigated and trocars are removed under direct vision, and the pneumopreperitoneum is then finally evacuated. If a small rent is made in the peritoneum during the course of this procedure, there are several options. A very small hole can be closed with an endoloop. A slightly larger hole can be managed by placing a trocar into the peritoneal cavity and opening the trocar to serve as a vent,

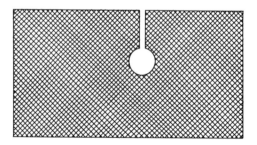

Figure 19.36. A 7.5 × 13 cm piece of mesh is prepared by making a keyhole 5 cm from one end with a 3.8 cm vertical slit.

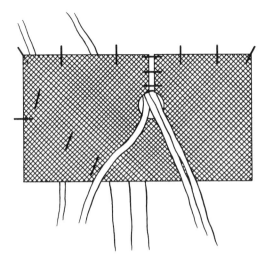

Figure 19.37. The mesh stapled in place behind the cord structures. No staples are placed near or below the iliopubic tract.

thus reducing the intraabdominal pressure. Lastly, a very large hole will require the procedure to be transformed into a transabdominal preperitoneal repair.

Transabdominal Preperitoneal Hernia Repair

As for extraperitoneal repair, the surgeon stands on the side contralateral to the hernia. Pneumoperitoneum is achieved and an initial 10-mm infraumbilical trocar placed, as is standard for most laparoscopic procedures. A major difference between transabdominal preperitoneal hernia repair and extraperitoneal repair is the trocar positions. A 10-mm trocar is placed on the right and left sides approximately halfway between the umbilicus and the anteriosuperior iliac spine. It is sometimes helpful to move the ipsilateral trocar position slightly cephalad at this point, and the contralateral trocar position slightly caudad. This allows the distance between the trocars and the deep inguinal ring to be approximately equal (Fig. 19.38).

With the patient in the Trendelenburg position, any intraabdominal adhesions are cleared off the region of the deep inguinal ring. The hernia is usually readily visible and the pneumoperitoneum will cause it to pouch outward. Occasionally, with large direct inguinal hernias, the defect may be somewhat subtle and difficult to appreciate.

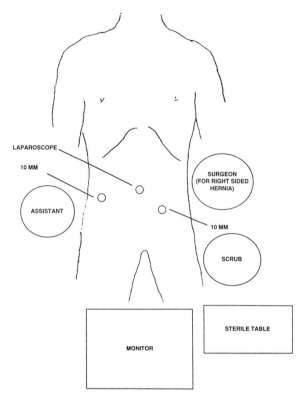

Figure 19.38. Operating room setup and trocar positions for transabdominal preperitoneal hernia repair.

The next maneuver involves a transverse incision in the peritoneum immediately above the deep inguinal ring. The incision extends from the medial umbilical ligament medially to a position approximately 3 cm lateral to the deep ring (Fig. 19.39). A flap of peritoneum is developed inferiorly. If there is an indirect hernia sac that can be separated easily from the cord structures, the sac is transected and controlled with an endoloop. If the sac is small, the entire defect can be reduced into the abdomen, requiring no further attention. Again, the cord vessels are dissected out, which will allow the mesh to be placed beneath them. A vessel loop or Penrose drain can be placed around these vessels for retraction.

The medial dissection, through the peritoneal flap, is identical to that performed for extraperitoneal hernia repair (see above). The mesh is cut

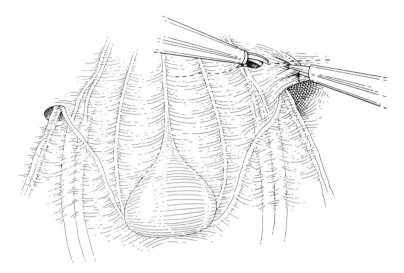

Figure 19.39. A transverse incision is made in the peritoneum and a flap of peritoneum developed inferiorly.

in an identical fashion and placed beneath the vessels with the keyhole in the same position as above. The mesh is secured with an endoscopic stapling device as mentioned above. The peritoneum is then closed over the mesh. This peritoneal closure may be accomplished with staples, but this often leaves gaps exposing the mesh to intraabdominal contents and

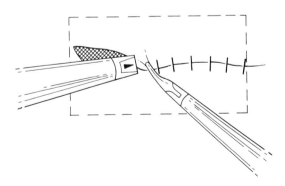

Figure 19.40. Peritoneum closed over the mesh using either staples or sutures.

possible adhesion formation. If it is desired to completely extraperitone-alize the mesh, it is advisable to use a suture closure of the peritoneum (Fig. 19.40). Upon removal of the left and right flank trocars, the trocar sites are closed, preferably with full-thickness sutures to prevent Richter hernias from developing through the hernia defects. The pneumoperito-neum is evacuated, the midline trocar removed, and the umbilical site fascia closed with a single suture.

Postoperative Care

Patients are generally discharged from the hospital on the day of surgery and allowed to return to full activity or work as soon as the pain abates. This usually occurs 5–7 days following laparoscopic surgery.

Index